A Practical Guide to Family Therapy

Grounded in systemic family therapy and drawing on a variety of other models to enhance skills development, this book is a comprehensive, practical guide to working with families.

This second edition is thoroughly updated and includes new chapters that cover working with First Nations Families, diversity and family therapy, understanding emotions, and dialogical reflective processes. The book begins with a focus on the therapeutic relationship and use of self as a foundation, and from there provides the reader with practical, skill-oriented guidelines for working with families. From the first session to addressing the complexities of separated parents, parent-child relational breaches, family of origin issues, wider systems, managing emotions, diversity, and much more, the book takes the reader through core practices that will become essential skills for family work.

Written by an expert team of authors committed to innovative and contextual practice, this book is for experienced clinicians who want to learn to work with families and for beginning therapists to learn from a structured approach to developing complex skills.

Andrew Wallis is a clinical social worker and systemic family therapist. He has worked with adolescents and their families for more than 30 years. Andrew's clinical and research work at Sydney Children's Hospitals Network has primarily focused on family therapy approaches for eating disorders, clinical supervision, and teaching.

Kerrie James, MSW, MLitt, has taught and supervised family therapists for over 30 years in postgraduate programs at Relationships Australia and the University of New South Wales Sydney. Her research and publications have focused on the intersections between family therapy, gender, family violence, and trauma.

Paul Rhodes is an Associate Professor at the University of Sydney with a wide range of clinical and research interests including family therapy, ecological emotions and the climate crisis, post-structural and New Materialist research methods, and the decolonisation of psychology.

A Practical Guide to Family Therapy

Structured Guidelines and Key Skills

Second Edition

Edited by Andrew Wallis, Kerrie James, and Paul Rhodes

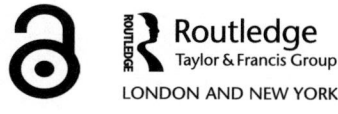

Routledge
Taylor & Francis Group

LONDON AND NEW YORK

Designed cover image: © Getty Images

Second edition published 2024
by Routledge
4 Park Square, Milton Park, Abingdon, Oxon OX14 4RN

and by Routledge
605 Third Avenue, New York, NY 10158

Routledge is an imprint of the Taylor & Francis Group, an informa business

© 2024 selection and editorial matter, Andrew Wallis, Kerrie James and Paul Rhodes; individual chapters, the contributors

The right of Andrew Wallis, Kerrie James and Paul Rhodes to be identified as the authors of the editorial material, and of the authors for their individual chapters, has been asserted in accordance with sections 77 and 78 of the Copyright, Designs and Patents Act 1988.

First edition published by IP Communications 2011

British Library Cataloguing-in-Publication Data
A catalogue record for this book is available from the British Library

ISBN: 978-1-032-78984-2 (hbk)
ISBN: 978-1-032-78983-5 (pbk)
ISBN: 978-1-003-49010-4 (ebk)

DOI: 10.4324/9781003490104

Typeset in Galliard
by KnowledgeWorks Global Ltd.

Andrew

I dedicate this book to my partner, Katrina, and almost grown-up children, Jack and Emilea, who have supported my work and study over so many years and remind me to put 'theory into practice' at home. I would also like to thank the many young people and their families I have worked with since the early 1990s, and for all I have learnt in that process. I also want to thank my past, present, and especially long-standing colleagues at Sydney Children's Hospitals Network, where family therapy approaches have always been, and continue to be, the foundation for our work.

Kerrie

I dedicate this book to Laurie MacKinnon. Laurie has travelled the world of therapy with me since our paths crossed at the University of Calgary, Canada, in 1979 where we discovered a shared interest in Gestalt therapy and psychodrama. Our joint Master's thesis tried to make sense of the magic of Gestalt therapy by distilling it into over 200 teachable skills. During that time, we also both trained at the Family Therapy Program, in Calgary, and were irrevocably converted to the systemic view. In the ensuing decades, Laurie and I collaborated extensively, working and writing together. Often through a critical or feminist lens, we contributed to the fields of trauma, domestic violence, and systemic family therapy.

I also extend my heartfelt acknowledgment to Carmel Flaskas, a colleague and friend who has profoundly influenced my thinking and work. Our collaboration for over three decades at the University of New South Wales in Sydney involved developing and teaching two master's programs. Carmel's exceptional contributions to family therapy, both in Australia and internationally, have been an inspiration, and it has been an honour to work alongside her.

Paul

I'd like to dedicate this book to specific role models and teachers who demonstrated the possibility of activist-relational practice. My lecturers Daphne Hewson and Carol Boland, and in particular Margaret Condonis who believed in me with such certainty and was the first to teach me 'live' in the classic reflecting team. I'm also indebted to Maureen Crago who first recognised my potential as an author and encouraged my first paper.

Contents

Figures and Tables

Figures

Tables

Foreword

A Practical Guide to Family Therapy for the 21st Century

Andrew Wallis, Kerrie James, and Paul Rhodes are all seasoned and highly respected Australian family therapists, educators, and academics who in this revised book project family therapy well into the 21st century. In doing so, they capture the latest developments in the profession translating systemic ideas into practice for beginning and experienced family therapists alike. They have crafted the latest thinking about what it means to practice as a systemic family therapist while being mindful of the challenges of integrating ideas and practices both from within and outside the discipline. This acknowledges that family therapy is at an exciting point of development forging significant new connections with other mental health disciplines such as clinical psychology, psychiatry, and more. This is evident when you look at journals and publications across the gamut of therapy disciplines where it is not uncommon to come across rich descriptions of integrative practice that combine family therapy with a range of psychological, psychiatric, and mental health interventions and approaches.

While the first edition of this book has been a mainstay for beginning and experienced family therapists for over a decade, this revised edition adds much more with several new outstanding chapters that address cultural, social, and gender issues, working with indigenous families and dialogical practice. As the title suggests, the book captures many aspects of the real-life practice of family therapy with all chapters written by experienced and well-known practitioners in their specialisation and in the field.

The strength of this book undoubtedly lies in its description of the nuts and bolts of how to *do* practice in family therapy in the contemporary systemic era. This is what it describes and illustrates best how to do the *practice* as a practical guide to family therapy from the beginning to the middle and the end. Each chapter provides a detailed description of theory that is illustrated by detailed practice examples and case studies including segments and transcripts of family interviews to clarify the practice of family therapy.

As such, this book will take a prominent space on the bookshelves in the everyday working offices of beginning and experienced family therapy practitioners alike. It is certainly on the prospective reading list for my beginning students in family therapy. Another strength of the book is the focus on a range of practice and cultural contexts including working with children, teenagers, and parents as well as First Nations people and families of origin. It will be an invaluable aid for teachers as well as beginning and seasoned family therapists keen to apply contemporary systemic practice across a variety of settings.

As this book recognises, systemic therapy today is very much an integrative enterprise and incorporates evidence-informed practice with systemic, narrative, social constructionist, and dialogical practices as all these frameworks are essential for the practitioner dealing with the complexities of practice in the 21st Century. It illustrates the broad spectrum of theory and approaches spanning the history of the profession and makes it easily available and accessible to practitioners. These include structural and strategic family therapy, post-Milan systemic therapy, social constructionist and dialogical frameworks, solution focused brief therapy and narrative therapy as well as the more recent evidence-informed approaches such as attachment-based family therapy.

Enough said! For now, I turn you over to the editors who will inspire you to go on the journey of reading and to put into practice the many wonderful ideas and approaches to family therapy described in the book.

Dr. Glenn Larner,
Editor-in-Chief Australian and New Zealand Journal of Family Therapy
Sydney November 2023

Preface

This book had its origins in the late 2000s when Paul and Andrew were running a family therapy research clinic for clinical psychology students, from the University of Sydney, at The Children's Hospital, Westmead, for families referred from the Departments of Psychological Medicine and Adolescent Medicine, where we also worked. Prior to the clinic, we had been teaching systemic family therapy and family therapy for anorexia nervosa since the early 2000s and recognised the need newer clinicians had for a high level of structure to learn before they could bring more of their own style and self to the work. It was Paul's idea to do a book and we contacted many of the people who had crossed our paths during our learning and invited their contributions. A first edition was published by a small Australian publisher in 2011.

Fast forward to 2021 and the first edition was out of print but people were still contacting us looking for copies, and a number of family therapy training programs were still using the book in their course material. At this point Kerrie enters, a luminary of Australian family therapy and author in the first edition; teaching family therapy to Masters students at the University of NSW and sees the need for an updated and contemporary second edition. And here we are, November 2023, and very grateful to have worked together again on another project, and it has been an absolute pleasure and privilege to have Kerrie join us and bring her experience and literary skills to the text.

Our hope is that *A Practical Guide to Family Therapy* supports your learning and capacity to help the families with whom you work.

Andrew Wallis

Contributors

David Allan has over three decades of experience as an individual, couple, and family therapist. He is a university medalist who completed both his undergraduate and post-graduate Social Work degrees at the University of New South Wales and trained as a psychotherapist with the Australian and New Zealand Association of Psychotherapy. He has held numerous senior clinical roles and established and managed a broad range of clinical education programs, including managing the adolescent family therapy program of Relationships Australia, NSW. He has developed and delivered a range of under-graduate and postgraduate clinical programs at the University of New South Wales, Macquarie University, Charles Sturt University, and the Australian Institute for Rela-tionships Studies. An ongoing area of interest and research has been common factors of therapeutic practice and the integration of psychodynamic, interpersonal, and neuro-biological models of therapy.

Dr Judith M. Brown is a clinical social worker and family therapist who has worked in tertiary level child and adolescent mental health, as well as with individuals, couples, and families in the non-government sector. She is now in private practice, offering therapy, su-pervision, and training, informed by systemic and dialogical approaches to family therapy. Judith has always had a particular interest in the theory and practice of couple and family therapy. Since observing Open Dialogue in Finland in 2011, she has engaged with dia-logical ideas, published and trained nationally and internationally on the dialogical ap-proach to clinical practice, and devised a dialogical research methodology. She was trained in Finland as a clinician, supervisor, and trainer in Open Dialogue and dialogical practice (Dialogic Partners & University of Jyväskylä). Judith's research and writing have included the grief of mothers of young adults with intellectual disability, the effect of psychological and emotional abuse on the family, and training in dialogical practice. More recent writ-ing is informed by her studies in Creative Writing Non-Fiction at Cambridge University.

Hugh Crago was born in Sydney in 1946. He has taught literature, human development, and counselling at Charles Sturt, Griffith, UNE, ACU, and Western Sydney and retired as Senior Lecturer in Counselling, at Western Sydney University, in 2012. He continues to practise part-time as an individual therapist. Hugh is the author of nine books, including *Couple, Family and Group Work* and *A Safe Place for Change: Skills and Capacities for Counselling and Psychotherapy*. He has also published many articles, including some on family therapy.

Dr Torrey Creed is an Associate Professor at the University of Pennsylvania's (Penn) Perelman School of Medicine and a licensed clinical psychologist. Her professional career began with the Center for Family Intervention Science (Diamond, Director) at the Children's Hospital of Philadelphia, followed by a faculty appointment at Penn. There, she founded the Penn Collaborative for CBT and Implementation Science which encompasses a large network of community partners, a program of training and implementation, and a rigorous complementary research agenda. Penn Collab's research leverages their large natural laboratory of community partnerships to develop and evaluate strategies to support the implementation of cognitive behavioural therapy and other evidence-based practices (EBPs), particularly in under-resourced public mental health settings. Dr Creed also has ongoing funding from NIMH to examine strategies to improve access, treatment fidelity, and sustainability of EBPs in community mental health. She serves as Health Policy Advisor to Partners in Health, implementing CBT and other EBPs in low- and middle-income countries. She is a Senior Implementation Consultant for Lyssn.io, leveraging artificial intelligence-based tools to improve the delivery of EBPs in routine care. She also serves on several scientific advisory boards, teaches, mentors students and postdoctoral fellows, and provides workshops and consultation around the world.

Dr Lisa Dawson is a Senior Clinical Psychologist, family therapist, and researcher who has been working with young people with eating disorders and their families for over a decade. She is currently the Team Leader of the Eating Disorder Intensive Program for Adolescents at Sydney Children's Hospital, a specialist tertiary, state-wide eating disorder service created to provide treatment to young people for whom standard treatments have not been sufficient. Lisa's clinical work has focused on responding to complexity in families experiencing eating disorders and considering how to respond when families experience 'stuckness' in treatment. Lisa is trained as an Open Dialogue trainer and her supervision and clinical work emphasises the values of dialogical practice where openness, social inclusion, and genuine user and family involvement in decision-making processes are emphasised. Lisa's research has focused on Open Dialogue, family-based approaches for eating disorders, and recovery from anorexia nervosa. She has provided supervision and training for clinicians in family therapy, Multi-Family Therapy, and Open Dialogue, as well as teaching and training for students from the University of Sydney, UNSW and UTS, where she is an Adjunct Associate Professor.

Dr Guy Diamond is Professor Emeritus at the University of Pennsylvania School of Medicine and was Associate Professor at Drexel University in the College of Nursing and Health Professions until he retired in 2023. At Drexel, he was the Director of the Center for Family Intervention Science (CFIS). His primary work has been in the area of youth suicide prevention and treatment research. On the prevention side, he has created a program focused on training, screening, and triage to be implemented in non-behavioural health settings. On the treatment side, he has focused on the development and testing of attachment-based family therapy (ABFT), especially for teens struggling with depression and suicide. ABFT has now been applied to children and young adults, LGBTQ youth and adults, and adopted in clinics all over the world where it is used as a transdiagnostic approach to patient mental health and ruptures in family attachment. Dr Diamond is now President of the ABFT International Training Institute which disseminates this model around the world.

Robyn Elliott is a Family Therapist and Mental Health Social Worker in the Department of Psychology, Counselling and Therapy, the Bouverie Centre, La Trobe University in Melbourne where she has worked for more than 25 years. She is Senior Lecturer and Course Coordinator of the Master of Clinical Family Therapy, a course that includes a systemic approach to working with trauma. She was a member of the sexual abuse team at the Bouverie Centre for 10 years. She is a Consultant with the EMDR Association of Australia and a trainer in The Havening Techniques. Her main area of interest is in integrating a systemic approach with various individual approaches to trauma and interpersonal challenges including narrative therapy, schema therapy, IFS, EMDR, and Havening. She delivers non-award training in addressing trauma, provides secondary consultation to individuals, groups, and organisations, and engages in clinical work with individuals, couples, and families.

Dr Carmel Flaskas, a social worker and family therapist, worked for many years as Associate Professor in the School of Social Sciences, University of New South Wales while continuing her therapy and supervision practice. She drove the development of the Master of Couple and Family Therapy and the Master of Counselling Social Work at UNSW and sustained a long-term teaching commitment in both these programs. Carmel's writing focussed on the therapeutic relationship, on psychoanalytic ideas in the systemic context, and on knowledge in family therapy. Her most recent work explored the balance of hope and hopelessness, thirdness and reflective processes, and contemporary frameworks in family therapy practice theory. During her career, Carmel was awarded an Honorary Doctorate by the Tavistock Clinic in London for her contributions to systemic psychotherapy and received the ANZJFT Award for Distinguished Contributions to Australian Family Therapy. Carmel's many publications are widely used in the training of family therapists and her contribution to family therapy internationally and in Australia has been outstanding. She is now happily retired and living in Sydney.

Roxanne Garven is a clinical social worker and systemic psychotherapist with postgraduate qualifications in Systemic Therapy (UK). She has over 30 years of experience working in a range of contexts, such as child and adolescent mental health, drug and alcohol services, child protection, and adult psychiatry. Roxanne is the Director of the Systemic Consultation Centre, Perth, WA, which provides training in systemic therapy. She has led training in systemic practice in the UK, Spain, and Australia and was involved with training initiatives to enhance collaborative work practices with families for the Victorian and Western Australian state governments from 2007 to 2009. Roxanne was the president of the board of the *Australian and New Zealand Journal of Family Therapy* and is currently on the board.

Roxanne consults to mental health organisations, provides supervision to clinicians working with adolescents and their families, and continues to work as a systemic psychotherapist in her own clinical practice.

Kerrie James has worked in the field of family therapy in Australia for over 40 years. In her role as Clinical Director at Relationships Australia NSW, she was instrumental in introducing family therapy services and establishing one of the first training programs in this field in Australia. As a lecturer in social work at UNSW Australia, she played a significant role in developing the Master of Counselling Social Work program, a distinctive qualification in Australia, and has been involved in training social workers and other professionals in counselling and family therapy throughout her career. With a publication count exceeding 30, Kerrie has contributed to the field of couple and family therapy, focusing on issues related to gender and domestic violence. In 1999, she was recognised with the *Distinguished Contribution to Family Therapy Award* from the *Australian and New Zealand Journal of Family Therapy*. Kerrie continues her academic involvement at UNSW and practices at Insite Therapy and Consulting.

Robyne Latham is a Yamatji/Caucasian woman from Western Australia. She has lived and worked in Melbourne for the past 35 years. Robyne's career traverses two distinct paths, that of an artist of national and international renown and as a university academic/researcher. Her art practice explores several mediums, from ceramics and works on canvas to performance art, set design, and bronze sculptures. Robyne has won the tender for several public art commissions (www.robynelatham.com). For the past 14 years, Robyne has also worked in the Bouverie Centre's First Nations Team at La Trobe University (LTU). This team has delivered a Post Graduate Degree in Family Therapy to Aboriginal and Torres Strait Islander child and family workers across Victoria and Northern Queensland. To date, there are some 183 graduates from this landmark training program, and several have attained a Clinical Master's in Family Therapy. Robyne holds a B.A. Fine Art, Curtin University, a Post Graduate Diploma in Education, Edith Cowen University, and a Master's in Fine Art, by research, Monash University. She has worked in the faculty of fine arts and education at Curtin and Edith Cowen Universities in Perth, WA, and of fine arts and allied health at Deakin and La Trobe Universities in Melbourne, Victoria.

Dr Suzanne Levy is an internationally renowned licensed clinical psychologist and Co-Developer of ABFT. She is the CEO and Co-Owner of ABFT International Training Institute, LLC. Formally she was the Executive Director of Strategic Initiatives and Training for the ABFT Training Program at Drexel University. ABFT is a manualised, empirically informed, and supported family therapy model specifically designed to target family and individual processes associated with adolescent suicide and/or depression. Since 2007, Dr Levy has been conducting ABFT training workshops and supervision for therapists nationally and internationally. She has presented regionally, nationally, and internationally on ABFT, emotion coaching, child and adolescent therapies, resilience, adolescent depression, adolescent development, and adolescent substance use. Along with her colleagues, Drs. Guy and Gary Diamond, Dr Levy has written the first book on ABFT, *Attachment-Based Family Therapy for Depressed Adolescents*, published by the American Psychological Association.

Dr Laurie MacKinnon, originally from Calgary, Canada, completed her BSW and MSW degrees at the University of Calgary. In Canada, she worked as a therapist and social worker in hospitals and non-profit community settings. Her experience included working at the University of Calgary's Family Therapy Program, where she learned from international family therapists. She earned her PhD from the University of Sydney, Australia. Laurie has published widely within the field of family therapy and is the author of the book *Trust and Betrayal in the Treatment of Child Abuse* (1998). For over 30 years, Laurie has been in private practice as the Director of Insite Therapy and

Consulting in Sydney. Her work involves providing therapy to individuals, couples, and families, training and supervising therapists, and consulting to Sydney's counselling and government organisations. Since 2012, she has been developing and training therapists in Radical Exposure Tapping, a trauma processing model. Dr MacKinnon received the Distinguished Contribution to Family Therapy Theory and Practice Award from the American Family Therapy Academy in 2012. In the same year, the *Australian and New Zealand Journal of Family Therapy* awarded her for her distinguished contributions to family therapy.

Banu Moloney is a Family Therapist, Social Worker, and Psychologist. Banu recently retired from La Trobe University/the Bouverie Centre as a Senior Lecturer. Over the years, she has worked in multiple roles as a teacher, supervisor, and clinician. She had key responsibility for La Trobe's Graduate Certificate in Family Therapy: First Nations. This course has been successfully delivered to Aboriginal and Torres Straits Islander Child and Family Workers for the last 15 years with over 170 graduates to date. Banu continues to remain as a consultant to the First Nations team. Prior to that, she was a member of the HIV and AIDS team from 1990 to 2000, working with HIV affected and infected people and their families. It was a significant period not only because being HIV infected was often a death sentence but also because at that time many gay men were coming out to their families for the first time. Banu has an interest in supervision training and practice and developed the curriculum for the six-day supervision training at the Bouverie Centre. Banu also has a small private practice in which she works as a family therapist and as a supervisor.

Dr Lawrence (Lawrie) Moloney worked in family mental health in Scotland and on returning to Australia at Bouverie Clinic. In 1976, he joined the then new Family Court of Australia and for 10 years was Director of Court Counselling. After three years in student services at Swinburne, Lawrie joined La Trobe University, teaching counselling psychology for 20 years and becoming Head of the Department. Before 'retiring', Lawrie spent several years as a Senior Research Fellow at the Australian Institute of Family Studies. Lawrie has published widely, mainly in the area of family-related interventions, family law, and family policy. He has a special interest in processes that promote child and family welfare in the context of parental separation.

Dr Jane Mowll holds a BSW and PhD from the University of NSW (UNSW), Australia. With over 23 years of experience, Jane is a practising social worker with expertise as a therapist. Her extensive career includes a significant role as a senior social worker at the Department of Forensic Medicine Sydney for 16 years, leading a team of social workers providing support and counselling to family members after a death reported to the NSW State Coroner. Jane currently convenes the Master of Counselling Social Work program in the School of Social Sciences at UNSW, where she is also involved in teaching counselling and the supervision of social work practitioners. Her academic research is primarily focused on the experiences and support needs of individuals navigating bereavement, grief, and loss, making substantial contributions to the field through both her scholarly work and teaching in undergraduate and postgraduate social work programs.

Lyndal Power is a social worker and family therapist with over 30 years of clinical experience. Her early experience involved working with families and children of all ages on Child, Youth, and Family Teams. She was the Clinical Coordinator of an adolescent family therapy program at Relationships Australia, NSW for nearly two decades. She has taught undergraduate subjects in the University of New South Wales' Bachelor of Social Work course. She has also taught theory and practice subjects in Relationships Australia's Graduate Diploma of Couple and Family Therapy course and the University of New South Wales' Master of Couple and Family Therapy program. She has developed and delivered training on couple and family therapy and adolescent family therapy for workshops and conferences. She provides private practice supervision of family therapists' work. She is currently the coordinator of a family therapy service for students and their families in the western suburbs of Sydney.

Dr Paul Rhodes is an Associate Professor of Clinical Psychology at the University of Sydney where he teaches family therapy, community-based approaches to mental health, multiple discourses in mental health, qualitative methods, and cultural responsiveness. His research interests include open dialogue and climate emotions, lived experience co-design, youth suicide prevention, arts-based translation, and the decolonisation of psychology. He practices at Uspace, St Vincents Private Hospital, and is a practising fine artist at Lennox St. Studios in Sydney.

Catherine Sanders is a distinguished clinical psychologist and family therapist, serving as the Co-Director of Bower Place in Adelaide, South Australia. This innovative centre combines clinical practice with training and knowledge generation. She plays a pivotal role at the Bower Place Complex Needs Clinic, where her work contributes to the development of original materials for the Bower Place Knowledge Site and forms the foundation of the Bower(method) and Bower(note) practice protocols. As an accredited supervisor, Catherine is actively involved in the AAFT-accredited Family Therapy and Systemic Practice Training Programme. Her expertise extends to conducting workshops and professional development sessions both within Bower Place and for external agencies, including international programs. Recognised for her contributions to the field, she has presented at various national and international forums and has a robust publication record. Her leadership roles include serving as the president of the Family Therapy Association of South Australia and the Australian and New Zealand Journal of Family Therapy. She has also been a key member of the Australian Association of Family Therapy and the Convener of State, Territory, and Regional Branches. Her significant contributions were honoured in 2011 with the ANZJFT Award for Distinguished Contribution to Family Therapy in Australia.

Dr Andrew Wallis is a clinical social worker and systemic family therapist. He has been working with adolescents and their families for more than 30 years. For most of that time, Andrew has been in a leadership role at Sydney Children's Hospital Network Eating Disorder Service focusing on family inclusive service development, including family therapy, multifamily therapy, and an intensive treatment day program. Andrew has also been involved in research and academic work with more than 30 peer-reviewed papers and book chapters, including his PhD research on the impact of Family Based Therapy on family relationships in the treatment of anorexia nervosa. He is currently an Adjunct Assoc Professor at the University of Technology, Sydney. Andrew with Paul Rhodes edited the first edition of this book published in 2011 and was also an author of *Multiple Family Therapy for Anorexia Nervosa: A Treatment Manual* in 2021 and a book for parents in 2021, *Help Your Child Start to Recover from Anorexia Nervosa*. Since the early 2000s, he has provided consultation, clinical supervision, and training to numerous clinicians in private practice and public health settings across Australasia. Andrew was recently awarded the Australia and New Zealand Academy of Eating Disorders 2023 Distinguished Achievement Award for his contribution to the Eating Disorder Sector in Australasia.

Anne Welfare has worked as a Clinical Psychologist and Family Therapist since the early 1980s. She worked for more than 35 years at the Bouverie Family Therapy Centre where she pioneered work with families where there had been sexual assault from a trusted family member. She was also one of the first Lecturers appointed in 1996 by La Trobe University and was deeply involved for 30 years in the training and teaching of family therapy skills at a master's and PhD level. In addition, Anne provided expert witness and reports to the Children's Court Clinic in Victoria and provided systemic investigative reports to the Child Safety Commissioner following a child death in the Child Protection System. Anne's PhD was in the area of sibling sexual abuse and incorporated the development of ideas for recovery for the families, for the victim, and for the young person with sexually harming behaviours. In 2011 Anne moved to work as a Principal Practitioner in the Child Protective system and has continued in this role with Anglicare Victoria. In both these roles, she has continued training and teaching Child Protection workers and therapists in the area of family violence and sexual harm.

Introduction

The Craft and Values of Contemporary Systemic Family Therapy

Andrew Wallis, Kerrie James, and Paul Rhodes

At the heart of family therapy lies the notion of empathically aligning with a distressed family, collaborating to navigate and transform the challenges they face; 'a difference that makes a difference' (Bateson, 1972, p. 459). This approach is deeply rooted in values that guide our engagement as therapists and shape our interactions with families. This book embodies this significant approach. In addition to the practical focus on core skills found in many chapters, we have aimed not only to highlight the crucial role of the therapeutic relationship and interviewing skills but also to emphasise the importance of valuing and respecting diversity as a foundation for our practice. Family therapy, in many respects, has evolved in tandem with broader societal changes over the past decade, reflecting a growing awareness of issues related to privilege, equality, and structural disadvantages at both institutional and individual levels.

Systemic family therapy's history has always considered the social forces interacting and shaping people's lives. The integration of the critical idea that therapists cannot be objective observers in family therapy only came about with the second wave of theory. This wave, led by feminist scholars and advocates for marginalised groups, started to dismantle and critically examine issues of power within families and broader society. Naturally, family therapists' own internalised discourses and the dominant discourses of society had impacted their capacity for objective observation. This led to second order cybernetics which emphasised the therapist as a collaborator who was primarily interested in family members' stories and narratives and who presented as less of an expert (Dallos & Draper, 2010). Importantly, second order cybernetics also allowed issues such as family violence and sexual abuse to be seen not as part of an interactional process but also as abuses of power that therapists could not be neutral towards. This pivotal change in family therapy was accompanied by the influence of social constructionists, who emphasised the need to consider not just the social and cultural contexts of families but also how therapists themselves are shaped by their own social and cultural backgrounds. This perspective highlighted that the viewpoints and interpretations therapists hold regarding their clients are filtered through the lens of their own unique contexts (Dallos & Draper, 2010). Social constructionism influenced family therapy to address 'power' both inside and outside of the therapy room. The idea of power had been dismissed as a 'linear' concept, but now the power of the therapist and abuses of power occurring within families have finally become an important consideration in systemic thinking. As these influences evolved in the decade since the first publication of this book, 'third order' thinking has been proposed.

Third order thinking emphasises the necessity for therapists to consciously acknowledge and address the effects of societal systems, power dynamics, and the shared aspects of

DOI: 10.4324/9781003490104-1

culture and meaning-making (as discussed by McDowell, Knudson-Martin, & Bermudez, 2019, p. 2). This paradigm shift is pivotal as it encourages therapists to introspect about their own positions and privileges and understand the implications of these in their interactions and influence on clients. Third order thinking not only incorporates considerations of equity and justice into all family therapy but also advocates for tailored responses to each family, acknowledging that families from the same cultural background can have diverse experiences. For families affiliated with specific cultures or groups, this approach offers a liberating framework. It pairs relational and sociocultural attunement (as noted by Knudson-Martin, McDowell & Bermudez, 2020) with the therapist's skilfulness in guiding the therapeutic process.

The aim of this book is to bring together this contemporary understanding of family therapy and provide practical guidelines and key skills that enable family therapists and those new to the discipline to feel skilful and disciplined in their work with families. From a theoretical point of view, the book is centred around the theory and positioning of post-Milan systemic family therapy (Jones, 1993; Carr, 2012). Post-Milan systemic family therapy provides a solid foundation because of its tolerance of, and ability to integrate skills from a wide variety of practices in family therapy.

Throughout the chapters, you will find numerous references to seminal works from the 1970s, 1980s, and 1990s, including those by Minuchin, Rosman, & Baker (1978), Haley (1987), Boscolo, Cecchin, and Hoffman (1987), Tomm (1987, 1988), de Shazer (1985), White (1991, 1993), and White and Epston (1990). These are presented alongside more recent contributions from the 2000s and later, demonstrating an appreciation for both the historical and the contemporary. The early papers, groundbreaking in their time for pioneering ways of engaging in conversations with families, provide a depth and practical insight that, while now often assumed as standard, were once revolutionary. This blend of old and new perspectives enriches the understanding and application of family therapy.

Each chapter of the book focuses on a different component of the family therapy process, from the first session to the last. Special emphasis will be placed on the core practices required by a therapist when working with families, such as engagement, the questioning process, and use of the self in therapy, practices that have passed the test of time in the history of the field. Detailed examples of therapeutic interactions and case studies will also feature highly.

The first chapter, *The therapeutic relationship and use of self*, by Carmel Flaskas, serves as a critical foundation for the book, reminding us that despite the focus on family therapists as agents of change, we need to remain emotionally attuned to the complexities of the multiple relationships in the room, including the one that we have with ourselves. While this chapter speaks to the integration of systemic family therapy with psychodynamic ideas, it remains fundamentally practical, offering concrete advice regarding the maintenance of the therapeutic relationship during sessions. The second chapter, *Structured guidelines for the first session of post-Milan systemic therapy*, by Andrew Wallis and Paul Rhodes, provides a detailed structured approach to the first assessment/intervention, not only breaking down the process into distinct stages but also outlining specific questions for the therapist to use throughout. This chapter is one of the few published to provide such technical detail, providing an essential resource to those aiming to conduct contemporary systemic family therapy. The third chapter, *Deviation amplifying: The second session*, by Paul Rhodes and Andrew Wallis, provides a similar level of detail, with a focus on how the therapist can exploit small changes to family interactions that have been prompted by the first session.

Any changes, from the significant to seemingly inconsequential, provide an opportunity for amplification, with the aim of initiating a virtuous rather than a vicious cycle. The discussion focuses on how to employ solution-focussed and narrative skills for systemic and relational ends.

Chapters 4–10 serve as a guide for the continuing sessions of family therapy, each representing a specific yet common issue, a focus on meeting the specific needs of children or adolescents, or when and how to see couples or adult individuals on their own. In terms of common issues, we begin with *Establishing the parental hierarchy: An integration of Milan systemic and structural family therapy*, by Kerrie James and Laurie MacKinnon. This chapter is a must-read, providing a step-by-step account of how to combine Minuchin's ideas and Milan circular questioning in systemic practice, a fundamental yet sophisticated set of skills that can be applied to a significant number of cases seen by family therapists. *Working with abuse in families: The challenge of establishing safety while fostering therapeutic relationships*, by Anne Welfare and Robyn Elliott, is equally important, drawing on a wide range of theoretical principles, including attachment and feminism, to guide the therapist through the complex ethical and clinical dilemmas involved in working systemically with abuse. The advice presented here places safety above all other considerations, whilst demonstrating the need for curiosity and compassion.

Three chapters focus specifically on meeting the needs of children or adolescents within family therapy. *Including children in family therapy*, by Catherine Sanders, provides much needed advocacy for a more significant engagement with young children by therapists, a surprisingly neglected emphasis in the literature. She includes a substantial compendium of techniques and practices that can be used, each demonstrating how the family therapist must not forget their playful side when working with families in distress. *Improving relationship security for distressed adolescents*, by Suzanne Levy, Torrey Creed, and Guy Diamond, provides a road map for healing relationships between adolescents and their parents in conflict. Their detailed description of the tasks involved in relationship repair demonstrates the privilege of working with vulnerable parents and their children at risk. David Allan and Lyndal Power's *Family therapy with adolescents: Key ideas and their application* completes the focus on adolescents by taking on the challenging task of describing systemic practice for a very wide range of presenting problems, including aggression, self-harm, substance abuse, running away, and use of social media. This detailed chapter serves as an ideal 'how-to' for adolescent family therapy in general.

Two further chapters, *The why and how of separate parent sessions in family therapy* by Kerrie James and Laurie MacKinnon and *Family of origin session: Why, when, how* by Hugh Crago, focus on therapy that may deliberately exclude the children. The first fills an important gap in the literature, providing a host of practical and theoretical reasons for occasionally, but strategically seeing parents on their own, not simply when conducting couple sessions, but also for the purpose of responding to triangulation, parenting dilemmas, or clinical impasse. The second provides a sensitive account of when it might be important to focus on the early life of parents while maintaining an emphasis on facilitating relational change in the present.

Chapters 11 and 12 provide a foundation for integrating third order thinking alongside the skills and special populations focus of earlier chapters. *Embracing differences: Transforming family therapy through diversity and inclusion* by Kerrie James and Jane Mowll places a spotlight on family therapy's engagement with social issues. Initially, this engagement was driven by feminist critiques of gender and power and then more recently through considering the impacts of dominant cultural narratives on disadvantaged and marginalised communities. Importantly it also acknowledges the impact on clients of intersectionality and the compounding effect of multiple sources of disadvantage. This chapter brings into focus ways that therapists can acknowledge their privilege and bring cultural humility to their work. *Working systemically with Australian First Nation families* by Banu Moloney, Robyne Latham, and Lawrence Moloney skilfully explains the profound negative impact of colonisation on First Nations people and the need for family therapists to understand this and to thus make therapy 'culturally safe'. Through a case study and transcript, the authors highlight the nuances of putting cultural safety into practice in the room, as well as showing how the therapist's authenticity in relating to families is critical for engaging with First Nations people.

Dialogical reflecting processes and practices in family therapy by Judith Brown and Lisa Dawson connects the reflecting team process of early family therapy to the groundbreaking work of Tom Andersen (1991) in the early 1990s and then to contemporary practices in Open Dialogue. Dialogical practice equips therapists with a holistic approach to their work, emphasising deep listening that engages not only the ears but also the heart and body. This method utilises reflective techniques to encourage significant changes. It provides individuals who have personal experiences with mental health challenges a therapeutic journey that prioritises genuine listening and authenticity. Open dialogue has its roots in systemic family therapy and readers will appreciate the way that this chapter brings something additional to the other chapters that have provided guidelines and specific interventions. The last chapter in the book is about the final therapy session and addresses termination issues. Roxanne Garven and Paul Rhodes's *The final session* supports the therapist to know when to finish and outlines six specific tasks that help to 'finish well'.

While we have set out to provide a practical tool for learning and consolidating skills, at the same time this book is not meant to be a manual. New practitioners will need to hold a careful balance between a number of factors: their need for structure and a disciplined approach to learning specific skills; the harnessing and adaption of these skills within the therapeutic relationship and with the self-awareness required for sociocultural attunement. A balance that is *a difference that can make a difference*.

References

Andersen, T. (Ed.). (1991). *The reflecting team: Dialogues and dialogues about the dialogues*. New York, NY: W.W. Norton.

Bateson, G. (1972). *Steps to an ecology of mind: Collected essays in anthropology, psychiatry, evolution, and epistemology*. NJ: Jason Aronson Inc.

Boscolo, L., Cecchin, G., & Hoffman, L. (1987). *Milan systemic family therapy: Theoretical and practical aspects*. New York, NY: Harper & Row.

Carr, A. (2012). *Family therapy: Concepts, process and practice* (3rd ed.). West Sussex, United Kingdom: John Wiley & Sons Ltd.

Dallos, R., & Draper, R. (2010) *Introduction to family therapy: Systemic theory and practice*. Open University Press.

de Shazer, S. (1985). *Keys to solution in brief therapy*. New York, NY: W.W. Norton.

Haley, J. (1987). *Problem-solving therapy* (2nd ed.). San Francisco, CA: Jossey-Bass Pub.

Knudson-Martin, C., McDowell, T., & Bermudez, J. M. (2020). Sociocultural attunement in systemic family therapy. In K. S. Wampler, R. B. Miller, & R. B. Seedall (Eds.), *The handbook of systemic family therapy: The profession of systemic family therapy* (pp. 619–637). Wiley Blackwell. https://doi.org/10.1002/9781119790181.ch27

McDowell, T., Knudson-Martin, C., & Bermudez, J. M. (2019). Third-order thinking in family therapy: Addressing social justice across family therapy practice. *Family Process, 58*(1), 9–22. https://doi.org/10.1111/famp.12383

Minuchin, S., Rosman, B., & Baker, L. (1978). *Psychosomatic families: Anorexia nervosa in context.* Cambridge, MA: Harvard University Press.

Tomm, K. (1987). Interventive interviewing: II. Reflexive questioning as a means to enable self-healing. *Family Process, 26*, 167–183.

Tomm, K. (1988). Interventive interviewing: III. Intending to ask circular, strategic or reflexive questions? *Family Process, 27*, 1–15.

White, M. (1991). Deconstruction and therapy. *Dulwich Centre Newsletter, 3*, 21–40.

White, M. (1993). Commentary: The histories of the present. In S. Gilligan & R. Price (Eds.), *Therapeutic conversations* (pp. 121–135). New York, NY: W.W. Norton.

White, M., & Epston, D. (1990). Consulting your consultants: The documentation of alternative knowledges. *Dulwich Centre Newsletter, 4*, 25–35.

Chapter 1

The Therapeutic Relationship and Use of Self*

Carmel Flaskas

Introduction

This chapter gives an overview of the significance and place of the therapeutic relationship in work with families. There are particular practices and skills involved in inviting relationship in family therapy, and in the way you make use of yourself as a therapist in the interests of the therapy. Nonetheless, I am choosing to focus here not so much on practices and skills, but instead on the core issues in relating therapeutically in family therapy and on ways of thinking about (and orienting to) the therapeutic relationship (Flaskas, 2016, 2012).

In the first part of this chapter, I will outline the significance of the therapeutic relationship, and why it is important to think about therapeutic relating and attend to it in your practice. Practitioners learning family therapy usually already have a solid base of counselling practices that meet the conditions of working with people individually, so discussing the question 'what is different about the therapeutic relationship in the context of seeing families?' will help to locate some pragmatic and stylistic differences in work with families. The third part of the chapter will explore the realness of the therapeutic relationship and the specificity of wider contexts and the involvement and use of self. Finally, the importance of the discipline of reflective practice, and the accountability and challenge of reflective practice, will be considered.

The significance of the therapeutic relationship

In everyday practice, it is difficult to ignore the importance of the therapeutic relationship, or the extent to which having a good-enough therapeutic relationship is generally one of the minimum conditions of successful therapy. Therapy is a personal process, involving the therapist's use of self in making and holding a real relationship with families who come hoping for some help. Particularly when therapy becomes stuck or fails, most of us face very squarely the complexity and messiness of therapeutic relating, and the challenge to our own use of self. Indeed, the personal and messy nature of therapy, for both clients and therapists, is the stuff of our everyday informal collegial discussions and one of the main refrains of supervision.

---

* This chapter builds on ideas published in a number of previous papers. The first part – *the significance of the therapeutic relationship* – relies heavily on an introductory section in Flaskas (2004). Some of the ideas on impasse in the final part – *the discipline of reflective practice* – are drawn from Flaskas (2005). In the new edition, readers are referred to Flaskas (2012) and Flaskas (2016) which develop the themes from this chapter.

DOI: 10.4324/9781003490104-2

Thus, we can easily claim knowledge of the significance of the therapeutic relationship from the evidence of our own lived experience as therapists. However, we also have knowledge from the amassed evidence across four decades of empirical research exploring the common factors of successful therapy outcomes across different therapy models and different therapeutic modalities and contexts. This research has been brought together in a number of recent publications (Duncan, Miller, Wampold, & Hubble, 2009; Sprenkle & Blow, 2004; Sprenkle, Davis, & Lebow, 2009). Many counsellors and psychotherapists are by now familiar with the four groups of factors related to positive therapy outcomes: the strengths and resources that clients bring with them to the therapy, including all the fortunate factors promoting change outside the context of the therapy itself; clients' capacity for hopefulness about the therapy which allows a placebo advantage; the therapeutic alliance and relationship-mediated variables in the therapeutic process; and, finally, the specific techniques and models of therapy.

Hubble, Duncan, and Miller (1999) note that of these 'big four', client strengths and extra-therapeutic factors account for approximately 40% of the outcome variance, while the next biggest group of factors at 30% relate to the therapeutic alliance, and the remaining two groups of factors – clients' expectations and capacity for hope, and therapeutic techniques and models – account for about 15% each. Put another way, factors relating to clients themselves, what they bring with them to the therapy, the surrounding circumstances of their lives, and their hopes for change account roughly for about 55% of the outcome variance. Of the 45% variance which may be within our ambit as therapists, factors relating to the therapeutic alliance seem to be twice as important as factors relating to technique and model.

Sprenkle and Blow (2004) quite correctly warn against tightly holding onto these percentages, noting that they emerged in the research as 'guesstimates'. Nevertheless, even as a rough map, the empirical evidence for the 'big four' group of factors powerfully underlines the significance of the therapeutic relationship. It will be interesting to see the directions taken in the common factors research in the next decade, particularly with respect to the development of the relationship between the different groups of factors. One can wonder, for example, about the relationship between a therapist's confidence in her/his repertoire of skills and her/his capacity to be therapeutically present for clients – or indeed about the more general relationship between learned skills/techniques and our ability to use our selves sensitively and flexibly in engagement. Thus, I am suggesting that there are more complex interrelationships between the four groups of factors which further research may well illuminate.

In the meantime, alongside the current empirical research, we rely on knowledge built through systematic reflection about clinical practice, and theory ideas that emerge directly from the experience of practice. These understandings are built in a different way to those offered by empirical research. They appeal to therapists because they speak to practice experience and to the development of clinical knowledge and clinical wisdom and offer a richness of thinking that is often considerably ahead of the capacities of the current empirical research programmes.

What is different about the therapeutic relationship in family therapy?

Therapeutic relationships are crafted in context. Discussions of the therapeutic relationship in the counselling and psychotherapy literature commonly use the template of individual therapy, yet seeing a number of people in one room at the same time is different from seeing just one person in therapy. This different context shapes elements of therapeutic relating in family therapy. It is useful to map the difference and what it means in terms of the use of self and therapeutic style.

The anxiety generated by seeing families

There are a number of pragmatic issues here. When you see just one person in therapy, the therapeutic relationship is the only in-the-room relationship. When you see a family of three or four or five or six, the most intimate in-the-room relationships are between family members, and so the therapist is de-centred. This occurs in the intensity of the emotional action and in the intimate familiarity of the patterns the family has built up across time and even across generations. Coming for therapy by yourself, as a sole client, about to see a complete stranger (the therapist) can be anxiety provoking, but coming for therapy with your family in tow is often far more so. In individual therapy, you do have some control over what you talk about when, what you choose to disclose, and how you language and present your own story. In family therapy, you walk in 'showing' your closest relationships whether you want to or not; you have far less control over how you present yourself and what will be said when and by whom. Thus, the venue of family therapy itself shapes a particular kind of anxiety for clients.

It is perhaps not surprising, then, that this anxiety is mirrored in the therapist. Not every therapist would say this, of course, but those of us who would say it might offer the following consolation to beginning family therapists. Feeling more anxious about seeing families doesn't usually change with experience, for you can see hundreds of families and still note a nagging anxiety as you approach a first family meeting. But what does change is that you get used to it, you come to orient to your own anxiety as being just one part of the relational territory of family work, and it ceases to be any big barrier to your capacity to engage. Your own anxiety as the therapist can serve to remind you to think about what it might be like fronting up as a family for the first time and not to become blasé about what is, in fact, a very peculiar and unfamiliar social situation. Moreover, family therapy is a situation that many therapists themselves have only ever experienced from the therapist's 'end' of the therapeutic relationship. I usually ask beginning family therapy students about their own experience of being in therapy, and while many like me have experienced individual therapy, fewer have experienced couple therapy, and usually only a small minority of students approach learning family therapy with the advantage of having been a client in family therapy themselves.

Multi-engagement

The context of family work also presents different challenges in the processes of engagement and empathy, and these challenges strongly influence the style of therapeutic connection. Work with families requires continuous multiple engagement a difference between individual and family therapy. Let me lay out a series of implications for the therapist's use of self in meeting the challenge of multi-engagement.

It goes without saying that 'the family' is no homogeneous entity. When as therapists we talk about the task of relating to 'the family', this is a convenient, if somewhat misleading, 'shorthand' representation of the task of relating to all family members and to the family as a whole, including relating to the commonness and difference within and between family members. There are often major differences in how people within the family feel about coming to therapy, there are often major differences in developmental levels, and there are differences in the location of family members to the presenting problem, in emotional positions, in the meaning they each give to the presenting problem, and in the stories each person has to tell about significant events and times within the family's history. Families also usually encompass gender differences, and sometimes racial and cultural differences, and differences in physical and cognitive abilities. As therapists, we will find some families easier to relate to than others and, when we see a particular family, we usually find some family members easier to relate to than others. This last sentence could be repeated from the other side of the coin, highlighting that some families, and particular family members within families, will of course find us either easier or harder to relate to.

The upshot of this is that the generic therapeutic tasks of joining with clients, witnessing their stories, and trying to convey a desire to understand their predicament and their position all occur in a more complex field. When this is combined with the anxiety that families may be experiencing about therapy, particularly in its early stages, it becomes even more important for family therapists to be very careful about how they use themselves in inviting relationship with all family members.

Family therapy techniques are shaped by the demands of multi-engagement and the style of therapeutic relating also reflects these demands. One sees this from the first session, and usually a short formulaic 'social' engagement with each person in the family in turn marks the beginning of the first family meeting (see Rivett & Street, 2009). This ritual beginning can feel almost counter-intuitive to the beginning family therapist more used to individual work, as she or he learns to deliberately hold off any problem-talk until there has been direct eye-contact and some 'ordinary' talk with each person (for once problem-talk starts, the 'heat' of exposure usually settles on particular family members, most commonly the person with the presenting problem). This beginning ritual may feel quite awkward in itself, but it usually 'settles' the first wave of anxiety of both therapist and family as everyone gets used to being in the room and embarking on what is usually unfamiliar territory. From this first part of the first session, another important piece of information is conveyed: that the therapist is interested in hearing from everyone and relating to everyone. The technique of negotiating 'air space' to ensure the involvement of all family members, which is used in the first minutes, sets up the conditions for continuing multi-engagement.

Therapeutic style and empathy

A much fuller outline of the first session is the subject of Chapter 2, but I want to note here the therapeutic style that is shaped by this kind of beginning. Family therapy sessions, particularly in the earlier stages of therapy, are therapist directed, and the therapist uses herself/himself in a very 'present' and immediate way in inviting relationship. While family therapy sessions are more structured and therapist-led, therapists at the same time often use a low-key informality in how they relate. This more immediate, direct, and informal therapeutic style has the effect of balancing what otherwise could be experienced by the family as a rather high-handed management of the session. This potential 'high-handedness' needs to be ameliorated, as otherwise the effect would be to inhibit rather than create space for (all) family members to begin to convey their experience and their thoughts and their stories. This style also soothes anxiety and makes the therapeutic process more readily accessible across different age ranges, different family members, and different levels of class and cultural familiarity. Having said this, not every family therapist with every family would use this kind of therapeutic style, but it is a common practice shaped by the context of family work and the conditions of multi-engagement.

Empathy lies at the heart of the therapeutic process regardless of the modality of the therapy. Empathy from the client's side of the relationship is the experience of feeling understood, while from the therapist's side, it is the experience of trying to understand and trying to convey our attempts to understand (Flaskas, 2002, 2009). It should go without saying that empathy is a relational process. In family therapy, alongside our attempts to understand each different person's position and story and thoughts and emotions, we also hope to relate in a way that invites and strengthens mutual empathic connection between family members. Multi-engagement presents challenges for the development of emotional attunement and the expression of empathy – first, the challenge of how to be 'evenly' attentive in trying to be open to understanding different members' experiences; secondly, the challenge of how to negotiate what can be a highly contested field within the family.

Again, we see that the style of the therapeutic relationship is crafted within the context of these specific challenges. In therapy with sole clients, the therapist's attempt to understand is often conveyed using 'reflecting-back' comments, as in 'it seems that when your husband said X, you felt Y' or 'this must have been pretty excruciating, and it sounds like you found yourself thinking A and feeling B'. Indeed, introductory counselling training still routinely focuses heavily on the skill of reflecting-back as a way of developing the therapist's capacity for empathic communication. In family therapy, this form of reflecting-back communication can be at times intensely problematic. Particularly in the early stages, and particularly when the field of who-is-entitled-to-feel-or-think-what is heavily contested within the family, 'reflecting back' expressions from the therapist potentially raise anxiety about whether you will be open to appreciating the different experiences of different family members. And so, for example, an exquisitely understanding reflecting-back response to a mother about her pain and horror at finding her daughter in hospital after a drug overdose may ripple around the room, as the daughter feels overwhelmed with guilt/shame/anger, and the father feels sidelined in his more non-verbal distress and perhaps guilty about his distancing and failure to change things. While the mother may feel comforted by this form of empathic expression, both the daughter and the father may register a fear that you will not be able to relate so well to their experience, a fear that in turn may shape how they relate to you (and to the mother) in the next interactions in the session, as well as how free they feel to 'show' or not show their different experiences.

The upshot of this contextual challenge is that family therapists need to develop a broad repertoire of ways of expressing understanding that avoid unwittingly conveying alignment with one particular family member and so constraining the possibilities of empathic engagement with other members. Ron Perry (1993) draws out the empathic function of a range of family therapy techniques – from the skills of questioning, to the use of reflecting teams, to the form of opinions and therapist feedback, to the choice of tasks. I would add to this list the careful use of respectful non-aligning language that is often embedded in questions used in family therapy, language that nonetheless actively shows your attempt to understand (Flaskas, 2009). Orienting to context is one 'trick' of non-aligning language – '*and so, when you found yourself reacting to this, and of course as the father you would have found yourself feeling about it all pretty differently, what was this like for you?*.... (and later to the son) '*what was it like for you from where you were coming from, what did you find yourself doing'*.... (and later to the daughter) '*knowing your father and brother in the way that you do, what sense do you make of the difference between how they each found themselves reacting?*'

Because family therapists ask a lot of questions and rely quite heavily on them to express the (empathic) desire to understand, this also shapes the style of therapeutic relating. Often referred to as 'the stance of curiosity', the therapist invites relationship, expresses understanding, and maintains an even and open interest in the positions of all family therapy members. The idea of 'neutrality' is linked here too, in the sense of the therapist having a curiosity and openness to all family members. Rivett and Street (2009) give a succinct overview of these processes, and there will be a much fuller discussion in later chapters of this book about curiosity, neutrality, and questioning. However, I will still note something immediately about the kind of curiosity that invites a strong therapeutic relationship. Families should not feel objectified by questioning, or that the therapist is asking a series of questions from a mystifying and 'cool' distance. In terms of nurturing the therapeutic relationship, questions are better asked from a warm, curious, involved, and experience-near position. Though different therapists will have different ways within their own personal repertoires of doing this, I think the important generic relational imagination on the part of the therapist is of wanting to connect with family members and to try to understand their experiences (Flaskas, 2009). When questions (regardless of their content) are embedded in this kind of imagination of relationship, they will more powerfully build a good therapeutic connection. Of course, how clients experience the therapeutic invitation of questions is not always in line with our intention, and careful attention to clients' cues in non-verbal and verbal feedback is a common skill in all modalities of counselling and therapy and not specific to family therapy.

This second part of the chapter has explored some particularities of the context of family therapy and the way context influences and shapes the style of therapeutic relationship. I have drawn attention to what is obvious: that, in contrast to individual therapy, family therapy usually involves many people in the room, with everyone but the therapist already intimately connected in the relationship. These conditions can generate anxiety for both family and therapist, and this anxiety sits alongside the special challenges of multi-engagement and empathic connection in family therapy. An outline has been given of a 'general' style in which the therapist is present, immediate, and active in inviting relationship, using an open and even stance of curiosity that I have described as warm, involved, and experience-near. The therapist's imagination of the relationship with the family plays an important role in offering an empathic connection.

The realness of the therapeutic relationship: Wider contexts and the involvement and use of self

What I have just drawn is a broad-brush picture of the general style of the therapeutic relationship in family therapy, focusing first on the context that is simply the choice to see a family and not a sole client. Yet of course there is no such thing as 'the' (generic) therapist or 'the' (generic) therapeutic relationship. In all our work, our offer of relationship (and the way in which clients offer relationship to us) is grounded in the realness of the context of our agency/service and the realness of our own very specific personal presence and use of self.

Embedded and embodied

To start with the outer layer, I will note that when families walk through the door into the counselling room, or you walk through their front door, it is the context of the service in which you are located which has so far been the most specific 'known' factor for clients. This influences, sometimes powerfully, how they are already thinking about the idea of therapy and you-as-the-therapist. Experienced practitioners are usually quite aware of the clout, for better or worse, of the agency in which they work, and the significance of the referral route in affecting the task of engagement. In our own settings of work, we tend to develop routine ways of orienting to the common experiences clients may have when they front up to see you in the psychiatric hospital, the child and family mental health team, the early psychosis team, the specialist child protection treatment service, the juvenile justice centre, the private counselling practice, or the interview room attached to the oncology ward. Before you get to show your face or open your mouth, quite a lot has already gone on in terms of the meaning clients have given to the referral and the sense they have made of the kind of service that is the 'home' of the work. And, as has already been discussed, there will be a set of meanings within the family, with commonalities and differences within and between family members. On the other side of the coin, you will already know some things about the family and their predicament, and maybe even know the extensive history of their involvement with services in the past. Thus, there is no 'blank slate' on either side of the relationship in the first meeting.

Of course, you usually show your body before you open your mouth and this is the next layer of context influencing the therapeutic relationship. You are a woman or a man, you are brown or white or black, your race and culture are obvious or not obvious (your surname has perhaps already led to expectations), you are young or old, you look too middle class or not middle-class enough, you may be assumed to be heterosexual or homosexual, your clothes are cool or unutterably daggy, you are beautiful or unusually small or maybe you roll up in a wheelchair. In short, you carry into the room a whole set of social signifiers and when you look at your clients, they too carry a whole set of social signifiers for you. A jumble of unworded assumptions and expectations go with this on both sides, which may or may not help the relating between you to be therapeutic. And it is only then that you open your mouth and the talk begins.

Vivien Hardham (1996) has offered an elegant and succinct description of these layers when she says that the therapeutic relationship is 'embedded' (in the specific wider context of our service and its meanings) and 'embodied' (in the context of our own specific social being-ness and the meanings attached). These contexts are real, and though families and ourselves can construct a range of meanings about the kind of agency/service we work in, and what we make of our own and others' social being-ness, the range of meanings is not limitless, and they are constructed within a field of cultural and social constraints and possibilities.

There is also a realness in our experience of wider contexts and social-beingness, and in the immediate and very personal nature of the therapeutic relationship. I am inclined to think that the realness of the therapeutic relationship, the extent of the involvement and use of self, and the personal nature of our work all lie at the heart of the pleasure of being a therapist. Those of us who are attracted to family therapy often enjoy the spontaneity and at times the humour and the chaos of sessions, the quickness of the interactional happenings, the creativity (especially of children), and the messiness and ambiguities of direct work with multiple relationships. Some of us are perverse enough to enjoy even the sheer lack of dignity that can go with family work.

Therapeutic 'fit' and the good-enough therapeutic relationship

The realness of the therapeutic relationship and the specificity of contexts mean that the issue of therapeutic 'fit' between therapist and family is important. I have suggested in other places (Flaskas, 1997) that one should be aiming not so much for a 'good' therapeutic relationship, but rather a 'good-enough' therapeutic relationship. I am not using 'good-enough' here to suggest 'less than ideal', but rather to signal the pragmatism of therapeutic fit within a constellation of factors. A therapeutic relationship needs to be 'good-enough' in terms of the possibilities and constraints of the agency context. It needs to be 'good-enough' so that the commonalities and differences between therapist and family in terms of class, race, culture, age, and sexuality are mutually negotiated. In intercultural work, special attention is needed in forging a 'good-enough' connection which both allows the space for an appreciation of difference and yet finds and holds the commonness of the therapist's and family's hopes for the therapy. At the other end of the spectrum, intra-cultural therapeutic relationships, when the therapist and clients see each other as very alike, also demand attention to the issue of a good-enough fit. A taken-for-granted cosy familiarity does not necessarily make for a therapeutic relationship. And as the joke about the new grounds for gay divorce reminds us, irreconcilable sameness may turn out to be as corrosive of a relationship as irreconcilable difference!

Another set of factors in the constellation of the good-enough therapeutic relationship is emotional and interactional style. Within the same culture and class, there can be enormous differences, with some families very serious, some very jokey, some more formal, some more informal, some more intense, some perpetually 'light', and so on. Similarly, as therapists, we have our own personal preferred style of relating, which may or may not be a good fit with the family we have sitting in front of us. Precisely because family therapy is a therapist-active and therapist-present process, it is especially important in this modality to develop flexibility in your in-the-room use of self, and bit-by-bit broaden your personal repertoire of ways of relating which attune to greater difference with your clients. I am not suggesting here that one is aiming for a 'match' with the family's way of relating, for this may not be congruent for you nor is it likely to be experienced as genuine by your clients – and anyway, as noted above, commonality is not the goal of therapeutic fit. Rather, I am suggesting that as therapists we actively modulate our use of self in the room with different families, in the interests of finding a meeting space for the possibility of (empathic) connection. I feel the need to add here that this is what clients also do with us, and so this finding a fit in terms of interpersonal style is by no means a one-way process.

But perhaps the most universally significant set of factors in the constellation of the 'good-enough' therapeutic fit is the therapeutic work itself, for it is the therapeutic work that sets the frame for what is required in a good-enough therapeutic relationship. At the risk of saying the obvious, families and therapists build a relationship and therapeutic environment in order to do something, and so the therapeutic relationship is primarily shaped by the needs of the work. Even in the same practice context, the work can vary enormously. In a child and adolescent mental health setting, working with parents around developmental behavioural challenges needs a different kind of relationship to working with a family after the son has sustained brain damage from an overdose. Or seeing a family in an oncology setting immediately after diagnosis is different from working with them around the mother's desire to mother her children as well as she can both leading up to her death and in relation to the foreshadowed loss. Intimacy and closeness in the therapeutic relationship are modulated by both the complexity of the work and the demands of emotional 'holding' generated by the therapy that the family wants to do. Moreover, what is required of the therapeutic relationship will be different in the early and middle stages as the work develops, and at critical times of relapse and impasse.

After presenting a 'broad-brush' picture, this part of the chapter has added detail about the specificity of the therapeutic relationship. Beginning with the ideas that the therapeutic relationship is always embedded in the wider context and always embodied in the social being-ness of our clients and ourselves, I moved to the idea of the 'good-enough' therapeutic relationship, with good-enough being constituted in a constellation of factors relating to therapeutic fit between the therapist and the family. Three themes have been woven through all this: the realness of contexts, the realness of the experience of the therapeutic relationship, and the importance of the use of the self of the therapist.

The discipline of reflective practice: Using the richness of the therapeutic relationship

We come then to the last part of this chapter. Here I want to extend the discussion of the richness of the therapeutic relationship, underline the importance of the discipline of reflective practice, and gesture to multiple lenses and practices for therapist reflection.

Impasse and anti-therapeutic relating

While my main purpose has been to explore the particularity of therapeutic relating in family therapy, the therapeutic relationship is, on one level, just a relationship like any other. As therapists we have reactions and counter-reactions to our clients (and they to us), we co-construct and respond to the emotional climate of the therapy, and we are continually making meaning, doing things, and feeling things in the micro-interactions of every session. The lens we use to understand our own thinking about the meaning, emotion, and behaviour embedded in our relating is as applicable to us as it is to our clients in orienting us to our own involvement in the therapeutic relationship.

Engagement has already been explored in some detail, for it is a critical time in inviting and forming the therapeutic relationship. However, impasse, those times within the therapy when the change process feels stuck, also presents important challenges to navigate in therapeutic relating, not the least because impasse often precedes therapeutic failure (Flaskas, 2005). Precisely because the therapeutic relationship exists (and is experienced) as a personal and real relationship, it is always affected by the difficulties of impasse. In these times, the emotions of frustration, anger, shame, blame, anxiety, hopelessness, and fear of failure can come to the fore, as the family feels bad about the lack of change. While almost invariably these periods are much more difficult for clients, they are also difficult for the therapist.

I have written before (Flaskas, 2002, 2005) about our vulnerability during periods of impasse to 'anti-therapeutic sequences' in the therapeutic relationship, when we begin to relate to clients in ways that are more likely to make change harder rather than easier. One could think of this as temporarily losing the 'therapeutic' part of our relating, for we have no special immunity against becoming rattled in the process of therapy. Impasse is an ordinary experience in therapy because the process of change is rarely neat and unilateral; it is an ordinary experience for the family to find themselves in a fraught emotional and interactional territory during an impasse; and it is an ordinary experience for the therapist to become rattled during times of impasse and to find herself/himself unwittingly beginning to relate 'anti-therapeutically'.

Reflecting on the therapeutic relationship

The discipline of reflective practice is both a safety net and a holding framework for the use of self and the therapeutic relationship. Reflective practice should be continuous throughout the therapy process. Precisely because the attention in family therapy is about context, relationship, and connection, family therapy has generated a range of reflective practices, including practices that are finely tuned for direct conversation with families about their experiences.[1] At this point, though, I am interested in the discipline of reflection that therapists use themselves in the therapeutic relationship, especially during times of engagement and impasse.

Robust practice in family therapy requires a multiplicity of forms of reflective practice. Different practitioners will build up different sets of lenses for reflective practice in relation to their own use of self in the therapeutic relationship, crafted to their own contexts of practice and particular ways of working. Here I will point towards a number of orientations that can be used specifically for the purposes of reflection about the therapeutic relationship.

A sample repertoire of ideas for use in reflection

I have already foreshadowed the notion that we can simply use ideas for understanding family relationships as a basis for our reflection on the therapeutic relationship and our own relating. And so, alertness to the circularity of unhelpful repetitive sequences within the therapeutic relationship may free us up to behave differently towards the family, and in the discipline of behaving differently, we may find ourselves eliciting different responses from family members and in the process begin to generate different meanings and respond differently ourselves.

Narrative theory draws attention to the way in which 'problem-saturated' and fixed narratives powerfully maintain problems and constrain the space for change. It can be useful when we are stuck as therapists to think about what kind of narrative we have come to have about the family and their dilemmas. The question here is whether our narrative has become stubbornly fixed and increasingly unhelpful, thus closing rather than opening space for the family to approach things differently. At times, we may even find ourselves coming to have a problem-saturated narrative about the entrenchment of difficulties in our own relating to clients. In our reflective practice, we can challenge our own meaning-making and the fixedness of our narratives about our clients, their situations, and our relationship with them.

While narrative ideas draw attention to what may be happening to the story we have constructed about the family during the impasse, the idea that we are vulnerable to losing our capacity for curiosity is angled more towards the conditions of meaning-making and story development. Narratives are likely to become fixed when the capacity for curiosity is lost. In this sense, holding onto the capacity for curiosity and holding an openness about our narratives about the family and the therapy are two sides of the same process. Curiosity has already been discussed in this chapter with respect to the need for multi-engagement. As a theory, the idea of curiosity is most closely associated with Milan therapy (see Cecchin, 1987), having as part of its evolution the earlier Milan idea of neutrality (see Selvini Palazzoli, Boscolo, Cecchin, & Prata, 1980). The notion of the therapist's position of curiosity signals the therapist's openness to meaning, and particularly to the construction of meaning which recognises the integrity and sense of the family's dilemma and possibly the integrity of the presenting problem itself as an expression of the family's and/or individual's struggle (Flaskas, 2005).

Though curiosity has its background within the Milan framework, it has become part of a more general configuration of theory and practice ideas within family therapy. For example, one sees a strong commitment to the therapist's curiosity in the techniques of narrative therapy (White, 1997, 2007), and Harry Goolishian and Harlene Anderson also very deliberately developed the allied idea of the therapist position of not-knowing in their therapy framework informed by postmodernist and social constructionist ideas (see, for example, Anderson, 1997; Anderson & Goolishian, 1992).

Psychoanalysis provides other sets of ideas that may be borrowed for reflective practice in family therapy about the therapeutic relationship. Glenn Larner (2000) has noted the resonance between the ideas of curiosity and the position of not-knowing in family therapy and the idea of not-knowing in psychoanalysis. He writes of the tension of knowing-not-to-know and explores the historical shift in psychoanalysis from a primary interest in an individualised concept of mind to an interest in the relational context of knowing and being known and indeed the relational concept of the capacity to think (Larner, 2000). Larner singles out the work of Wilfred Bion, which has been particularly important in this shift as well as influencing broader therapy discussions. Bion's notion of (emotional) containment within the analytic relationship and his ideas about the space for thinking that the analyst tries to create through her/his immersion in the analytic work have been translated for use in wider therapeutic contexts, including family therapy. These ideas are tied very closely to his understandings of the emotional and relational processes of the capacity to think (Flaskas, 2002).

I have also been interested in using the psychoanalytic ideas around transference, countertransference, and projective identification as part of the repertoire of reflective practice in family therapy (Flaskas, 1997, 2002). These ideas actively orient to the complexities of the therapist's experience of self and the immediacy and specificity of the therapeutic relationship. They also orient to unconscious and unlanguaged processes of the family's relating and the therapist's relating. Transference, countertransference, and projective identification are all about patterns in relationship and can sit relatively easily alongside the standard attention we give to patterns and sequences within the therapy.

Using self: A sample reflective process

So far, I have simply been listing a sample repertoire of ideas that can be used in reflective practice drawn from the narrative, systemic, and psychoanalytic traditions of therapy. I will conclude the list by referring to the reflective process offered by Peter Rober, a Belgian systemic family therapist who places dialogue at the centre of his understanding of therapy and relating. Rober (1999, 2002) draws the distinction between the 'inner conversation' the therapist finds herself having during the process of therapy and the 'outer conversation' she has with the family or with colleagues and in supervision. In an article on the impasse, he offers a four-step process for reflective practice that uses the richness of the involvement of self and of your inner conversation during therapy (Rober, 1999), which I will summarise as:

Step 1: Accept that your personal experiences arising in therapy are not meaningless … they may be a result of your own personal history, but they are nevertheless shaped 'by the context in which they arise' (p. 219)

Step 2: Be sceptical about your experience….ask yourself: 'is this experience more connected to my own personal story than the context of this therapeutic conversation?' (p. 220)

Step 3: Formulate hypotheses of ways in which your experience might be meaningful for the conversation, and if they might open out space for the not-yet-said (p. 220)

Step 4: Search for a 'constructive and respectful way' to bring your experience into the 'outer' conversation of the therapy (and if you find yourself struggling to think of any constructive or respectful way, this is an especially good time to use conversation with colleagues and/or the supervisor) (p. 220)

This process outlined by Rober is enduringly useful as a guide to reflective practice about the use of self in the process of therapy, all the more so because it allows the possibility of drawing on a broad repertoire of lenses in the way in which you might formulate hypotheses in Step 3.

There are many excellent discussions within family therapy of reflective practice with respect to the therapeutic relationship, exemplifying a much broader repertoire of ideas beyond my sample list (see, for example, the breadth of contributions in Flaskas, Mason, & Perlesz, 2005). The main message of this last part of the chapter has been the value of using the richness of the therapeutic relationship, and that the discipline of reflective practice is not an optional add-on in the process of therapeutic relating, but rather sits at the centre of all good practice in the therapeutic relationship and use of self.

Conclusion

The discussion has been layered, beginning with the significance of the therapeutic relationship for good therapeutic outcomes. The context of seeing families shapes the form of therapeutic relating, and so the challenges of managing anxiety, multi-engagement, and (multiple) empathic connections tend to produce a relational style in which the therapist is present, immediate, and active in an inviting relationship, using a stance of warm 'involved' curiosity. In the third part of the chapter, this general description moved to the specificity of therapeutic relationships as always embedded in wider contexts and embodied in what I called 'social-beingness'. We aim for a 'good-enough' therapeutic fit with families, as we meet a constellation of factors relating to commonalities and differences with our clients, alongside the emotional and relational demands of the work itself. The final part of the chapter continued the themes of the realness of the therapeutic relationship and our use of self, and the richness of therapeutic relating, this time underscoring the discipline of reflective practice and the need for multiple lenses for reflection.

There are many kinds of therapeutic contexts in family therapy, many kinds of families, many kinds of people within families, many kinds of family therapists, and many kinds of good therapeutic relationships. Attending to your use of self in therapeutic relating is part and parcel of all family therapy, and so the ideas offered here can now sit as background as the further chapters map core topics in family therapy practice.

Note

1 Examples of reflective practices used within family therapy sessions include narrative witnessing (White, 2000, 2007) and reflecting teams (see Chapter 2 in this book; Anderson & Jensen, 2007; Dallos & Draper, 2000; Vertere & Dallos, 2003).

References

Anderson, H. (1997). *Conversation, language and possibilities: A postmodern approach to therapy.* New York, NY: Basic Books.

Anderson, H., & Goolishian, H. (1992). The client is the expert: A not-knowing approach to therapy. In S. McNamee & K. J. Gergen (Eds.), *Therapy as social construction* (pp. 25–39). London, England: Sage.

Anderson, H., & Jensen, P. (Eds.). (2007). *Innovations in the reflecting process: The inspiration of Tom Andersen.* London, England: Karnac Books.

Cecchin, G. (1987). Hypothesizing, circularity and neutrality revisited: An invitation to curiosity. *Family Process, 26,* 405–413.

Dallos, R., & Draper, R. (2000). *An introduction to family therapy: Systemic theory and practice.* Buckingham, England: Open University Press.

Duncan, B. L., Miller, S. D., Wampold, B. E., & Hubble, M. A. (Eds.). (2009). *The heart and soul of change: Delivering what works in therapy* (2nd ed.). Washington, DC: American Psychological Association.

Flaskas, C. (1997). Engagement and the therapeutic relationship in systemic therapy. *Journal of Family Therapy, 19,* 263–282.

Flaskas, C. (2002). *Family therapy beyond postmodernism: Practice challenges theory.* Hove: Brunner-Routledge.

Flaskas, C. (2004). Thinking about the therapeutic relationship: Emerging themes in family therapy. *Australian and New Zealand Journal of Family Therapy, 25,* 13–20.

Flaskas, C. (2005). Sticky situations, therapy mess: On impasse and reflective practice. In C. Flaskas, B. Mason, & A. Perez (eds). *The Space Between: Experience, Context and Process in the Therapeutic Relationship* (pp. 111–125)/ London: Karnac Books.

Flaskas, C. (2009). The therapist's imagination of self in relation to clients: Beginning ideas on the flexibility of empathic imagination. *Australian and New Zealand Journal of Family Therapy, 30,* 147–149.

Flaskas, C. (2012). The space for reflection: Thirdness and triadic space in family therapy. *Journal of Family Therapy, 34,* 138–156.

Flaskas, C. (2016). Relating therapeutically in family therapy: Pragmatics and intangibles. *Journal of Family Therapy, 38,* 149–167. https://doi.org/10.1111/1467-6427.12108

Flaskas, C., Mason, B., & Perlesz, A. (Eds.). (2005). *The space between: Experience, context and process in the therapeutic relationship.* London, England: Karnac Books.

Hardham, V. (1996). Embedded and embodied in the therapeutic relationship: Understanding the therapist's use of self systemically. In C. Flaskas & A. Perlesz (Eds.), *The therapeutic relationship in systemic therapy* (pp. 71–89). London, England: Karnac Books.

Hubble, M. A., Duncan, B. L., & Miller, S. D. (Eds.). (1999). *The heart and soul of change: What works in therapy.* Washington, DC: American Psychological Association.

Larner, G. (2000). Toward a common ground in psychoanalysis and family therapy: On knowing not to know. *Journal of Family Therapy, 22,* 61–82.

Perry, R. (1993). Empathy – still at the heart of therapy: The interplay of context and empathy. *Australian and New Zealand Journal of Family Therapy, 14,* 63–74.

Rivett, M., & Street, E. (2009). *Family therapy: 100 key points and techniques.* London, England and New York, NY: Routledge.

Rober, P. (1999). The therapist's inner conversation in family therapy practice: Some ideas about the self of the therapist, therapeutic impasse and the process of reflection. *Family Process, 38,* 209–228.

Rober, P. (2002). Constructive hypothesizing, dialogic understanding, and the therapist's inner conversation: Some ideas of knowing and not-knowing in the family therapy session. *Journal of Marital and Family Therapy, 28,* 467–478.

Selvini Palazzoli, M., Boscolo, L., Cecchin, G., & Prata, G. (1980). Hypothesizing-circularity-neutrality. *Family Process, 6,* 3–9.

Sprenkle, D. H., & Blow, A. J. (2004). Common factors and our sacred models. *Journal of Marital and Family Therapy, 30,* 113–129.

Sprenkle, D. H., Davis, S. D., & Lebow, J. L. (2009). *Common factors in couple and family therapy: The overlooked foundation for effective practice.* New York, NY: Guilford Press.

Vertere, A., & Dallos, R. (2003). *Working systemically with families: Formulation, intervention and evaluation.* London, England: Karnac Books.

White, M. (1997). *Narratives of therapists' lives.* Adelaide, Australia: Dulwich Centre Publications.

White, M. (2000). *Reflections on narrative practice: Essays and interviews.* Adelaide, Australia: Dulwich Centre Publications.

White, M. (2007). *Maps of narrative practice.* New York, NY: W. W. Norton.

Chapter 2

Structured Guidelines for the First Session of Post-Milan Systemic Therapy

Andrew Wallis and Paul Rhodes

Introduction

This chapter will outline a structure for the first session of systemic family therapy. Whether you are working on your own or in a therapy team, these guidelines will be useful. This structure is also well suited to single session therapy models (Hymmen, Stalker, & Cait, 2013). Structured guidelines provide a useful place to begin developing skills and can provide an anchor to manage the complexity of interviewing a family. They can also support learning and provide an important developmental step for new therapists (Rhodes, Wallis, & Nge, 2008).

We will begin by covering some key theoretical ideas that lay a foundation for the structure of session one. This will not be an exhaustive discussion of theory as this is not the purpose of the book. Further suggested reading to build firm foundations can be found at the end of the chapter. At its most basic family therapy is about trying to understand and support change to occur by viewing the situation in its context. Context considers many factors and aspects such as who is living together, extended family, family of origin, and the psychosocial context, such as school or work, plus the influences that society and culture bear upon the family. This contextual emphasis on people's problems has its roots in systems theory but in the post-Milan systemic frame also encompasses broader social and psychological theories (Pocock, 1995).

Key theoretical ideas in systemic family therapy

Contemporary family therapy models encompass a broad range of theoretical influences including attachment, psychodynamic theories, neurobiology, and developmental theory, but developed in the 20th century through two primary influences: systems theory and cybernetics. Systems theory describes the mutual influence that parts of a system have on each other, and the larger systems of which they are a part. Central tenets of systems theory include the importance of system stability and that systems operate based on feedback loops (communication) between the parts to navigate change with the goal of returning to and maintaining stability (Bateson, 1972). These ideas were originally applied to the functioning of biological systems (Von Bertalanffy, 1968) but were utilised by family therapists to understand and explain family systems. A second related influence came from the field of cybernetics. Cybernetics (Weiner, 1961) was the study of communication and control, particularly as it applied to self-regulated systems or mechanical systems in which feedback in one part of a system generated an action in another part of the system automatically.

DOI: 10.4324/9781003490104-3

Cybernetics' most important contribution to family therapy theory was the notion of circular rather than linear causation. That is, influencing and being influenced happen recursively in a system. Applied to human systems, these ideas can start to help us to identify and understand interactions between family members that come to therapy. Seven questions are proposed below to translate this theory into practice.

What influence do family members exert on each other?

Family members engage in processes of mutual influence. Some of these processes are overt, such as rules around family routines, behavioural expectations, or who is the decision-maker for particular issues. Some are more implicit or covert, such as who you can share difficult feelings with or which issues to avoid in order to manage conflict. These rules, be they explicit or implicit, are recursive in that they influence people's behaviour, thoughts, and feelings towards others in the family and vice versa. This process of mutual influence occurs through feedback loops (verbal or non-verbal communications) which either increase or decrease certain behaviours in family members. Over time many of these feedback loops become habitual and awareness of them is not necessarily conscious. Mutual influence via feedback loops can help us start to understand how systems remain stable or change because the feedback loops try and regulate what is occurring for the system (Jones, 1993).

The concept of mutual influence implies that influencing between people in a system is equal. However, a moment of thought into the types of problems families present with for therapy makes it clear that some members of a system are, or act, more powerfully than others. Adults, for instance, usually have more power than children. A perpetrator of family violence exerts unequal power. Feminist critiques have written extensively about these issues emphasising the weakness of systems theory in this area and noting the importance of understanding power issues in interpreting family dynamics (Mackinnon & Millar, 1987). Other chapters in the book will deal with this issue in detail, but it is important to think about when a theory, such as systems theory, can help our understanding or hinder seeing things appropriately (Carr, 2000).

What happens when a family is faced with change?

Systems theory emphasises the importance of stability (homeostasis) as a primary goal for a system (Jackson, 1968). Applied to a family system, this means members will respond to their circumstances in a way that strives to keep stability. Challenges to stability are normal and come from within as people need to make developmental or life cycle adjustments or can come from the influence of social networks or culture or via an unexpected event. If an event occurs that has a significant impact on the family system, it is often referred to as a nodal point (Vetere & Dallos, 2003) whether an expected event like a life cycle change or an unexpected event like a crisis.

When confronted with a change or a challenge, the family will endeavour to maintain stability via their feedback loops. If the change is manageable for the family, a new homeostasis will develop through the process of natural growth or morphogenesis (Dell, 1982). However, if the change is unmanageable or threatening, then feedback loops will develop to try and maintain stability; for example, a parent spends large amounts of time at work due to the threat of losing a job. This may cause anxiety for the child who perceives this absence as related to the parent's relationship difficulties. The child may respond by having behavioural difficulties to invite the absent parent to return so the parents can work together to help the child. So, in this way, a problem may develop that helps solve a bigger problem for the family system, thus striving to bring stability, i.e. reduce the impact of the stressful change.

Why do problems develop for some families and not others?

All family systems face points of change and challenge and many of the changes families confront are similar to families in all walks of life. However, not all families need to seek clinical help when they get stuck. Given this, why then do some families get stuck? This question is not easy to simply answer without seeming to dismiss the complexity of family experiences; however, we do have some clues from the theory discussed so far. If we leave aside for a moment the personal, economic, and cultural resources that families have, such as their pre-morbid stability, strengths, and psychosocial factors such as wealth and education, it seems that a key issue is the flexibility of the family system to make the required adjustments when confronted with a particular change (Tomm, 1984). Of course, all those other factors we mentioned previously will play a role, but the issue of family adaptability and flexibility helps us to think about why some families get stuck and others do not (Carr, 2000). It may help to visualise a map where some families can see a path through the issue, even though challenging, and others are stuck finding directions for the territory they need to navigate.

Who or what is to blame if problems develop?

You will remember earlier that the key contribution of cybernetic theory to family therapy was the notion of circularity. Problems cannot be seen in linear ways as simple cause and effect if we hold to a circular way of seeing interactions. The strength of seeing interactions between people as circular is that blame cannot be attributed to one person's behaviour per se. Circularity allows you to think beyond surface appearances and descriptions of how the interactions between people are connected. In effect, the pattern of interactions can become the problem rather than an individual person. This notion allows us to develop systemic empathy as we consider each person's perspective on the family's concerns and how it makes sense to them. Circularity can help us appreciate that even illogical, seemingly hurtful behaviour can make sense and have a purpose from another's perspective. These notions of circularity directly influence how we will interview the family in therapy and the types of questions we will ask as we aim to help family members understand each other's point of view and behaviour and importantly the meaning they are ascribing. More on this later in the chapter.

How does change occur in family therapy?

Given the theory we have highlighted so far, we can expect change to be triggered when the meaning around the symptom or situation changes for one or more people in the system, which leads to a "difference that then makes a difference" (Bateson, 1972). Once this occurs, the feedback loops maintaining the problem can no longer stay the same, so something must shift. From an individual's point of view, each person in the family holds an explanation that makes sense to them for the situation, and that is only one description of the problem. When stress builds, capacity to think of alternate explanations usually diminishes. With each person holding a different explanation or meaning, the family ends up in what Tom Andersen (1991) described as a "stand still situation". If new meanings are to emerge that lead to change, then conversation between people is the conduit for shifting meaning. Whether the conversation helps trigger a change or it is a conversation that consolidates or notices a change, meaningfulness is at the heart of systemic family therapy. So, change can be thought of as occurring via one or more of these pathways.

1 Firstly, by one or more family members acting differently and thus changing the pattern around a problem. Because of mutual influence, a change for one person should lead to a change for others. Thus, we may ask people to act differently and try out new ways of doing things to disrupt a pattern and we can then get them to reflect on the impact to understand the meaning of the new behaviour.
2 Secondly, change can occur via insight into the meaning of the problem. This is a change at a level of meaning about interactions between people and the problem and therefore can lead to a change in interaction around the problem. This news of difference might come from thinking, feeling, or behaving differently in oneself or in the experiencing of another.
3 Thirdly, change can occur through re-remembering (Madigan, 1997) past strengths and interactional patterns that the family preferred but have been lost because of the challenging nature of a change they have had to navigate. Re-remembering can of course lead to news of difference as the family recognises they can find a way through difficult situations.

Change in the presenting symptoms is a first order change and change that is deeper and involves a change in the underlying pattern of a problem is referred to as second order change (Carr, 2000). With a second order change comes the hope that the capacity to navigate future changes and challenges has increased.

Do therapist's views exert an influence?

Early systemic thinking and first order cybernetics concentrated on the observable patterns in the family. The therapist was considered an outside observer of the family system, an expert in the objective analysis of family processes and able to determine how to change the system. This perspective had some critical flaws. How do we separate our own family experiences, culture, and social position from what we observe? First order cybernetics has been challenged by both constructivism and social constructionism. Proponents of constructivism have argued that people actively construct meaning from what is around them; that is, everyone develops their own reality or truth. In addition, our individual constructions are made within our social world with all its influences (Gergen, 1994). Our ideas are shaped by receiving and expressing ideas via language (verbal, non-verbal, or written). These influences have led to a reconsideration of the therapist's influence in family therapy via second order cybernetics (Atkinson & Heath, 1990).

Second order cybernetics (Keeney, 1982) asserts that the therapist is not separate from what is observed, but plays an active role in constructing the observation (Jones,

1993). This viewpoint acknowledges that the therapist does exert influence and has to be careful not to think they are acting objectively or without power. The second order cybernetic perspective shapes the interview process in contemporary systemic therapy leading to a more curious and "not knowing" stance with a strong emphasis on reflexive questions as the primary tool to help the family discover their own solutions (Tomm, 1987a, 1987b, 1988). The most important application of second order cybernetics is for the therapist to ensure that they balance their perception of what is happening with a curiosity that helps the family work out what is true for them (Hoffman, 1985). While at the same time, we need to recognise we have experience and insights that may be useful to the family and power from our role that needs to be managed effectively (Gibney, 1996).

What influence does the family have on its social systems and vice versa?

Family therapists need to be mindful, both of the relationship between family members and the relationship of the family to its wider context. Just as people in a family influence each other in a reciprocal way, a similar exchange occurs between the family and its social systems. Patterns or problems in the family can be replicated in different parts of the system (Carr, 2000). In this way, the family can influence the therapy team's functioning and vice versa (Hardwick, 1991) or a school context may replicate the dynamics of the family. For example, the school may be inconsistent in applying behavioural strategies in a similar way to the parents. Similarly, the social constructionist position reminds us that societal structures and discourses influence us all deeply (Gergen, 1994). Families often accept "truths" that reflect these influences, accepting cultural, gender, and socio-economic expectations that affect their capacity to solve their difficulties.

The first session

What is the purpose of this session?

There are three main purposes for session one. The first is to engage the family in the process. The second is to assess and understand their difficulties. The third is to begin to invite change. While engagement or joining is typically thought to occur at the beginning of each session, it is an ongoing process throughout the process of therapy. The first session is critical to ensuring that a family returns, providing hope that things can change and developing their commitment to work with the therapist towards their goals (Weber & Levine, 1996).

The second purpose is to assess the difficulties the family is bringing to treatment. The initial referral information often provides a description of the "problem" from the family's or referrer's point of view but Session One allows this to be explored in detail. The goal is to bring an interactional context to bear on the information that is being reported so that the therapist and the family come to recognise the circular nature of the problem and the interactional patterns that maintain the problem. This is achieved from an empathic position that does not ascribe blame to any one person or event, but via the process of the session helps the family gain insight into how the problem functions.

The third purpose is to prompt the beginnings of change by introducing alternative ways for the family to think and feel about the problem. In systemic family therapy, there is not a separate assessment and intervention process but both processes are reciprocal throughout the therapy process.

What is the theory behind this session?

In the first section of the chapter, some key concepts have been articulated that are meta-concepts embraced by several family therapy models to varying degrees. The session structure that follows is most closely aligned with post-Milan systemic family therapy. This model emphasises some additional concepts that provide a foundation for the first session structure. They are briefly outlined here and detailed in the session description.

Hypothesising is a way for the therapist to think about the meaning of the presenting problem for the family. Hypotheses should be relational and create a notion about the function of the presenting problem. Hypotheses guide the therapist to ask questions to determine which hypothesis fits for the family's situation and is useful to them. In a post-Milan framework, the ideas from many psychological and family models can be utilised to understand the family's problem (Brown, 1994; Sadler & Hulgus, 1989; Palazzoli, Boscolo, Cecchin, & Prata, 1980; Cecchin, 1987; Carr, 1997; Cecchin, Lane & Ray, 1992).

Circularity refers to how problems are explained, as mentioned before, but extends to describing how the interview process is conducted. This is done by using circular questions that draw connections and distinctions between people (Brown, 1997a, 1997b). The assumption is that this circular approach to interviewing releases information about relationships and this information creates a difference that redefines relationships, thus allowing for changes (Palazzoli, Boscolo, Cecchin, & Prata, 1980).

Neutrality describes the disposition of the therapist in the interview process. The therapist should be in a meta-position to the family in terms of their beliefs and interactions (MacKinnon & James, 1987). The purpose of this position is to not be drawn into siding for or against a person or an issue so that the family can consider their own beliefs and patterns (Tomm, 1987a). Neutrality is maintained by a *curious position* that invites openness, and therefore information is shared between family members, and with the therapist. Neutrality does not imply that the therapist has no viewpoint but is utilised to put the focus on validating the family member's views (Campbell, 2003). Neutrality is not meant to suggest that the therapist is morally neutral about safety issues such as violence and abuse in the family or wider social system (Campbell, 2003; Jones, 1993).

Strategising implies an active and interventive role for the therapist and differentiates family therapy from non-directive counselling (Tomm, 1987a). The therapist is informed by the principles of hypothesising, circularity, and neutrality but acknowledges a clear role as a change agent, albeit through collaborative conversations with the family.

Relational ethics in post-Milan systemic therapy involves remaining true to systemic thinking as the underlying framework for therapy but importantly recognises the feminist and social constructionist critiques of systems theory (Brown, 1994). Therefore, post-Milan systemic therapy emphasises the therapist taking an active position against violence, abuse, and power dynamics and being attuned to larger sociocultural narratives and their own power and privilege.

What are the steps and questions to use for this session?

While the aim of this chapter is to detail Session One, the thinking and skills used can be employed across future sessions. The Session One structure outlined tries to achieve a balance between content and process. This balance is important so that it is not just assessment but remains therapeutic. The session plan outlined is designed to support a transition from the least to the most intense subject matter over the course of the interview. For example, a discussion of the presenting problem occurs first, and more sensitive relationship issues are left to near the end of the session.

The structure also provides a scaffold for the therapist to stay focused and not become overwhelmed by one aspect of the family's presentation. Without this, it is very easy to get lost in one issue and then a systemic focus does not develop. This session format takes about 1.5–2 hours to complete but is well worth it given the foundation it creates. It could also be done across two meetings if needed.

Step one – Pre-session preparation

The first step is to draw a genogram of the family so that you can get a visual picture of how people fit together from the referral information. Clearly, the amount of information can vary greatly but you need to have enough to start thinking about how the presenting problem might make sense or function for the family. Once you have drawn up the genogram, the next step is to hypothesise.

Hypotheses are about trying to understand systemically what the problem means or what the relational function is for the family. Hypotheses should try and include all parts of the family so that it is systemic (Palazzoli, Boscolo, Cecchin, & Prata, 1980). A useful way to think is how the problems might be "helping" the family with their situation (Brown, 1994). This is a key premise in systemic therapy that people act with good intentions even when their behaviour seems unhelpful. For example, we may see a father's withdrawal from home to work as a way of reducing conflict in the marriage, thus preserving the family. Hypothesising also functions to get our own biases out in the open. Without hypothesising, we are more likely to join the family system unwittingly by being caught in our own blind spots. For example, we might over empathise with the mother and take a position against the father because the father's withdrawal reminds us about our own family dynamic as a child.

Hypotheses are ideas that help guide and organise the interview. The therapist should mediate against becoming attached to specific ideas, by generating more than one hypothesis, including those in direct opposition to each other. Hypothesising serves to tune the therapist into interactional processes that might otherwise get missed in a session and should be constantly revised throughout the session as the family describes their experience. If you are struggling with the specific hypothesis, then thinking about a theme that unifies the information you have can be a useful starting point like adjustment, transition, grief, disconnection and then develop a greater understanding of the specifics with the family in the interview.

A strength of the post-Milan systemic framework is that hypotheses can be developed from a multitude of different traditions or lenses. These can include:

- Developmental and life cycle theories
- Cultural perspectives

- Psychodynamic theory
- Attachment theory
- Sociological/feminist perspectives
- Previous clinical experience
- Other family therapy models constructs.

Some key questions to begin hypothesising include:

What effect is the problem having on the family?
Does the problem help the family in any way?
What might it mean for them at this particular point in time?
Are there wider systems issues that relate to the presenting problem?

It can be useful to shift your language and think about people "showing" behaviour or feelings rather than "being" their behaviour or feelings. For example, if we say Mary is *showing* sadness rather than Mary is sad, it allows relational meaning to become more prominent because it prompts us to ask, who is she showing (Jones, 1993)? We can generate hypotheses utilising the following format:

Tom shows increasing misbehaviour (symptom) at home as a way to invite firmer boundaries (outcome) by his parents to make him feel more secure (meaning) because he is worried about his mother's apparent sad mood and his father's increasing work hours (relational connections).

Hypotheses should be written in a way that positively connotes the symptom or presenting problem as helping in some way. With the example above, we would be thinking about the need to test ideas including the parent's relationship, parenting style, and the relationship quality between the parents and the child. While the hypothesis is written from the viewpoint of the symptomatic person, there is circular intent. For example, did the misbehaviour lead to the mother's low mood and the father's withdrawal, or did the mother's low mood reduce her parenting capacity, thus leaving the child to need to draw in the father, etc.

Step two – Providing a format for the session to the family

Step two is to give the family a sense of structure for the session. This is important because it is the start of setting some rules for the therapy sessions. Families are often very anxious about what is going to be discussed, so settling things quickly is important. Essentially you want to communicate that

- Everyone will have the opportunity to participate.
- Session will go for approximately x amount of time and what the end of the session will involve, such as a reflecting team or end of session break before feedback.
- Discuss confidentiality and its limits.
- Any other housekeeping items such as a team behind a one-way screen or that the meeting is being recorded, etc.
- If a team is involved, provide an opportunity for the family to meet the team.

Step three – Engaging all family members

The third step is to engage or join with each family member. The aim is to make a personal connection with each family member. Some key questions you can use include the following:

Parents

What do you do during the day?
How do you find that?
Do you have anything you do just for you?

Children

Where do you go to school, what is it like?
What do you spend time doing outside school?

Aim for questions to be open and neutral so that you can lean in the direction of the client's response. For instance, the questions *What do you do during the day? How do you find that?* allow you to avoid judging whether a parent is working or is home with children and allows them to say whether they like or dislike something. Given that the goal is engagement, following the person's lead is key. If you ask, "how do you find school?" and the person responds negatively, exploring that response will be more engaging than responding with a positive like "what do you like about school?" If the response is ambivalent, then we can ask about both likes and dislikes. You can also start to think about your hypothesis and gather information. For instance, if part of your hypothesis involves a parent being distant and unavailable, then inquiring about work hours may provide some helpful information.

Another important aspect of engagement is to start setting some implicit rules for the session. This is done by creating a structure for the family, for example, speaking to one person at a time, interrupting other family members who interject during the process, and having people answer the question you have asked. In this way, people are learning that the session will be orderly, that everyone will get a turn, and that people will be treated fairly. An effective way to deal with interruptions is to say – *I know you have things you want to say but at the moment just let me ask x? or I'm going to get around to everyone?*

Similarly, if people are not answering your question or being tangential, redirect them back to the question. If we do not manage these process issues early on, the session can get out of hand quickly and your position as the conductor of the session can easily be undermined. Essentially, we want to take a position where the family owns the content, but setting up an effective and safe process is the therapist's responsibility. If we can manage these sorts of process issues, we also send a message to the family that we are competent, confident, and can handle difficult discussions and dynamics. This is the beginning of creating a safe space that contains emotional vulnerability (Bion, 1962).

Other issues to consider in this part of the interview are who do you engage with first and what about missing family members? An effective way to decide on whom to speak to first is to choose the parent that you have not had contact with before the appointment. This can help maintain your neutrality. You can also think structurally and begin with the parent who seems to hold the greatest influence or the parent who may need this recognition to engage and then the other parent and then the children in age order. It is important to recognise that this choice is not about gender per se, if choosing to speak to the father first for instance, but should be about the family's values or culture, with the aim to make engagement easier in the initial stage of the interview. There is plenty of time to challenge gender roles and other social constructions as therapy proceeds. Family members or other important adults not in the session should also be introduced. You often get a sense of this in the referral information, and they may feature in your hypotheses. There may be a parent, siblings, or grandparents not living in the current household. Children often enjoy introducing these people. One can ask – *are there any other people in the family that are important to introduce to me?*

Finally, despite all these issues, engagement should not be a large part of the session. A beginning therapist often spends too much time on this part of the session. We do not want to inadvertently convey the idea that we are not ready to talk about why the family has come.

Step four – Exploring concerns of family members

The fourth step is to explore the family's concerns. The aim of this part of the session is to get a rich description of the presenting problem. It requires persistence to get past behavioural descriptions to their meaning, effect, and relational contexts. One should start with the adults when exploring concerns to emphasise the authoritative role of the parents. It may also be useful to commence with the least reserved parent, breaking the ice for others to follow, or the parent who you feel will put "issues on the table" more easily. Criticism or high expressed emotion must also be managed at this early stage, by stepping in to manage interruptions or help family members explore and take responsibility for their own emotions.

The process of exploring concerns starts with an open question, such as – *what is concerning you most at the moment?* It seems to work more effectively to leave it this open and just see what the response is. The response may be about an individual or can be relational from the start. To resist joining the family system, we would not start with, *what is concerning you about (child)?* With this question, you can easily end up with a description that is directed at the identified client and the wider context is diminished. Anything that you do not understand should be followed up. The simplest way this can be done is to ask – *what do you mean or can you help me understand?* A useful principle that applies here, but throughout the whole session, is to use simple questions where possible and keep more complicated question types for when they are really needed. This can make our questioning more impactful and effective and the tone of the session more conversational for the family.

From the initial question, it is then a matter of getting underneath the voiced concern to more relational issues. This is done by taking each concern and listening to the response for information that contains either affect or relationship material and then focusing in with follow-up questions such as – *what concerns you most about x? What is your worst fear about it continuing?* If there are a range of concerns, you can ask that they be ranked from least to most worrying or use a forced choice question to create a hierarchy between two, for example – *are you more concerned about the fighting or the effect it is having on the relationship?*

The aim is for each person in the family to speak about their worries. It is not enough for the second parent to say they agree with the first parent who spoke. If this occurs ask – *can you describe the concern in their own words?* The mechanism of change in systemic therapy is to create new perspectives for each person in the family and this can only happen through the injection of information. The simplest way to help a parent who is happy to agree with their partner is to ask them to describe their concerns in their own words.

It is common in the initial stages of the interview for family members to be reluctant to speak. This is most often the identified client. A useful way around this is to employ a particular questioning style synonymous with systemic therapy, namely dyadic and triadic circular questioning. Dyadic and triadic circular questions (Tomm, 1985; Brown, 1997a, 1997b) can be used to help with resistance but they also release information into the system because they are inviting one person to comment on how they think another person or pair is thinking. Triadic circular questions have a format that asks one person outside a relationship about two people in a relationship and dyadic circular questions ask one person about another person. A dyadic circular question in this context would have the following format:

Therapist asks person A

If I was to ask B what his concerns were at the moment, what do you think he would say?

Therapist asks person B

How does what A said fit for you?

To employ this technique, it is essential that the therapist interviews person A until enough information is released that person B feels that they can respond. The interviewer needs to keep an eye on person B while talking with person A and to look for body language that indicates a shift. Most noticeably person B may get a tear in their eye if very emotive, or it is usually much more subtle at this stage in the session and be just a small shift in the seat or some eye movement. It is important when you ask a circular question to find out from the person who was spoken about what they think about what was reported. This should be done as neutrally as possible, rather than asking if they agree or disagree. This gives a more open flow and allows for new information to come out. We tend to rely a lot on using the simple question – *how does that fit for you?*

Finally, as the sensitivity of material in the session increases, it is important that the therapist is monitoring content and process. Where possible, we want to get underneath any high expressed emotion or criticism and connect it with relational descriptions. For instance, if people are showing anger, they may also be feeling sad about a change or situation. A mantra for managing the process is to "lean into any affect", following emotions where possible. When emotion or affect is occurring, it is useful to consider whether you are hearing or seeing a surface emotion (secondary) or deeper emotion (primary emotion). A surface emotion is often the emotion that covers the more vulnerable emotions. For example, anger is often an easier emotion to show than sadness. A second way to lean into relational descriptions is to listen for attachment orientated words like lonely, missing, caring, connected, etc. and then highlight those words to recognise their significance – *"Missing your mum, can you say more about that?"* The "rules" that were set up in engagement, such as having people answer your question and interrupting without upsetting people, become even more crucial as the session goes on.

Step five – Understanding the start and effect of the problem

The fifth step is to try and understand the onset of the presenting problem. Theoretically, this is the point at which the family's map or rules could not adjust to changing circumstances or a challenge that was upon them. Identifying nodal points punctuates the family's

Table 2.1 Four categories of onset events

Onset type	Examples
1 Life cycle/ developmental change	These are natural changes that happen for all families such as births, deaths, marriages, adolescence, and leaving home but they can be times of incredible stress
2 Relational break	These are changes or challenges that are relational such as attachment disruptions, relationship breakdowns, separation/divorce, and specific events such as infidelity. They can occur in the family living together or across generations
3 Trauma/crisis	Traumatic onset events can range from involvement in natural disasters, accidents, intentional trauma such as violence and abuse, unexpected deaths, or other losses, such as work, financial, or the onset of health difficulties
4 Chaos	Families who have a chaotic lifestyle often have no specific onset events per se. They have always lived with difficulties, relational stress, and tragedy of one kind or another. Their difficulties are often intergenerational with common themes and patterns in their family of origin. There can be a connection between social disadvantage and this type of family experience

story and helps them begin to think about why things changed when they did. This starts to reframe the problem away from the symptomatic individual and locate it in the wider family or system. Onset events often fit into four categories that can overlap. While not exhaustive, Table 2.1 provides a way to organise your thinking and thus help the family think through the effect of various onset events.

There are two steps to exploring onset. The first is to identify events or issues. This is often very clear, especially if it involves a crisis or identified trauma event, but on other occasions may require some curiosity on the part of the therapist to help the family identify possible changes or events (words like stresses, strains, challenges built into an open question is often a good prompt). For example, the impact of a developmental change may be hard to identify or if a historical change, like a separation, that children coped with at the time, it may now seem insignificant to parents, but impact in a new way now the children are older. Step two is to explore the effects of the various onset events on family members and relationships. This process can of course happen reciprocally. Step two is enhanced by employing circular questions as these continue to expand the interactional frame that is likely to help people think and feel differently about their and other people's positions.

The following questions can be used to explore onset events:

When did you first notice what was happening or that things had changed?
Why do you think the problem began then and not at (another time)?
What else was happening for you as a family at that time?
Were there other stresses/strains/challenges for the family at that time?

The effects of onset events can be explored using the dyadic and/or triadic circular questions. The benefit of using circular questions at this point in the interview is their capacity to release information not previously known or considered by family members. Remember, it is the experience of hearing new information that can make create the opportunity for change in systemic therapy, i.e. the difference that makes a difference (Tomm, 1984).

This is another part of the interview where we want to lean into affect and relational descriptions as noted above.

Dyadic circular questions ask one person about another person such as:

Therapist asks person A

If I was to ask B what effect x had on him, what do you think he would say?

Therapist asks person B

How does what A says fit for you?

Triadic circular questions ask one person outside a relationship about two people in a relationship, for example:

Therapist asks person A

What effect do you think (event) had on things between person B and person C? What did you see or hear that makes you think that?

Therapist asks person B

How does what A says fit for you?

Therapist asks person C

How does what A says fit for you?

The flow in this part of the interview depends on integrating the information you are hearing, with the process occurring between people in the room, the affect generated, and the hypothesis you are exploring. It can be challenging for the family to have to connect events and feelings together. It can be useful to explore the intentions behind why people acted the way they did and the meaning ascribed to the onset events. This often creates news of difference because it begins to loosen up the meaning of events for family members.

An enduring concept for this session and the whole of therapy is that empathy and understanding have to match the level of challenge. In other words, the more you want to put difficulties or issues on the table or help people face up to behaviours or events, the more the engagement and warmth of the therapist are relevant to holding the space for the conversation. This helps the family feel safe and mediates against the family rejecting the connections you are trying to help them make.

It is important to note that while the aim in this part of the interview is to mediate against scapegoating or blame in the family by creating a more circular view of problems, this is to be actively avoided if there is violence or abuse of any kind. These issues are discussed in detail in other chapters but if safety issues, or violence, or abuse are disclosed, family therapy may need to go on hold until safety is restored.

Step six – Eliciting a sequence of interactions around the problem

Step six aims to elicit information about the interactions that occur around the problem. The previous section of the interview focused on the start and effect of the problem, and step six focuses on the interactions that maintain it. Sequences of repeated actions and behaviours are an aspect of all interactions between people. Breunlin and Schwartz (1986) identify four time periods in which sequences can occur. The first are sequences that range from seconds to hours (S1), the second from a day to a week (S2), the third from several weeks to several years (S3), and the fourth across at least one generation (S4). Here we are concentrating on the exploration of S1 sequences. In simple terms, the sequence imbeds the interactions or behaviour in a wider context. The sequence explores behaviour but also the intentions behind behaviour and thus releases information about the meaning people in the family have ascribed to each other's actions.

There are some rules of thumb for setting up the sequence.

1 Identify a specific incident that is directly related to the main presenting problem. To start ask a question that focuses on the behaviour in question such as, *Can you tell me about a specific incident when x was at its absolute worst?* Without asking about the worst occasion, you are likely to get the fragment of a sequence. This is because when behaviour or a sequence of behaviour is entrenched, some steps are not necessary as they become automatic over time. We may miss an important step to understanding if we explore one of these more low-key occasions.

2 Sequences involving as many family members as possible are likely to be the most useful. Even if family members were not present, their absence may still be indicative of an interaction with others. Siblings are often a rich source of observation in a sequence and so endeavour to help the family choose a time when more rather than less people were involved.

3 Start the sequence when things were calm and track it through until calm has returned. Understanding the situation before the sequence starts can provide important context. An argument with a teenager at bedtime, for example, may create resentment expressed as school refusal in the morning. The time in the latter stages of the sequence as the escalation diminishes often elicits information about communication patterns in the family. For example, do people apologise, do they withdraw, do they pretend it did not happen, or do the difficulties cease on the surface, but the feelings remain unresolved until the start of the next sequence. If you visualise a clock from 12-3 is the pre-sequence context, 3-9 is the sequence in focus and 9-12 is what happened after the event in focus (to return to normal routine or not).

4 The sequence should focus on behavioural descriptions and avoid generalisations. The questioning style should be curious but seek to make the behaviour concrete in the context of the example given. It can help to think about the sequence being on video and you have the remote control so you can slow all the interactions down frame by frame.

Endeavour to show interest in everyone's view, minimise interruptions and side tracks. It is crucial to linger over inconsistencies in how people describe what happened and help them reflect on what they were thinking, feeling, and trying to achieve or communicate through their actions. It is in the inconsistencies where new information is most likely to reside and the place where people's intentions or the message they were trying to send may be more important than their actual behaviour.

The following questions are a starting point for working with the sequence.

What did x say/do?
If I was a fly on the wall watching, what would I have seen you do next?
What happened next?
What effect did that have?
What did you see happen?
Where were you when that took place?
How would you describe it from your point of view?
What were your intentions in doing that?
What were you trying to say/communicate?

Step seven – Exploring family relationships

Step seven is to explore the relationships between people. Relationship discourses should occur every session (MacKinnon, 1998) because changes in closeness often begin problems and conversely can be the solution. The specific investigation of relationships is intentionally towards the end of the session for two reasons. The first is that we may have understood certain relationship patterns in the interview to this point and can therefore make this part of the interview more precise in exploring specific relationships. The second reason is that relationship-specific discussions are usually the most emotionally intense, and the session format is designed to warm people into discussing more difficult issues as they get more comfortable in the process.

Relationships can be explored with a technique called a relationship scan[1] that is built around the use of triadic circular questions. Start with the relationships that are the easiest and move towards the relationships we see as most problematic or hottest. This allows the family to warm into the task but also gets the relational language in use before more difficult issues are explored. You would normally start with the nature of relationships in the present, but you can also collapse time (White, 1986) and move from the present to the past and the future depending on the information gained, the hypothesis, or how interventive you intend to be (Tomm, 1987a, 1988). The questions in Table 2.2 can be adjusted depending on the time period.

In the case of larger families, it may not be possible to explore every relationship. Time can be reduced by either scanning a limited number of key relationships or by ranking them in order of difficulty. Ranking can still be done using circular questions in the following way:

To mother: If I was to ask father who he is closest to in the family at the present moment, what do you think he would say? Who next? and then who, etc.

To father: How does your wife's ranking fit for you? How would you rank who you are closest to?

To father: If I was to ask mother who she is closest to in the family at the present moment, what do you think she would say? Who next? and then who, etc.

To mother: How does your mother's ranking fit for you? How would you rank who you are closest to?

Table 2.2 Exploring family relationships

Format	Question
1 Setting up	"I would like to get an idea about relationships in the family. I'm not asking about how much people love each other but rather how close people are at the moment"
2 Triadic circular question to a person outside the relationship	To mother How would you describe the relationship between Mary and father?
3 Make description concrete	What do you see or hear happening between them?
4 Use the scaling question to make the description concrete	On a scale of 0–10 where 0 is not close and 10 is very close where would you put their relationship?
5 Check with people inside the relationship and make their observations concrete	To father How does mother's description fit for you? How would you describe the relationship in your own words? To daughter How does mother's description fit for you? How would you describe the relationship between you and your father now?
6 Move to next the dyadic relationship	To father If you were to describe the relationship between Mary and mother, how would you describe it?
7 Repeat the steps for each relationship in the family	

Step eight – Closing the session with reflection and feedback

Step eight involves reflecting on the session and giving the family feedback. The aim is to bring all the parts of the interview together providing a reflection and feedback that is both systemic and interventive for the family. This may have several aspects such as a reflection on how the problem the family brought to the session might make sense or invite the family or a particular family member to engage in a task. Reflections or feedback are going to generally align with how we are expecting change to occur as discussed earlier. A reflection will generally be quite tentative and will invite the family to reflect on their situation. Feedback has a more direct quality and often involves giving an opinion or requests that the family do something more specific. Reflections need to be given tentatively because from a second order cybernetic position we cannot know if what we are thinking will fit or resonate with the family. Remember the "difference that makes a difference" is the difference that the family responds to not what the team or therapist holds on to. This will be reflected in the language we use – *"I wonder if..., What comes to mind is..., I am not sure if this is on the right track but I was thinking..., I hope this is a helpful thing to say .... This might seem a bit strange but...".* Any reflection and feedback are an offering to the family to get them to reflect and make a 'change'. Table 2.3 outlines the key points to cover.

A feature of system family therapy is to positively connote or reframe the problem (Jones, 1993). For example, we may frame behaviour problems as inviting the parents to work together to increase the child's security and strengthen their relationship, rather than saying the child is misbehaving and they need to take control. It can also be useful to think about what is the immediate need that has evolved from the session, such as the focus above on

Table 2.3 Key points for giving feedback

Key point	Rationale	Reflection
1 Affirmations	There should be a compliment for each family member about their participation or character that came through in the session. It is essential to be able to say something positive to everyone as this is part of having systemic empathy for the family	*What strengths have different family members demonstrated today?*
2 Concerns	The concerns of each family member should be revisited. Primarily this is to let the family know you have been listening. However, you can also use this to help them see common issues they share	*What concerns have the family got at the present moment?*
3 Onset	Reflect on any events/experiences that were significant nodal points emphasising the effect these events had on relationships and problem development	*What were the significant nodal points that contributed to problem development?*
4 Message	In this part of the feedback, it is important to link the concerns with the onset events/ circumstances, the sequence, and the relationship scan, in order to explain the presenting problem to the family. It is important to only say things that there is evidence for from the interview. Where you can, remembering the family's actual words or metaphors really helps communication to occur	*How do you make sense of the presenting problem and why?* *Is there a metaphor that would be useful to communicate the ideas?*
5 Positive connotation	This is the point where the meaning you have made of the problem needs to be delivered back to the family. This may not make sense to them when they first hear it and that is okay. It is meant to be "news of difference" and perturb the current family system in order to stimulate change. It is important that the message and positive connotation are given tentatively such as "…in a funny kind of way it's almost like…". This helps the hearing of the message but also reflects the theoretical position of systemic therapy where reality is constructed through interaction and cannot be observed by the therapist. Hence, a tentative and curious stance allows ideas to be put forward – some will resonate and others will not	*How is the presenting problem "helping" the family?*
6 Task/ritual	Giving a task or a ritual is not essential but can often be helpful in assisting the family to think through the information you are feeding back. They can be very simple or complicated. For example, a common task may be to set up an activity between two people who need to improve their relationship. It is not really important whether the task is done or not; it is just another way of injecting new information and often the family will take an idea you have given and change the task to suit them better	*Is there an activity that would highlight the positive connotation for the family between sessions?*

reconnection or safety, but also give feedback on what might be the "bigger picture" such as the need to develop more open emotional expression and communication as a unit. This signalling can help the family feel that you have understood the spectrum of issues that may have occurred in the discussion. The reflection and feedback can be given in several formats, depending on the availability of a co-therapist, a reflecting team, or a sole therapist.

Sole Therapist

On many occasions a therapist will conduct the first session without the luxury of a co-therapist or reflecting team. This places pressure on the therapist to conduct the session, engage in a process of progressive hypothesising during the session, and then provide feedback at the end without assistance. It may be useful instead to take a short break of 15–20 minutes, taking time to reflect on the initial hypotheses, how they have changed throughout the session, and how you want to reflect to the family.

Reflecting Teams

Two types of reflecting teams are used in systemic family therapy. Originally, a team would observe the session behind a one-way screen and consult with the therapist at the end of the session away from the family, and then the therapist would return and give feedback, so the family would be on their own for 15–20 minutes. As giving feedback evolved, this was seen as lacking transparency and reflecting teams changed to have the family (and their therapist) swap rooms with the team and observe the team giving feedback through a conversation together (Anderson, 1995). This approach is more transparent and allows for the family to be provided with a wider range of ideas to stimulate change. Once the team discussion is complete, the two groups swap rooms again and the family can then reflect on the reflections with the therapist. Each family member should be invited to respond briefly rather than engage in any further long therapeutic conversations. Further conversation at this point can risk diluting the effect of the reflections and extending the first session unnecessarily.

Interestingly, families recognise positive effects from either model of reflecting (Mitchell, Rhodes, Wallis, & Wilson, 2013) with the presence of a team heightening the experience and supporting change. Training teams may find it useful to follow the guidelines for reflecting teams provided in Table 2.4. The lead team therapist should begin the

Table 2.4 Training therapists in reflecting team conversations

Training therapists in reflecting team conversations	
1 Affirmations	What impressed you about the family today?
2 Concerns	What concerns do you think they brought to the meeting?
3 Message	How do we make sense of the difficulties they are experiencing?
4 Positive connotation	In a funny kind of way … It is almost like … I'm not sure but … (then deliver positive connotation)
5 Task	What ideas did we have about where to from here?
Post-reflecting team with therapist and family	
6 Family impressions	What stood out to you from what the team said? Or what struck you about the feedback?

conversation and use similar questions to those below to keep some structure in the feedback by asking other team members questions. Ways of reflecting with families continue to evolve and reflections throughout the session, rather than at the end, is a more recent development outlined in detail in Chapter 13.

Step nine – Post-session reflection

Step nine should involve processing the interview, reflecting on the family's response to feedback, and contemplating future sessions. Reflecting teams should also review their own interactions and any parallels with the family system. Sole therapists or teams may recognise new strengths in their work or uncover biases that had led to a particular response by the family. In some cases, these biases may reflect an attachment to one specific hypothesis, and on other occasions they may reflect blind spots emanating from the specific culture of a therapist, their values, or their own experience of family life.

Step ten – Optional – Therapeutic letter to the family

The use of therapeutic letters has been documented by both systemic and narrative therapists (Morgan, 2000; Kindsvatter, Nelson, & Desmond, 2009; Wojcik & Iverson, 1989; White & Epston, 1990a; Wood & Uhl, 1988). As a way of intervening at the end of Session One, we routinely use such a letter. A therapeutic letter to the family should reiterate the feedback. It is a very useful way to stimulate further thought and reflection. This can be pivotal in helping the family remember what was said during the interview and feedback. Many families will be overwhelmed by the feedback and just will not remember the details. The letter format does not need to be any different from the live feedback that was given. The written tone should be similar to the way the feedback was given. Address family members by first name. It is not meant to be like a professional letter you would write to the referrer. To receive the letter before the second session often provides a very useful starting point for the next meeting as you can ask the family, *from the feedback or letter what stood out to you from the feedback last session?*

Conclusion

This chapter has outlined eight key theoretical ideas that describe systemic family therapy in the post-Milan tradition. Rationale and structured guidelines for conducting the first session of post-Milan systemic family therapy have been detailed that include a number of core skills that can be utilised in all sessions of therapy. A clear, structured approach to interviewing can aid therapist development (Rhodes, Wallis, & Nge, 2008), help manage anxiety, and lead to increased confidence to be more spontaneous and responsive to family needs in session. It can also provide a means of ensuring basic competencies for therapists working together, students in training, and those engaging in research. This format would complement the guidelines already published in the Systemic Family Therapy Manual (Pote et al., 2000). A competency chart for this session is given in Table 2.5.

Table 2.5 Post-Milan systemic family therapy first session competency chart

Step	Aims	Key questions/notes	Competency	Achieved
1 **Pre-session preparation** a. **Genogram** b. **Hypothesis**	Draw a map of the family and note key relationships Develop systemic understanding to guide the therapist's thought and interview process • Bring thinking biases out into the open Note: Hypotheses are progressive and will change with the information gathered in the interview	What effect is the problem having on the family? Does the problem help the family in any way? What might it mean for them at this particular point in time? E.g. life cycle and developmental stage Are there wider systems issues? E.g. school Are there sociocultural issues to attune to? E.g. racism or other discrimination	Correctly construct the genogram Develop more than one hypothesis Convey hypothesis utilising systemic thinking with possible positive connotations Consider personal blind spots	
2 **Provide a format for the session**	Outline format for the session Outline confidentiality Outline team (if appropriate) and end of session process	I will ask everyone some questions Meeting is confidential with a few exceptions, e.g. risk of harm Meet for approx. 1.5–2 hours "I want to start by getting to know you outside of the problem"	Convey a clear structure with key items covered – format, confidentiality, end of session process Respond to family anxiety appropriately to contain it as needed	
3 **Engage all family members**	Engage family members Begin to set ground rules for the therapeutic process – one person talking at a time, everyone to participate, answering a question when asked	What do you do during the day? What do you like most/least about it? When you have free time, what do you like to do?	Use open questions as much as possible Make a personal connection with each person Demonstrate warmth and interest in each family member Contain family members by conveying you are confident with the process Deal with interruptions appropriately without damaging engagement	

(Continued)

Table 2.5 (Continued)

Step	Aims	Key questions/notes	Competency	Achieved
4 Explore concerns of family members	Understand concerns Develop a focus on relational concerns Deepen engagement through discussion of difficult issues Maintain neutrality Monitor evidence for hypotheses	*What is concerning you for the family at this point in time?* *What is concerning you the most?* *How concerned are you?* Start with broad open questions and narrow them down to specifics Spend equal time with all family members Interruptions are best dealt with by saying something like *"I can see you have a lot to say and I will ask you about it in a minute"* Use circular questions – circular questions create an atmosphere of openness and *"news of difference"* Show empathy by asking a question rather than with individual therapy oriented active listening skills	Elicit each family member's concerns Get underneath stated concerns to relational concerns Follow affect as required by leaning into deeper emotions Use questioning styles effectively and correctly E.g. circular questions, forced choice questions, ranking questions, focusing questions Maintain neutrality by demonstrating curiosity Continue to manage the process For example, interruptions and high expressed emotions	
5 Understand when the problem began	To understand the point of change (nodal point) Explore the effects of onset effects on individuals and relationships Build empathy in family members for each other through creating new perspectives on events and their effects Look for connections between the onset events and the presenting problem Move the presenting problem from the individual and locate it in the wider family system either due to circumstances or specific actions Monitor hypotheses with evidence	*Why do you think it happened then and not now?* *Why do you think the problem is worse now rather than a year ago?* *What else has been happening for you as a family since the problem began?* Be curious about the problem and its place in the family Remember four types of the onset to consider • Life cycle/developmental change • Relational breaches • Trauma/crisis • Chaos	Demonstrate curiosity regarding onset effects Show capacity to consider events related to the four categories Explore the effects of events on individuals and relationships Use circular questions effectively to develop news of difference for events and meanings Follow affect as required	

(Continued)

Table 2.5 (Continued)

Step	Aims	Key questions/notes	Competency	Achieved
6 Elicit a sequence of interactions around the problem	Understand the influence of the presenting problem/primary concern in the present Imbed behaviour in a context Identify patterns in family interactions Monitor evidence for hypotheses	Sequence focus on behaviour: 1 Start a sequence from when things were calm through the problem and back to calm 2 Get a behavioural description but in interactional terms (avoid generalisations) 3 Show interest in all family members' views 4 Stop interruptions as necessary 5 Find out what all family members' actions were *Can you help me understand what it is like when things are at their worst?* *Has there been a time in the last week or so when it has been particularly difficult?* *What do you see happening at that time?* *What did x say/do?* *What did you see happen?*	Facilitate the family choosing an appropriate event for the sequence Stay focused on the event and avoid generalisations Elicit concrete descriptions of behaviour Explore the message and intentions behind people's behaviour	

(Continued)

Table 2.5 (Continued)

Step	Aims	Key questions/notes	Competency	Achieved
7 Exploring family relationships and connections	Exploring family relationships to place relationships centre stage for the family Identify strong and weak family connections Identify relationship changes over time Monitor evidence for hypotheses	The basic premise of family therapy is that changes in relationships create and solve problems. This also includes relationships outside the family, e.g. school, etc. *"I would like to get an idea about relationships in the family. I'm not asking about much people love each other but rather how close people are at the moment"* Ask open questions first following up with closed questions • To mother – *how would you describe the relationship between Mary and father?* • *What do you see happening between them?* • Then ask a scaling question to represent the relationship • On a scale of 1–10 where 1 is not close and 10 is close, where would you put their relationship? • Now ask the people in the relationship • To father – *how would you describe the relationship between you and your daughter now?* • On a scale of 1-10, etc. Move to the next relationship, etc. Collapse time as appropriate	Set up the relationship scan appropriately Scan relationships from coldest to hottest Utilise triadic circular questions effectively Elicit rich descriptions of the relationship dyad under focus Demonstrate an appropriate use of scaling questions Recognise when to collapse time and seek description either in the past or future to intervene	

(Continued)

Table 2.5 (Continued)

Step	Aims	Key questions/notes	Competency	Achieved
8 Closing the session with feedback	Summarise the session content and process Provide systemic feedback for the family problem Punctuate the meanings around family problems Invite candidate "news of difference"	1 Affirmation – one for each family member 2 Concerns – outline concerns as you have heard them 3 Onset – outline events/issues and effects on family/relationships 4 Message – is what you want to say to the family that pulls together the elements of the interview in a coherent way. Note: the evidence has to come from the interview 5 Positive connotation – this is the final comment at the end of the message that redefines the problem for the family. That is, it should be experienced as a "new" for the family about how it connects people's feelings/behaviour so the focus is not just on the symptomatic family member. This final part of the message needs to be tentative, e.g. "It's almost like.../I don't quite understand but.../In a funny kind of way it's like..." This helps the message to be reflected on by the family. Plus the reality is we cannot know the "truth" only what think we observed and heard 6 Task – this is not essential, but it is a way to get the family experimenting with a new position/role, etc.	Cover the main points of the session so that the family knows the therapist/team was listening Provide a message that is systemic and links presenting problem with new information from the session Ask each family member what they think about the feedback Terminate the session effectively without entering further discussion/debate	

Table 2.5 (Continued)

Step	Aims	Key questions/notes	Competency	Achieved
9 **Post-session reflection**	Review family response to interview process and message Evaluate initial hypotheses post session Conceptualise what future issues may need to be focused on Identify any practical issues to follow up on. Evaluate team processes/supervision issues.	Six key questions for self-reflection 1 *What did I/we learn from the interview about the meaning of the family's difficulties?* 2 *What would I/we like to see change for the family over the course of therapy?* 3 *What was my personal response to the session? And are there any issues of transference/countertransference to consider? Are there any safety/risk issues that need to be followed up on?* 4 *Are there areas for further reflection for me as a therapist from seeing this particular family?* 5 *What is one question I/we would take to supervision regarding this family?*	Demonstrate capacity to reflect on family interview Identify interview strengths and learning edges for further work Identify personal/professional issues that need to be brought to supervision	
10 **Therapeutic letter**	Reinforce the message from the session Stimulate further reflection and possible deviations for session 2	Words on a page do not fade from consciousness as easily as the words in the session The letter should be personally written without professional jargon. Use a similar format as the feedback after the session	Demonstrate a personal writing style Write a message in a tentative way that matches the verbal feedback given	

Acknowledgements

We want to acknowledge our early training internships with Relationships Australia at RAPS Adolescent Family Therapy and Mediation Service where similar structured guidelines were taught.

Resources

The following books provide excellent overviews of family therapy theory. The key papers referred to in the text are listed in the reference list.

- Carr, A. (2012). *Family therapy concepts, process and practice* (3rd ed.). Chichester, England: Wiley.
- Dallos, R., & Draper, R. (2015). *An introduction to family therapy – Systemic theory and practice* (4th ed.). Berkshire, England: Open University Press.
- Rivett, M., & Buchmüller, J. (2017). *Family therapy skills and techniques in action* (1st ed.). Routledge.
- Vetere, A., & Dallos, R. (2003). *Working systemically with families, formulation, intervention and evaluation*. London, England: Karnac.

Note

1 Based on The Relationship Scan developed by Laurie MacKinnon. See Chapter 4 (James & MacKinnon). The format in Table 2.2 deviates from the original by checking with people inside the relationship about whether the description fits.

References

Andersen, T. (Ed.). (1991). *The reflecting team: Dialogues and dialogues about the dialogues*. New York, NY: W. W. Norton.

Anderson, T. (1995). Reflecting processes; acts of informing and forming, you can borrow my eyes, but you must not take them away from me! In S. Friedman (Ed.), *The reflecting team in action* (pp. 11–37). New York, NY: Guilford Press.

Atkinson, B., & Heath, A. (1990). Further thoughts on second-order family therapy – This time it's personal. *Family Process, 29*, 145–155.

Bateson, G. (1972). *Steps to an ecology of mind: Collected essays in anthropology, psychiatry, evolution, and epistemology*. New York, NY: Ballantine Books.

Bion, W. R. (1962). *Learning from experience*. London, England: Karnac Books.

Breunlin, D. C., & Schwartz, R. C. (1986). Sequences: Toward a common denominator of family therapy. *Family Process, 25*, 67–87.

Brown, J. (1997a). The question cube: A model for developing questioning repertoire in training couple and family therapists. *Journal of Marital and Family Therapy, 23*, 27–40.

Brown, J. (1997b). Circular questioning: An introductory guide. *Australia and New Zealand Journal of Family Therapy, 18*, 109–114.

Brown, J. E. (1994). Teaching hypothesising skills from a post-Milan perspective. *Australia and New Zealand Journal of Family Therapy, 16*, 133–142.

Campbell, D. (2003). The mutiny and the bounty: The place of Milan ideas today. *Australia and New Zealand Journal of Family Therapy, 24*, 15–25.

Carr, A. (1997). *Family therapy and systemic practice*. Lanham, MD: University Press of America.

Carr, A. (2000). *Family therapy concepts, process and practice*. Chichester, England: Wiley.

Cecchin, G. (1987). Hypothesizing, curiosity, and neutrality revisited: An invitation to curiosity. *Family Process, 26*, 405–413.

Cecchin, G., Lane, G., & Ray, W. A. (1992). *Irreverence: A strategy for therapists' survival*. London, England: Karnac Books.

Dell, P. F. (1982). Beyond homeostasis: Toward a concept of coherence. *Family Process, 21*, 21–41.

Gergen, K. (1994). *Realities and relationships. Soundings in social constructionism*. Cambridge, MA: Harvard University Press.

Gibney, P. (1996). To embrace paradox (once more with feeling): A commentary on narrative/conversational therapies and the therapeutic relationship. In C. Flaskas & R. Draper (Eds.), *The therapeutic relationship in systemic therapy* (pp. 90–107). London, England: Karnac.

Hardwick, P. J. (1991). Families and the professional network: An attempted classification of professional network actions which can hinder change. *Journal of Family Therapy, 13*, 187–205.

Hoffman, L. (1985). Beyond power and control: Toward a "second order" family systems therapy. *Family Systems Medicine, 3*, 381–396.

Hymmen, P., Stalker, C. A., & Cait, C. A. (2013). The case for single-session therapy: Does the empirical evidence support the increased prevalence of this service delivery model? *Journal of Mental Health (Abingdon, England), 22*(1), 60–71. https://doi.org/10.3109/09638237.2012.670880

Jackson, D. (1968). *Human communication, vol.1. Communication, family and marriage*. Palo Alto, CA: Science and Behaviour.

Jones, E. (1993). *Family systems therapy, developments in the Milan-systemic therapies*. Chichester, England: Wiley.

Keeney, B. (1982). What is an epistemology of family therapy. *Family Process, 21*, 153–168.

Kindsvatter, A., Nelson, J. R., & Desmond, K. J. (2009). An invitation to between-session change: The use of therapeutic letters in couples and family counselling. *The Family Journal, 17*, 32–38.

MacKinnon, L., & James, K. (1987). The Milan systemic approach, theory and practice. *Australia and New Zealand Journal of Family Therapy, 8*, 89–98.

MacKinnon, L., & Millar, D. (1987). The new epistemology and the Milan approach: Feminist and sociopolitical considerations. *Journal of Marital and Family Therapy, 13*, 139–155.

MacKinnon, L. K. (1998). *Trust and betrayal in treatment of child abuse*. New York, NY: Guilford Press.

Madigan, S. (1997). Re-considering memory-re-remembering lost identities back toward re-membered selves. In C. Smith & D. Nylund (Eds.), *Narrative therapies with children and adolescents* (pp. 338–355). New York, NY: Guilford Press.

Mitchell, P., Rhodes, P., Wallis, A., & Wilson, V. (2013). A comparison of two systemic family therapy reflecting team interventions. *Journal of Family Therapy, 36*, 237–254.

Morgan, A. (2000). *What is narrative therapy: An easy to read introduction*. Adelaide, Australia: Dulwich Centre Publications:.

Palazzoli, M., Boscolo, L., Cecchin, G., & Prata, G. (1980). Hypothesizing, circularity, neutrality: Three guidelines for the conductor of the session. *Family Process, 19*, 3–12.

Pocock, D. (1995). Searching for a better story: Harnessing modern and postmodern positions in family therapy. *Journal of Family Therapy, 17*, 149–173.

Pote, H., Stratton, P., Cottrell, D., Boston, P., Shapiro, D., & Hanks, H. (2000). *Systemic family therapy manual*. Leeds Family Therapy and Research Centre; UK: University of Leeds.

Rhodes, P., Wallis, A., & Nge, C. (2008). Can you teach compassion? *Context, 97*, 24–26.

Sadler, J. Z., & Hulgus, Y. F. (1989). Hypothesizing and evidence-gathering: The nexus of understanding. *Family Process, 28*, 255–267.

Tomm, K. (1984). One perspective on the Milan systemic approach: Part 1. Overview of development, theory and practice. *Journal of Marital and Family Therapy, 10*, 113–125.

Tomm, K. (1985). Clinical interviewing: A multifaceted clinical tool. In D. Campbell & R. Draper (Eds.), *Applications of systemic family therapy* (pp. 33–45). New York, NY: Grune and Stratton.

Tomm, K. (1987a). Interventive interviewing: Part 1. Strategising as a fourth guideline for the therapist. *Family Process, 26*, 3–13.

Tomm, K. (1987b). Interventive interviewing: Part II. Reflexive questioning as a means to enable self-healing. *Family Process, 26*, 167–183.

Tomm, K. (1988). Interventive interviewing: Part III. Intending to ask lineal, circular, strategic, or reflexive questions? *Family Process, 27*, 1–14.

Vetere, A., & Dallos, R. (2003). *Working systemically with families, formulation, intervention and evaluation.* London: Karnac.

Von Bertalanffy, L. (1968). *General systems theory: Foundation, development, application.* New York, NY: Brazillier.

Weber, T., & Levine, F. (1996). Engaging the family: An integrative approach. In R. H. Mikesell, D. Lustman, & S. H. McDaniel (Eds.), *Integrating family therapy* (pp. 45–71). Washington, DC: American Psychological Association.

Weiner, N. (1961). *Cybernetics.* Cambridge, MA: MIT Press.

White, M. (1986). Negative explanation, restraint, and double description: A template for family therapy. *Family Process, 25*, 169–184.

Wojcik, J., & Iverson, E. (1989). Therapeutic letters: The power of the printed word. *Journal of Strategic and Systemic Therapies, 8*, 77–81.

Wood, D., & Uhl, N. (1988). Postsession letters: Reverberations in the treatment system. *Journal of Strategic and Systemic Therapies, 7*, 35–52.

Chapter 3

Deviation Amplifying

The Second Session

Paul Rhodes and Andrew Wallis

What is the purpose of this session?

In this first session, the primary aim of therapy is to engage in a conversation with the family that allows both therapist and family to recognise the circular patterns of interaction that maintain the presenting problem in the child (MacKinnon & James, 1987). In this sense, a new perspective on the problem is developed, one that is circular, rather than linear, mediating against the blaming of the child without resorting to the blaming of the family. Once the interview is completed, the reflecting team provides feedback to the therapist in conversation (Andersen, 1987), with the aim of perturbing or disrupting these problem maintaining interactions. In this sense, the first session is concerned with homeostasis. The conversation with the family is aimed at isolating and making sense of the negative feedback processes, developing a reflective capacity that allows room for small deviations to be possible.

The aim of the second session of therapy is to conduct this assessment in a very similar fashion, but with a focus exclusively on processes of change, rather than homeostasis. Instead of asking the family about their concerns, the therapist asks each family member to describe any small deviations in interactions that might have occurred between the two sessions. Instead of plotting a problematic sequence or vicious cycle, the therapist aims to plot a virtuous cycle that includes the deviations described. Each person's contribution to this cycle is amplified using skills from solution-focussed and narrative therapy, thus supporting the transition to a new and more adaptive form of family organisation.

When should I use this session?

In most cases the use of deviation amplifying is recommended for every second session. This is critical, as it takes full advantage of any outcomes from the first session, an opportunity that would be lost if a further problem-oriented session were to be conducted. Deviation amplifying can be conducted at any stage in therapy, following a wide variety of interventions. This chapter provides a comprehensive guide to the process for the second session; the therapist can select and extend specific practices described here for use in future sessions.

There are, however, several situations that would not be suited to deviation amplification in the second session. Firstly, it will be less appropriate if the family has experienced a crisis or a breach of safety of some sort between first and second sessions. A problem-oriented session would be required in these cases. Secondly, it may be prudent to repeat

DOI: 10.4324/9781003490104-4

parts of the initial intervention if new family members join the second session. This provides an opportunity to clarify, fine-tune, or modify the systemic case formulation and feedback.

What is the theory behind this session?

One of the primary concepts in the development of family therapy was that of homeostasis, derived from the study of biological and social systems (Ackoff & Emery, 1972; Bertanalffy, 1968) and adapted by theoreticians to families by the pioneers of family therapy (Bateson, 1972; Jackson, 1957). This concept implies that families regulate their own interactions to preserve equilibrium via corrective feedback mechanisms. While these processes are essentially adaptive, they can also lead to dysfunction when symptomatic or maladaptive behaviour is incorporated into these change-resistant patterns. This concept was so critical in the development of family therapy that the formal recognition of patterns of change in families, or morphogenesis, did not emerge until more than a decade after Jackson's original article on homeostasis (Dell, 1982; Hoffman, 1981; Speer, 1970). Homeostasis was seen, in isolation, as a potentially limiting concept for family therapists one that did not recognise the natural processes inherent in family adaptability to change. These authors drew on the work of the psychiatrist, Maruyama (1963), in differentiating between negative feedback, which counteracted deviations, and positive feedback, which both enabled and amplified them. For Maruyama (1980), changes can occur in leaps, but more often occur gradually. He positioned homeostasis and morphogenesis as two metatypes of causality.

The concept of morphogenesis is most relevant to the second-order cybernetic revolution in systemic therapy in the mid-1980s (Carr, 2006). While the original Milan school can be accused of being somewhat deterministic about the nature of symptom-maintaining interactional patterns (Boscolo, Cecchin, Hoffman & Penn, 1987; Selvini-Palazzoli, 1988; Selvini-Palazzoli, Boscolo, Cecchin, & Prat, 1980;), a social contructionist critique allowed for some irreverence concerning these cherished ideas (Cecchin, 1987) and prepared the ground for a focus on the integration of models in family therapy that was to come (e.g., Breunlin, Schwartz, & Mac-Kune-Karrer, 1992; Pote, Stratton, Cottrell, Shapiro, & Boston, 2002; Carr, 2004).

The concept of morphogenesis provides the ideal vehicle for the integration of systemic practice with solution-focussed and narrative therapy. Solution-focussed therapy (De Shazer, 1985, 1988) emphasises the strengths of the family over aetiological considerations and builds on exceptions to the problem to build a better future. Narrative therapy aims to thicken preferred and liberative stories to help people break free from problem saturated lives (Nicholson, 1995). These models allow the therapist access to familial resources that can be used to promote interactional change, if married theoretically to the principle of circularity.

What are the steps and questions for this session?

A series of steps and related interventive questions are provided below, as guidelines for the second session (see Table 3.1). In some cases, solution-focussed and narrative questions have been employed in a circular question format. From a solution-focussed perspective, this allows one family member to affirm the strengths of another. From a narrative perspective, one can serve as the outsider witness to another. This can be more effective than direct questioning by the therapist, promoting feedback loops that can accelerate the process of change.

Table 3.1 Steps and questions for the session

Steps	Models of therapy
1 Isolate news of difference recalled from the first session	Milan Systemic
2 Identify one or more deviations in familial interactions	Brief Solution Focussed
3 Plot the virtuous cycle	Milan Systemic
4 Use triadic circular questions to explore the circular effects of interactions	Milan Systemic
5 Employ dyadic circular questions to help family members identify strengths in each other responsible for these interactions	Milan Systemic Brief Solution Focussed
6 Employ dyadic circular questions to help family members to situate new behaviours and relational messages in longer standing personal narratives	Narrative
7 Introduce outsider witnesses to consolidate the recognition of preferred stories	Narrative
8 Collapse time regarding the presenting problem, relationships, and the significance of the current deviations	Strategic
9 Use scaling questions to identify current progress and stimulate further deviations	Brief Solution Focussed

Before proceeding, it is important to emphasise that the therapist may have to persist when employing these guidelines, maintaining his/her faith in the possibility of deviations and in the capacity and adaptability of the family in the face of familial anxiety or resistance. Some family members may find the recognition of change anxiety provoking or may experience difficulty in the recognition of their own competence. Persistence in amplifying deviations needs to be balanced with the continued establishment and maintenance of therapeutic relationships and may not be indicated when a presenting problem or family interactions have worsened between sessions one and two.

Step one: Isolate news of difference recalled from the first session

The first step is to reconnect family members with the feedback from the first session. This serves to prime the family to be open to questions about change and can mediate against the presentation of new concerns, or the re-enactment of behaviours that are part of vicious cycles of interaction.

Ask each family member:

- *Can you tell me one thing that most interested you from the feedback last session?*
- *What in particular caught your attention about these comments?*

Step two: Identify one or more deviations in familial interactions

Family members should then be asked to recall any small changes in the presenting problem or interactions since the last session. It may be useful to first ask family members who are most likely to recognise these small changes.

Has there been any time in the last two weeks, when you thought (the presenting problem) would happen, but it didn't?

Or

Has there been any time in the last two weeks where you thought (a change in interaction or relationship identified in session 1) would happen, but it didn't?

Or

Have you noticed any family member doing something slightly different in their interactions in the past two weeks?

Step three: Plot the virtuous cycle

The aim of step 3 is to help the family position one of these deviations in a wider context of interactions. Small changes in behaviour should serve as one step in a sequence of interactions that may have occurred over an hour, a day, or the entire week. The interviewer should aim to plot this sequence with the family in detail, avoiding any attempts to generalise, focussing instead on developing a consistent view of actual events across the relevant time period.

- *Can you tell me about this example in more detail?*
- *If I was a fly on the wall at your house, what would I have seen happen as a lead up to this example?*
- *What happened next?*
- *What happened after that?*
- *Continue to prompt for information until a distinct pattern emerges.*

Step four: Use triadic circular questions to explore the circular effects of interactions

The interviewer should then develop a richer view of these interactions with family members, exploring the relational messages that individuals were giving through new behaviours and the effects of those messages on recipients. In the example below one person is asked to explore the meaning of an interaction between two others. This may be employed with a variety of triads in this step, depending on the number of family members, the nature of the sequence, and the potential significance of interactions.

For example, ask person A the following and then check person A's impressions with persons B and C.

If I asked person B what message he was trying to give to person C, what do you think he would say?

Or

If I asked person B what his intentions were in interacting with person C in this way, what do you think he would say?

If I asked person C what effect person B's behaviour had on him, what do you think she would say?

Or

How important do you think person C would tell me this was to her?

Step five: Employ dyadic circular questions to help family members identify strengths in each other responsible for these interactions

Once a specific sequence and the relational messages have been identified, they can be further amplified by asking family members to identify strengths in each other that made them possible.

Ask person C

- *How do you think person B managed to interact in this way on this occasion?*
- *What advice do you think he was giving himself?*
- *What strengths do you think person B was relying on in interacting in this way?*

Ask person B
- *What was it like for you to hear person C's impressions about what you did?*

Step six: Employ dyadic circular questions to help family members to situate new behaviours and relational messages in longer standing personal narratives

Changes in behaviour can also be amplified by engaging in conversations that demonstrate their consistency with the person's preferred identity and values and the preferred story of their life to this date.

- *What does it tell you about him/her as a husband/wife/son/daughter?*
- *What does it tell you about him as a man/woman/child?*
- *How do you think it relates to his values or what he feels is important in his life?*
- *Can you tell me some other examples in the past of when he has demonstrated these qualities?*
- *Is there any one particular experience in his life that most contributed towards the development of these qualities?*

Step seven: Introduce outsider witnesses to consolidate the recognition of preferred stories

The introduction of witnesses to these changes serves to further thicken preferred stories, providing further solidarity to family members and introducing information to further support deviations.

- *Of all the people you have known, who would be the least surprised to see you taking these steps?*
- *What would this person tell me if they were here and I asked them to tell me a story about how they came to believe in you in this way?*

Step eight: Collapse time regarding the presenting problem, relationships, and the significance of the current deviations

Once small exceptions have been amplified in this way, it is important to return to the reality of the family's progress, not as an established significant amelioration of their concerns in the present, but rather as an event that has the potential to gather momentum if the family commits to further change. One way of achieving this is to collapse time, causing them to reflect on the significance of changes that could take place if they were to continue to interact in these ways.

- *If I met you in three months and these developments had continued, what would you tell me could have happened regarding the problem you initially came to see us about?*
- *If I met you in three months' time and these developments had continued, what would you tell me about the relationships between you?*
- *If I met you again in three years, how significant would you tell me the changes you had made in the past two weeks were? In the life of the identified client? In the life of your family?*

Step nine: Use scaling questions to identify current progress and stimulate further deviations

Scaling questions can also be employed to support the momentum of virtuous cycles, in particular between the second and third questions. Future-oriented scaling questions can also serve as substitutes to the therapist's prescription of systemic tasks.

- *Imagine a scale of 1 to 10, where 1 is how things were in the family at their most difficult and 10 is how you would like them to be. Where would you rate things at the moment?*
- *Imagine that when I see you in two weeks' time, you have progressed by half a point. What would you tell me had happened? What would you tell me had been involved in achieving this?*

The nine steps above provide a template to assist the therapist in amplifying small deviations in family interactions after the first post-Milan interventive interview. This is achieved through the rigorous contextualisation of a small deviation, in a sequence of interactions, in intentional efforts to enhance relationships, in a series of strengths and preferred narratives, and in the history of these preferred narratives. The amplification process is then extended into the future, thus allowing for the self-selection of specific systemic tasks.

Case vignette and transcript

Session one: Assessment and intervention

Daniel is a six-year-old boy referred because of oppositional behaviour and encopresis. He attends the first family therapy session with his mother Mari, aged 46, and her sister Rose, aged 56. Mari has become increasingly frustrated with her son's behaviour and expressed resentment regarding the amount of stress he is causing her. She describes his encopresis as one of many frustrations she has with him. He fails to respond to bowel movements on time and soils himself approximately twice per week. Daniel is somewhat difficult to engage, but after some circular questions involving Rose, he states that he is worried about his mother who 'cries all of the time'. Mari then describes how her frustration with Daniel started when he was two years old. At this time, they both relocated to another state with Daniel's father, Roberto, due to her mother's diagnosis of cancer. Mari spent nine months caring for her mother until her death. The family then relocated back to their current home. Three weeks later Roberto died from a massive heart attack in front of his wife and son. Mari stated that she cannot recall the 12 months following these incidents, adding that she simply survived on a day-to-day basis. She stated that the severity of her grief has subsided somewhat over the past two to three years, but that she still often feels depressed and teary. Mari was also able to respond to inquiries concerning the effect of these events on Daniel. She felt that he may have been traumatised by seeing his father die and that she had not been able to be available to him emotionally for the past four years. Mari and Daniel were then asked to describe a detailed example of his soiling behaviour. They described a recent incident where he soiled his pants and went to the bathroom to try and clean it up without telling his mother. When his mother found him, he was trying to clean his faeces in the sink. She became very distressed, shouted at him for over 15 minutes, and reported that she walked away because she was afraid of what she might do. Rose was then asked to describe the relationship between Daniel and his mother. She felt that they were very close on the inside, but that the events of the past four years and his behaviour meant that they often did not get on very well. Both Mari and Daniel agreed with this view, with Rose crying and expressing a desire to learn how to be close to him again.

Session two: Deviation amplifying

Mari and Daniel returned for a second session two weeks later. Mari had some difficulty recalling the feedback from the first session but felt that the team was able to understand what the family had been through. She recalled feeling some hope that she would be able to find a way through the problems she was having with Daniel (Step one). Mari found it very difficult to identify small instances in the past two weeks when she had been able to be close to Daniel. She expressed some resentment concerning his continued soiling behaviour. Persistence by the therapist, however, revealed one 20-minute period before school, when Mari had been able to play a card game with Daniel and had fun with him (Step two). Daniel reported that he had really enjoyed this exchange and he left for school feeling happy. Mari stated that she had managed to do this because she had been out with friends the night before and felt happier than normal in the morning. This was the first time she had socialised with friends since her husband's death (Step three). She felt that this interaction had made Daniel feel more secure, a statement that he then reflected in a drawing of his mother sitting together watching TV in their lounge room (Step four). Further persistent inquiry assisted Mari to recognise that this could be a small sign of her beginning to reconcile herself with the trauma of the past four years. She was able to isolate several strengths that enabled her to prioritise her own needs on this occasion (Step five). She stated tentatively that she had been a more extroverted and independent woman before her marriage (Step six). Mari chose her mother as the person who would be the least surprised to see her taking these steps in her life. Her mother had also been a sole parent and had been a 'pillar of strength' to her throughout her life. The therapist then consulted with her mother, asking Mari to state what she might have told us about her daughter's character if she had been present. Mari was less tentative during this part of the interview and very emotional. She recalled being a fun-loving and mischievous child, who sometimes got into trouble at school (Step seven). Mari responded well to the therapist's questions regarding the possible future effects of these developments on her relationship with Daniel. After some prompting, she expressed a desire to rediscover her capacity as a mother, modelling herself from her own experience of motherhood. Despite these developments, Mari felt that this was only the very beginning of their recovery from the trauma they had both experienced in the past four years (Step eight). She stated that she hoped to tell us that she had spent more quality time with Daniel at the next session (Step nine).

Transcript

Therapist:	Hi, good to see you, how's your trip in today?
Mari:	Good, Danny's missing sport, so he's a bit cranky, but we'll do it next time.
Therapist:	What sport was it, Danny?
Daniel:	Soccer
Therapist:	You play it much?
Daniel:	Yeah, I play on Sundays, with the Wombats.
Therapist:	Let's start with what interested you most from our last meeting. If there's one thing that struck you most, Mari, from then, what would it be?
Mari:	Good, good, you seemed to see lots of what we'd been through; it's been tough. Rose is the only one I talk to.
Therapist:	What interested you the most about the feedback?
Marie:	Well, maybe I and Danny can work things out. I know I've been focussed on other things. I know he's had a pretty hard run.
Therapist:	Have there been any times in the last two weeks where you thought there'd be trouble between you both, but even for a short time there wasn't?
Mari:	He's still soiling, one really gross one at the mall. I had nowhere to clean him; it stinks the car out.
Therapist:	I'm sure that was pretty awful, and we'll work very hard on it together, but have there been any times, maybe, where things between you were a bit different?
Mari:	(silence)
Therapist:	Despite the stress and everything you showed, that side of you that desperately wants to be closer to him.
Mari:	I tried before school one day; he likes cards.
Therapist:	Do you remember this, Danny?
Daniel:	We played snap and things.
Therapist:	What do you mean?
Daniel:	Mum played snap with me, and I won.
Therapist:	Wasn't mum very good at snap?
Daniel:	We played who could say 'snap' the loudest and I won.
Therapist:	Mari, what exactly would I have seen happening between the two of you if I had been a fly on the wall?
Mari:	We had fun; we forgot about things.
Therapist:	Forgot about things? What do you mean?
Mari:	Life's been so stressful for so long; we just played.
Therapist:	What effect would Daniel tell me it had on him?
Mari:	He was happy; he left for school well; he turned and waved to me, you know? Daniel has finished drawing a picture of himself sitting next to his mum watching TV.
Therapist:	Gee, that's a great picture, what are you doing?

Daniel: We're watching Saturday Disney; it's the weekend and we're watching the Disney shows on Saturday.

Therapist: Mari, how did you manage to do this given you're often not feeling all that great in the morning; I imagine it can be hectic too? What we're your intentions?

Mari: Actually, I went out with friends the night before. I saw two girlfriends I hadn't seen in a long time; we just went for dinner.

Therapist: How long since you'd been out socialising?

Mari: None. It's the first time since Roberto died. I just didn't feel like it before. I thought I'd lost touch.

Therapist: So what effect do you think Daniel would say it had on him, seeing you so happy in the morning?

Mari: Good. I know he feels better; he feels it's normal.

Therapist: What do you think this is a sign of Mari? What's happening to your own relationship with the past?

Mari: I don't know, maybe it's time to think about things?

Therapist: What do you mean?

Mari: To think about what's happening now, to start to move on a bit.

Therapist: How did you manage to give yourself permission to put your own needs forward the other night, to go out, to feel it was time?

Mari: I used to be social, so fun and extroverted, before Roberto. I loved him but he controlled me. I used to love life and do my own thing.

Therapist: Who would you pick who knew this side of yourself the best?

Mari: My mum, she was a single parent, a pillar of strength (crying). I was mischievous and naughty as a kid, into everything. I got into trouble at school, but you couldn't hold me back.

Therapist: Danny, your mum's saying she used to be a bit naughty when she was your age.

Daniel: What did you do mummy?

Mari: (laughing) I remember climbing trees with the boys in the bush and cooking cans of beans on a fire we made in the backyard, and mum used to go spare.

Therapist: If these changes continue where will you both be in six months' time?

Mari: We've moved on I hope. We need to make our own little life. He can be naughty too. I don't want him to be sad.

Therapist: How much do you miss you're son?

Mari: (silence)

Therapist: You're his pillar of strength.

Mari: (silence)

Therapist: If three months from now you are ten out of ten close and you used to be 1, where do you feel now? The last week?

Mari: Maybe four, things have still not been great.

Therapist: If you tell me you are three and a half when I see you next session, what will you tell me you had done to bring this about?

Mari: Not sure. I know we need to spend more time together; maybe we'll do some naughty things together (laughs). I'll show him some of my tricks from when I was young....

Conclusion

The aim of this chapter has been to provide trainees in family therapy with guidelines for conducting the second session of post-Milan systemic family therapy, one that aims to amplify small deviations in family functioning. These guidelines integrate solution-focussed and narrative practices with systemic, thus allowing for the mobilisation of morphogenic processes in the family. Conducting effective family therapy can be seen as a dance between the therapist and family members. Hopefully, these guidelines can provide trainees with a degree of confidence regarding the steps for the first session, increasing the likelihood that they will lead the dance and contribute towards the development of change. A competency chart for this session is given in Table 3.2.[1]

Table 3.2 Deviation amplifying competency chart

Stage	Aims	Key questions	Competency	Achieved
1 **Isolate news of difference recalled from the first session**	Reconnect family members with the feedback from the first session Prime the family to be open to questions about change	*Can you tell me one thing that most interested you from the feedback last session?* *What has caught your attention about these comments?*	Commence the position of being firmly consistent in your curiosity regarding change	
2 **Identify one or more deviations in familial interactions**	To support the family to recall any small changes in the presenting problem or interactions since the last session	*Has there been any time in the last two weeks when you thought (the presenting problem) would happen, but it didn't?* Or *Has there been any time in the last two weeks where you thought (a change in interaction or relationship identified in session 1) would happen, but it didn't?* Or *Have you noticed any family member doing something slightly different in their interactions in the past two weeks?*	Be persistently curious about change, even if faced with some 'resistance' Maintain your faith that changes have occurred, no matter how small	
Plot the virtuous cycle	To help the family to position one of these deviations in a wider context of interactions	*Can you tell me about this example in more detail?* *If I was a fly on the wall at your house, what would I have seen happen as a lead up to this example?* *What happened next?* *What happened after that?* *Continue to prompt for information until a distinct pattern emerges*	Plot this sequence with the family in detail, avoiding any attempts to generalise, focussing instead on developing a consistent view of actual events	

(Continued)

Table 3.2 (Continued)

Stage	Aims	Key questions	Competency	Achieved
3 **Use triadic circular questions to explore the circular effects of interactions**	Develop a richer view of these interactions with family members, exploring the relational messages that individuals were giving through new behaviours and the effects of those messages on recipients	For example, ask person A the following and then check person A's impressions with persons B and C *If I asked person B what message he was trying to give to person C, what do you think he would say?* Or *If I asked person B what his intentions were in interacting with person C in this way, what do you think he would say?* *If I asked person C what effect person B's behaviour had on him, what do you think she would say?* Or *How important do you think person C would tell me this was to her?*	Be aware that this conversation may provoke some initial anxiety, given it begins to challenge homeostasis	
4 **Employ dyadic circular questions to help family members identify strengths in each other responsible for these interactions**	To amplify deviations even further, develop interactive feedback loops based on mutual affirmation	Ask person C *How do you think person B managed to interact in this way on this occasion?* *What advice do you think he was giving himself?* *What strengths do you think person B was relying on in interacting in this way?* Ask person B *What was it like for you to hear person C's impressions about what you did?*	Use the meaning of specific questions but blend them into a more informal and varied conversational tone	
5 **Employ dyadic circular questions to help family members situate new behaviours and relational messages in longer standing personal narratives**	To deepen the process of amplification by demonstrating the consistency of new interactions with preferred identities and values of family members	*What does it tell you about him/her as a husband/wife/son/daughter?* *What does it tell you about him as a man/woman/child?* *How do you think it relates to his values or what he feels is important in his life?* *Can you tell me some other examples in the past of when he has demonstrated these qualities?* *Is there any one particular experience in his life that most contributed to the development of these qualities?*	Use the meaning of specific questions but blend them into a more informal and varied conversational tone	

Table 3.2 (Continued)

Stage	Aims	Key questions	Competency	Achieved
6 **Introduce outsider witnesses to consolidate the recognition of preferred stories**	To further thicken preferred stories, providing further solidarity to family members and introducing information to further support deviations	*Of all the people you have known, who would be the least surprised to see you taking these steps?* *What would this person tell me if they were here and I asked them to tell me a story about how they came to believe in you in this way?*		
7 **Collapse time regarding the presenting problem, relationships, and the significance of the current deviations**	Return to the reality of the family's progress, not as an established significant amelioration of their concerns in the present, but rather as an event that has the potential to gather momentum if the family commits to further change	*If I met you in three months and these developments had continued, what would you tell me could have happened regarding the problem you initially came to see us about?* *If I met you in three months' time and these developments had continued, what would you tell me about the relationships between you?* *If I met you again in three years, how significant would you tell me the changes you had made in the past two weeks were? In the life of the identified client? In the life of your family?*	Be sure to ask the questions in a pretend time frame or the family may feel that you are challenging them to change too directly	
8 **Use scaling questions to identify current progress and stimulate further deviations**	To support the momentum of virtuous cycles, in particular between the second and third sessions To encourage the family to develop their own solutions to problems rather than rely on therapists' prescriptions	*Imagine a scale of 1 to 10, where 1 is how things were in the family at their most difficult and 10 is how you would like them to be. Where would you rate things at the moment?* *Imagine that when I see you in two weeks' time, you have progressed by half a point. What would you tell me had happened? What would you tell me had been involved in achieving this?*	Keep the expectations low so that they are both achievable and surpassable	

Note

1 Part of this manuscript was previously published as Rhodes, P. (2008). Amplifying deviations in family interactions: Guidelines for trainees in post-Milan family therapy, *Australian and New Zealand Journal of Family Therapy*, 29, 34–39. Permission has been granted by the Journal.

References

Ackoff, R., & Emery, F. (1972). *On purposeful systems*. New York. NY: Intersystems.

Andersen, T. (1987). The reflecting team: Dialogue and meta-dialogue in clinical work. *Family Process, 26*(4), 415–428.

Bateson, G. (1972). *Steps to an ecology of mind: Collected essays in anthropology, psychiatry, evolution, and epistemology*. Chicago, IL: University of Chicago Press.

Bertanalffy, L. (1968). *General system theory. Foundations development, applications*. New York, NY: George Brazille.

Boscolo, L., Cecchin, G., Hoffman, L., & Penn, P. (1987). *Milan Systemic family therapy: Conversations in theory and practice*. New York, NY: Basic Books.

Breunlin, D., Schwartz, R., & Mac-Kune-Karrer, B. (1992). *Metaframeworks: Transcending the models of family therapy*. San Francisco, CA: Jossey-Bass.

Carr, A. (2004). *Family therapy: Concepts, process and practice*. West Sussex, UK: Wiley Series in Clinical Psychology.

Cecchin, G. (1987). Hypothesizing, circularity, and neutrality revisited: An invitation to curiosity. *Family Process, 26*(4), 405–413. https://doi.org/10.1111/j.1545-5300.1987.00405.x

De Shazer, S. (1985). *Keys to solutions in brief therapy*. New York, NY: Norton.

De Shazer, S. (1988). *Clues: Investigating solutions in brief therapy*. New York, NY: Norton.

Dell, P. (1982). Beyond homeostasis: Toward a concept of coherence. *Family Process, 21*, 21–41.

Habib, C. (2011). Integrating family therapy training in a clinical psychology course. *Australian and New Zealand Journal of Family Therapy, 32*(2), 109–123. doi: 10.1375/anft.32.2.109.

Hoffman, L. (1981). *Foundations of family therapy*. New York: Basic Books.

Jackson, D. (1957). The question of family homeostasis. *The Psychiatric Quarterly Supplement, 31*, 79–90.

MacKinnon, L., & James, K. (1987). The Milan systemic. Approach: Theory and practice. *Australian and New Zealand Journal of Family Therapy, 8*, 89–98.

Maruyama, M. (1963). The second cybernetics: Deviation-amplifying mutual causal processes. *American Scientist, 5*, 164–179.

Maruyama, M., Beals, K. L., Bharati, A., Fuchs, H., Gardner, P. M., Guilmet, G. M., ... & Van Esterik, P. (1980). Mindscapes and science theories [and Comments and Reply]. *Current anthropology, 21*, 589–608.

Murray, S. B., Wallis, A., & Rhodes, P. (2012). The questioning process in Maudsley family-based treatment. Part 1: Deviation amplification. *Contemporary Family Therapy, 34*, 582–592. https://doi.org/10.1007/s10591-012-9217-3

Nicholson, S. (1995). The narrative dance: A practical map for White's therapy. *Australian and New Zealand Journal of Family Therapy, 16*, 23–28.

Pote, H., Stratton, P., Cottrell, D., Shapiro, D., & Boston, P. (2002). Systemic family therapy can be manualised: Research process and findings. *Journal of Family Therapy, 17*, 149–173.

Richardson, K. (2016). Family therapy for child and adolescent school refusal. *Australian and New Zealand Journal of Family Therapy, 37*, 528–546. 10.1002/anzf.1188.

Selvini-Palazzoli, M., Boscolo, L., Cecchin, G., & Prata, G. (1980). Hypothesizing—circularity–neutrality: Three guidelines for the conductor of the session. *Family Process, 19*(1), 3–12. https://doi.org/10.1111/j.1545-5300.1980.00003.x

Selvini-Palazzoli, M. S. (1988). *The work of Mara Selvini-Palazzoli*. New York, NY: Aronson.

Speer, D. (1970). Family systems: Morphostasis and morphogenesis, or 'is homeostasis enough?' *Family Process, 9*, 259–278.

Chapter 4

Establishing the Parental Hierarchy

An Integration of Milan Systemic and Structural Family Therapy

Kerrie James and Laurie MacKinnon

Introduction

During the 1970s and 1980s, Structural/Strategic family therapists conceptualised family relationships as "family structure": triangles, hierarchy, and enmeshed or disengaged sub-systems (Haley, 1987; Minuchin, 1974). During the 1990s, the idea of family structure became controversial as newer "second order" approaches, underpinned by social constructionist ideas, notably Milan systemic family therapy and Narrative therapy, challenged the notion of family structure and its normative implications (Levy, 2006), instead emphasising individual experience, narratives, and the construction of meaning (Goldenberg & Goldenberg, 2008). These developments led to the use of "conversational" approaches evolving from structural family therapy and the Milan systemic approach and were regarded as occupying opposite ends on the continuum of family therapy models. Further, the last 20 years have witnessed an even stronger move away from the more goal-centred, directive therapies of the earlier years of family therapy towards a focus on processes in the session of listening, reflection, and dialogue (see Chapter 13). While not eschewing these developments, in this chapter and the other chapter in this book (Chapter 9), we preserve aspects of earlier structural and strategic approaches that we believe are useful in helping families resolve the problems that brought them to therapy.

While debates flourished within family therapy, further afield, family researchers were identifying family characteristics that correlated with optimal functioning in children, providing empirical evidence for parenting characteristics that correlated with children's internalising and externalising problems and supporting the structural concepts of "hierarchy" and "triangulation" (Baumrind, 1978; Fletcher, Steinberg, & Sellers, 1999; Marcone, Affuso, & Borrone, 2020). Researchers found that children who had "authoritative" parents (showing a combination of warmth, control, and tolerance) fared better academically, had fewer conduct problems, and were less anxious and depressed. On the other hand, children who had parents who were "authoritarian", "indulgent" or "uninvolved" fared less well (Baumrind, 1978; Fletcher, Steinberg, & Sellers, 1999). The importance of having an "authoritative" parent was, in fact, found to be so strong that researchers concluded that having one authoritative parent was more important to a child than having two parents who were consistent but not authoritative (Fletcher, Steinberg, & Sellers, 1999). This was also the case in several other cultures (Pinquart & Kauser, 2018). Family researchers also found significant empirical support for a correlation between unclear hierarchies, cross-generational coalitions, and children's conduct problems (see Baumrind, 1978; Diamond

DOI: 10.4324/9781003490104-5

& Liddle, 1999; Greenspan, 2006; Jiménez, Hidalgo, Baena, León, & Lorence, 2019; Sells, 1998; Shaw, Criss, Schonberg, & Beck, 2004).

This chapter illustrates how aspects of two apparently incompatible approaches, the Milan systemic approach and Structural/Strategic family therapy, can be integrated to address the two core dimensions of "authoritative" parenting: the dimension of parental "warmth" through enhancing attachment bonds and the dimension of "control" through strengthening the parental hierarchy. Specifically, from the Milan approach, hypothesising and circular questions are used to explore the complex web of family relationships. From Structural/Strategic family therapy, relationships are conceptualised in terms of coalitions and hierarchical patterns, and the technique of enactment is used to create change in relationships during the session.

Selected structural ideas and interventions

Structural family therapy originated with the work of Salvador Minuchin in the 1960s and 1970s. Jay Haley was an early contributor to the development of structural family therapy, while his later work, known as strategic family therapy, retained many structural concepts. Both approaches conceptualised family interactions in terms of power and hierarchy (Haley, 1986, 1987; Haley & Richeport-Haley, 2003; Minuchin, 1974; Minuchin & Fishman, 1981; Minuchin, Lee, & Simon, 1996; Minuchin, Montalvo, Guerney, Rosman, & Schumer, 1967; Minuchin & Nichols, 1993; Minuchin, Rosman, & Baker, 1978).

Hierarchy and coalitions

Haley defined "hierarchy" as family members' different levels of power and status conferred by generation, income, or other valued attributes. A "confused" or "unclear" hierarchy is one in which the "status positions are ambiguous as a result of one member at one level of the hierarchy forming a coalition with against a peer with a member at another level" (Haley, 1987, p. 110). A hierarchy is inferred by observing the behaviour between family members: a parent asks a child to do something, and the child refuses and the parent withdraws; a child is disrespectful and does not obey a parent; one parent supports a child in disobeying the other parent; a child looks after or dominates a parent.

Complementarity and "soft/hard" splits

In dyadic relationships, partners can fit together as two opposites as if in a mould that shapes their interactions (Minuchin & Nichols, 1993) such as in the complementary patterns of dominance/submission and over-functioning/under-functioning. In parenting, a complementary pattern is often manifested as a "soft/hard" split, an escalating difference between the parents where one parent's "softness" elicits the "toughness" of the other parent in a reciprocal manner. Feeling supported by a "soft" parent, the child increases their problematic behaviour. The "tough" parent, feeling isolated and on the outside of the triangle, escalates their critical or controlling behaviour, which in turn further elicits the softer parent to take the side of the child. The "soft" parent is either afraid of or unsuccessful in challenging the other parent and uses the coalition with the child to undermine him or her. Looking at it in another way, the structure of these family relationships is that of a confused hierarchy and interventions to increase parental consistency and promote authoritative parenting are warranted.

Thus "softness" and "toughness" are not simply personality characteristics but tendencies or traits elicited and reinforced when a parent has been dealing with the child's behaviour over a considerable time period. The parent is undermined by the other parent and there is concurrent actual or avoided marital conflict (Brown, 2023; James, 1989; Takeuchi & Takeuchi, 2008).

Structural enactment

An enactment is an intervention in the session where the therapist instructs two or more family members to interact, enabling the therapist to see the "family dance", elicit or coach new behaviours, and shift negative relationship patterns (James & MacKinnon, 1986; Minuchin & Fishman, 1981; Nichols & Fellenberg, 2000). Therapists can use enactments to support and coach parents to discuss and resolve difficult parenting and marital issues (Tsvieli, Lifshitz, & Diamond, 2022).

In setting up an enactment, the therapist explains the purpose of the enactment, specifies the specific content, and organises the physical space so that the partners are sitting close together and able to maintain eye contact. The therapist sits back, avoids eye contact, and stays out of the interaction until it seems useful or necessary to interrupt an evolving negative interaction. The therapist makes brief, specific, and process-oriented comments to help the couple stay on track, avoid interruptions, and maintain the content focus. When the couple have finished the dialogue, the therapist reviews with them the process of what has occurred, helping them notice what they did well and learn from what they did not do well (Butler, Davis, & Seedall, 2008; Davis & Butler, 2004; Nichols & Fellenberg, 2000). The therapist's directive style in creating an enactment contrasts with the therapist's more neutral and impartial position in the Milan approach.

Selected Milan ideas and interventions

The Milan systemic approach grew from the teamwork of four psychoanalysts in Milan, Italy, during the 1970s. Their work was shaped by the systemic ideas emerging from Gregory Bateson and the Mental Research Institute in the USA and they became known for their style of questioning, rigorous systemic conceptualisation, and paradoxical end of session interventions. The Milan approach was introduced to English speaking countries with the publication of *Paradox and Counter Paradox* (Selvini-Palazzoli, Cecchin, Prata, & Boscolo, 1978) and their seminal paper: *Hypothesizing, Circularity and Neutrality: Three Guidelines for the Conductor of the Session* (Selvini-Palazzoli, Cecchin, Prata, & Boscolo, 1980). When the group subsequently split and went in different directions, Selvini-Palazzoli and Prata began research into family functioning and Boscolo and Cecchin further developed the model of therapy and travelled internationally teaching their approach (Boscolo & Cecchin, 1982; Boscolo, Cecchin, Hoffman, & Penn, 1987; Pirrotta, 1984; Tomm, 1984).

Although the Milan approach was commonly considered a "strategic" approach, this view was mistaken for several reasons including, firstly, that the Milan approach, unlike Strategic family therapy, did not conceptualise family relationships in terms of hierarchy (MacKinnon, 1983). Secondly, while helpful for children with "internalizing" symptoms such as anxiety, depression, and psychosis, the Milan approach in its purest form was significantly less successful with "externalizing" symptoms such as children's acting out behaviour problems (MacKinnon, Parry, & Black, 1984). The elegant questioning process of the Milan approach and the therapist's neutral stance failed to empower parents to take charge of children who were "ruling the roost". This was a serious limitation for most family therapists whose work often involved children with behavioural difficulties. The Milan approach in its original form was also criticised for not considering the role of broader systemic issues such as the social context of gender, class, ethnicity, and the issue of violence and abuse (MacKinnon & Miller, 1987) and the importance of therapist warmth.

As originally defined by the Milan team, a hypothesis is the therapist's formulation "... based upon the information he (sic) possesses regarding the family he is interviewing. The hypothesis establishes a starting point for his investigation as well as his verification of the validity of this hypothesis..." (Selvini-Palazzoli et al., 1980, p. 4). Hypotheses are "more or less useful" and, if disconfirmed, new hypotheses are developed as the therapy progresses (ibid., p. 4).

Circularity is "the capacity of the therapist to conduct his (sic) investigation on the basis of feedback from the family in response to the information he solicits about relationships and, therefore, about difference and change" (ibid., p. 8). To solicit information about relationships, the therapist uses circular questions that ask one person about the interaction or relationship between two or more others (Brown, 1997a, 1997b; MacKinnon, 1988; MacKinnon & James, 1987; Tomm, 1987a, 1987b, 1988).

In this questioning process, the therapist maintains a neutral stance, balancing family members' participation in the session and remaining impartial but curious about each person's perspective. *Neutrality* is the "pragmatic effect ... (the therapist's) total behaviour ... has on the family... not his intrapsychic disposition" (Selvini-Palazzoli et al., 1980, p. 11).[1]

Case study

The therapist received the following intake information.

The mother phoned for an appointment.[2] She was in her early 50s and worked full time as a beautician. The father, in his 60s, had worked for many years in a struggling small business. Four children ranged in age from 13 to 26 with an age gap of eight years between the 13-year-old girl and the next eldest. The two eldest children, a male and a female, were not living at home. The maternal grandmother, in her 80s, had a terminal illness (Figure 4.1). The presenting problem was the behaviour of the 13-year-old girl, Sophie, who was failing school, truanting, and had been charged with stealing from a shop. The therapist noted that the family had an Italian surname.

Pre-session – Hypothesising

The benefits of pre-session hypothesising include the following:

- The therapist has clear hypotheses about family relationships in order to guide his or her questions during the session.
- The therapist retains flexibility in conceptualising the family, thus avoiding "marrying the hypothesis".

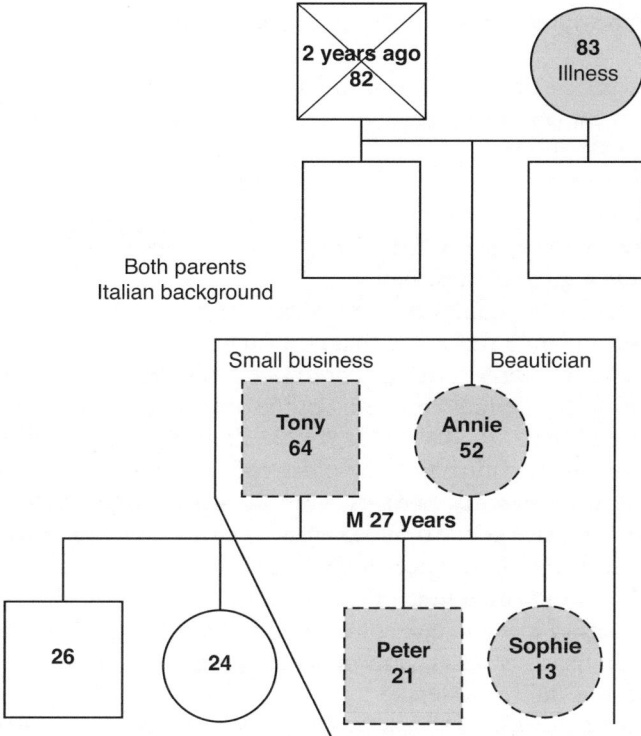

Figure 4.1 Genogram.

- The therapist prepares for the session, thus maximising the opportunities presented within each session and not overlooking important areas.

In the pre-session, the therapist draws on her understanding of individual and family development to formulate structural and systemic hypotheses about family relationships to guide her questioning in the session to follow. Using basic genogram information to hypothesise about boundaries, triangles, coalitions, and hierarchy, the therapist asked questions such as:

- What do the ages of family members tell us about their individual and family life stages?
- Given their life stage, what would we expect of the relationships between parents and children, between the father and the mother, and between this family and the parents' families of origin?
- How closely involved or autonomous are family members likely to be?
- Is there anything special or unusual about the number of children, the spread in ages between the children, and the difference in age between the parents or between the parents and children?
- What might be the impact of events on the family such as job loss, disability, illness, loss, separation and divorce, or death?
- What sense do we make of why this family would have this problem at this time?

In this case the therapist and her team speculated about:

- *Cultural stereotypes*, noting that in Italian families, relationships are close, often characterised by intense emotional expression and, under stress, emotional volatility. Families often privilege male children.
- *Life stage*, noting the age difference between the parents. The father may be nearing retirement and the mother may still see herself as relatively young. How much do they have in common at this stage of their lives? How able are they to cooperate in setting and following through with clear limits?
- *Sibling position*, noting a significant age difference between 13-year-old Sophie and her sibling, her position being more like that of a single child. Perhaps the parents did not expect to have their last child. Are they tired of parenting, giving up on having authority? Is one or are both parents softer with Sophie or treat her as special because she is the youngest of the children, "the baby"? Is Sophie closer to one parent than to the other?
- *Issues of loss and change*, noting that the older children have moved away. This is likely a loss for one or both parents, perhaps more for the mother. Perhaps it is also a loss for Sophie who may have tried to fill this gap by either a coalition with one parent or, alternatively, by investing in her peer network and pulling away from the family.
- *Family life cycle*, noting the illness of the maternal grandmother. The mother may be facing the anticipatory loss and current demands of caring for her own mother. If she is preoccupied, who feels her absence most acutely, her husband or her young daughter? Who do they turn to fill the absence?
- *The nature of the presenting problem*, noting that it is an "externalizing" rather than "internalizing" problem. This suggests a lack of consistent rules and boundaries and the likelihood that there is a coalition with a "soft" parent. A "soft" parent often perceives the other parent as too harsh and is trying to compensate. Perhaps the father, hurt and angry at his wife's preoccupation, is the soft one who turns to his daughter. Perhaps the mother is the soft one, left feeling overwhelmed with loss and family responsibilities and unsupported. Perhaps there is a shifting coalition with both parents, the girl intermittently receiving support for her misbehaviour from each parent.
- *The role of the older siblings*. Perhaps one of them sides with Sophie against her parents, enabling her misbehaviour. Alternatively, one of the siblings may have become "parentified", trying to take on the parent's role of disciplining Sophie.
- *The involvement of larger systems*. The family would have had news from the school and the police about the girl's behaviour. Perhaps they sided with the girl against the outsiders, forming a coalition that allowed the girl's misbehaviour. Alternatively, the parents may have felt criticised by the outsiders and has this decreased their confidence and effectiveness in setting limits for their daughter.

With these ideas in mind, the therapist began the first session with the family, curious to find out which of these ideas would find support as the interview unfolded.

Observing the family process as it unfolds in the room

As the family entered the room and sat down, the therapist took note of their spontaneous interactions – everyone talked at once and there was laughter. When they sat down, the father made a point of sitting beside the mother. The 13-year-old, Sophie, then moved to sit on the other side of the father, while the older 21-year-old son, Peter, sat in a chair next to the mother.

When the therapist asked about their concerns, the father took the lead, expressing concern for his daughter's "mental health", mentioning that in his own large extended family, there were others with mental health problems. The therapist noted that he framed the problem as involuntary and internal to the daughter.

The 21-year-old brother, his tone angry and critical, interrupted the father, "*You let her get away with murder. You never let us get away with anything. I wasn't out past 10 until I was 18*".

When it was the mother's turn to speak, her voice was hard, "*Sophie has embarrassed and humiliated us. Our older children were never like this. We've tried everything and I'm at my wits end*".

Sophie glared at her mother: "*You **hate** me, don't you? You wish I'd **never** been born*".

As the mother and Sophie began arguing, the father interrupted the mother, telling her not to get worked up, and then turned to Sophie, his voice softer, "Don't get like that now. We're here to help you. You know we love you". He turned to the therapist and said, "She's very upset. She has had a lot of trouble sleeping at night".

As the interview progressed, the therapist asked about the problem that brought them to therapy. While the parents described the problems with Sophie, the father mentioned that the mother was too harsh while the mother described how the father made excuses for Sophie, releasing her from consequences and talking to Sophie behind her back about the mother's moodiness.

In these opening minutes, the behaviour of family members already revealed a great deal. On the positive side, there was warmth, a sense of connection, and all family members seemed able to speak openly. There was evidence of a *complementary pattern*, a "hard–soft" split between the parents, and the possibility that the father was in a *coalition* with the daughter against the mother. The *hierarchy* was unclear – Sophie challenged her mother as though they were peers.

The triangle of mother, father, and daughter could be conceptualised as a cross-generational coalition, with the father and daughter aligned against the mother. The therapist wondered if there was also a coalition between the older brother and the mother against Sophie.

Scanning the relationship web

Using *circular questions*, asking one person about the relationship between two others, the therapist asked a series of overlapping questions using a technique the authors have termed the *relationship scan*. The relationships scan maps the intensity of dyadic relationship bonds and compares one relationship to another. The relationship scan gives an indication of key triangles of who is most central and who is most peripheral in family relationships (MacKinnon, 1998).

1. Scan of dyadic relationships

The therapist asked Peter, the brother, "*How do you see the relationship between your father and Sophie?*"

"*Quite close*", Peter said. "*She's always been the baby. He favours her over the rest of us*".

"If you gave their relationship a rating out of 10, 10 being the highest, what number would you give them?"

"Probably an eight. They're close", he said.

The therapist then asked the mother a similar set of questions about the father–Sophie relationship and she said that she also saw them as close, giving them a 7.

"How do you see the relationship between your mother and Sophie?" the therapist asked Peter.

"They used to be close when she was little but it's changed since she started high school", he said.

"What number would you give their relationship?"

"Now it's about a four".

The therapist then asked the father the same set of questions about the mother-Sophie relationship and he gave their relationship a 2, saying, *"They argue all the time"*.

"How would you compare your father and Sophie's relationship with your mother and Sophie's relationship?" the therapist asked Peter.

"The big difference is that Sophie and Dad don't argue that much because Dad gives into her", said Peter. *"And they talk more. With Mum, Sophie is rude back. She answers back and really stresses Mum"*.

The therapist then asked Sophie questions about the relationship between Peter and each of his parents.

"Dad and Peter argue a lot", said Sophie. *"Peter says he's too old for Dad to be telling him what to do"*. She rated the relationship a 5. On the other hand, she said that Peter and his mother were *"Much closer, a nine. He always takes her side. Even against Dad"*.

When the therapist asked the mother about the father-Peter relationship, she gave the relationship a 4, describing how Peter would often avoid his father who tended to criticise him. In contrast, the father described the mother-Peter relationship as very close, 8 out of 10. So far, the questions revealed that the mother was closest to the son while the father was closest to the daughter. The therapist went on to explore the sibling relationships, particularly interested in the relationship between Peter and Sophie. She started by exploring Sophie's relationship with each sibling.

"Sophie doesn't have much to do with them since they moved away from home", said the mother, *"but she used to be quite close to her sister who doted on her when she was little. They used to be a 9/10 but now it's probably only a five"*.

When the therapist asked about the relationship between Peter and Sophie, the mother said *"About a five. They don't have a lot to do with each other now that Peter is working and has a girlfriend"*.

"More like a three", said the father. *"Peter used to be kinder, like a big brother should be. Now he's critical and bossy and Sophie hates it. I wish he would spend more time with her and talk to her more"*.

"Why would I want to talk to him?" Sophie interrupted and sneered, tears welling up.

"How do you see your relationship with Peter?" asked the therapist.

"I don't want to talk about him. Alright?" Sophie said, turning her face away.

The therapist now understood that the relationship between Sophie and her brother was fraught. The parents, hearing this as well, also realised that this relationship was part of the problem. The therapist now wanted to explore how the children experienced their parents' relationship. She asked Peter and then Sophie: "How do you see the relationship between your mom and dad?"

Peter shrugged, "*All right. Maybe a 5*".

"*A six*", said Sophie. "*They argue but like don't most parents argue?*"

"*What do you see your parents arguing about, Sophie?*"

"*Me mostly. Sometimes about Nana and how much time Mum spends over there*".

The therapist then asked Sophie and Peter, "*When you compare your parents' relationship to other parents you know, say your friends' parents or your cousins' parents, how do you see their relationship?*"

Sophie rolled her eyes and said, "*How would I know? I don't have anything to do with my friends' parents*".

"*In some ways they're closer*", said Peter. "*Dad sticks up for Mom. But they do argue more than other parents do*".

The mother explained that her own mother was ill with cancer and her health had been failing in the last year. Tearing up, she said that three years ago her father, the grandfather, had died suddenly of a stroke leaving the grandmother bereft. As her only daughter, it was now up to her to support and care for the grandmother.

The therapist explored relationships in the family prior to the onset of Sophie's problems and before the death of the grandfather. They described the mother-Sophie relationship as much closer at that time, with Peter less close to the mother, and the parents arguing less. Sophie's older siblings had lived at home then and the older sister had had a particularly close relationship with the mother.

The therapist wondered about the effect of the grandfather's death and the grandmother's illness on both the mother's well-being and her emotional availability to Sophie. She knew it would be important to assess whether the mother was depressed and the degree to which the father was supporting her through this difficult time. She was concerned that if she were to ask these questions in the whole family session, the mother might not be completely open or might resent being exposed in front of her children. The therapist decided to wait and assess the mother for depression when she saw the parents alone.

2.   *Comparing and ranking dyadic relationships*

The therapist then asked relationship questions comparing one relationship to another and ultimately to rank order them in terms of closeness. This would give a clearer of idea of the degree to which Sophie was connected to each of her parents and an indication of relationships that could be improved.

First she asked Sophie, "*Of all the relationships in the family living at home now, which relationship would you say is the closest?*"

"*Peter and Mum*", said Sophie.

"*And then which relationship?*"

"*Dad and Mum*".

"*And then?*" asked the therapist.

"*Dad and Peter*".

"*And then?*"

"*Dad and me*".

"*And who after you and your Dad?*"

"*Me and Mum and very last of all me and Peter*".

Except for the father who challenged the notion that Peter was closer to the mother than he himself, family members agreed on the following ranking of relationships from closest (top) to the most distance:

Mother and Peter
Mother and Father
Father and Peter
Father and Sophie
Mother and Sophie
Peter and Sophie

From this, it became evident that all family members placed Sophie's relationships as less close than that of the parents with each other and with Peter. It confirmed the perspectives of family members that the least close relationship was between Sophie and her brother, Peter.

The therapist then asked Sophie where her older siblings fit into this picture. Other family members were asked similar questions to rank order the relationships. Compiling the multiple layers of their answers, the therapist developed her own picture of the relationship bonds within the family. Sophie seemed to have a distant and conflictual relationship with Peter and to be isolated from her other siblings. Once, before her grandmother's illness, Sophie and her mother had been close, and now Sophie seemed least connected to her mother. She had a closer relationship with her father, but this relationship was not nearly as close as the relationship between Peter and the mother or even between the mother and the siblings who had left home. Sophie was the "low man on the totem pole", the least important or lowest ranking person in the family, who had to answer to everyone above her.

At this point, the therapist conceptualised the key triangles as follows:

• Mother, father, and Sophie in which the father and Sophie are in a coalition against the mother. This could even be a shifting coalition, with the father sometimes siding with the mother against Sophie.
• Mother, Peter, and Sophie in which the mother and son are in a coalition against Sophie.
• Grandmother, mother, and father in which the father is on the outer.

The therapist could see that Sophie had no one who was clearly on her side.

Exploring hierarchy

To explore the hypotheses that the parents were polarised in a soft/hard split in their parenting of Sophie, the therapist needed to explore the hierarchy and control between Sophie, her mother, father, and brother. To do this, the therapist explored each of these relationships using the metaphor of "boss" and "friend".

To introduce this idea, the therapist spoke first to the father, saying, "*The relationship between children and parents is in some ways like that of friends – sharing special moments, talking, having fun together, and in other ways more like a boss-employee relationship where the parent must lead with directions and the young person must follow those directions. That tends to change over time as young people become more their own boss, making their own decisions and taking responsibility for themselves. When you look at the relationship between Sophie and her mother currently, what percentage is Anna a friend to Sophie and what percentage a boss?"*

"There isn't much friend, right now", said the father. *"Maybe 10% friend, 90% boss".*

"I see. And right now, given Sophie's age and stage in life, what would you think would be ideal percentage boss-friend in her relationship with her mother?"

"I'd say 70% friend, 30% boss".

The therapist asked the mother, *"How do you see your relationship with Sophie in terms of boss, friend?"*

"I guess we are not friends right now. But I'm not much of a boss either", she said. *"I try but I can't get her to do anything. Probably 90% boss and only 10% friend. That's not because that's how I want it to be. She pulled away from me and so it doesn't leave a lot of room for being friends left".*

"What would your ideal be?"

"At her age, right now, she still needs a lot of direction. So I'd say 50/50".

"And how do you see the relationship between Sophie and her father in terms of boss/friend?"

"Probably the exact opposite of mine. He tries to be her friend. 90% friend. Maybe only 10% boss".

"And your ideal? What should it be for Sophie and her father?"

"Same as mine. 50-50. Sophie needs her Dad to be stronger, a stronger leader not just a friend".

Turning again to the father, the therapist asked, "How do you see your relationship with Sophie? More boss? More friends? What percentage?"

"70-30. I think I'm 70% friend, 30% boss", said the father. *"And that's how I think it should be".*

"What about you, Sophie, how do you see your relationship with your dad in terms of boss and friend?"

"Like he says, about 70% friends."

"And how do you think it should be, at your age now?"

"Probably 60% friend. I don't think he should be a boss, though. Maybe he should be 40% leader".

"And with your mother?"

"She's a hundred percent boss or at least she tries to be".

"And how do you think it should be at your age?"

"60% friend, 40% boss".

"Was there a time it was more like that?"

"Before I went to high school. Before Nana got sick".

The therapist looked towards Peter and said, *"In all families one parent is a little bit softer or tougher than the other parent in terms of discipline with the kids. In your family, who is the softie and who is the toughie?"*

"Mum makes up the rules and Dad is softer. He just goes along with her", said Peter.

"What would you say, Sophie?" asked the therapist. *"Who do you think is the softie and who is the toughie?"*

*"Well isn't it obvious? Mum is a Sergeant Major and Dad is softer. He is **like normal**".*

*"He's a **marshmallow**"*, interjected the mother. *"He may not look it on the outside but that's what he is. He was that way with all the kids, but he's especially soft with Sophie".*

"Sophie, when you compare your parents to say the parents of your friends, do you think on average they are softer or tougher than your friend's parents?" the therapist asked.

"*Do I have to answer that one?*" Sophie sighed. "*Dad is way more understanding than my friends' dads so I guess you'd say a lot softer. Some of the other mothers are less strict than Mum. Some aren't.*"

The therapist then asked the mother, "*How do you compare yourself to other parents in terms of how soft you are about rules, consequences, follow-through?*"

"*I can yell up a storm*", she said. "*I guess if that makes me tough, then I am. But the reality is our kids have had it pretty easy. We were never big on rules and consequences. Until now. Until we were driven to this*".

"*What about between Peter and Sophie? How much is Peter boss and how much is a friend to Sophie?*"

"*I think Peter wants to be more of a friend but Sophie pushes him away*".

"*Just **answer** the question*", said Sophie.

"*Perhaps 40% friend. 60% boss*", said the mother.

"*And what do you think it should be ideally at their ages?*"

"*80% friend. 20% boss*".

The therapist turned to Sophie. "*And how do you see your relationship with Peter, Sophie?*"

"*He wants to be my boss, 100%. But I don't want him as my boss. I hate him*", said Sophie and she threw a cushion across the room at Peter. "*I hate you*". Then she turned to her parents and shouted, "*Why don't you tell her **the truth**. Tell her **the truth** about what he did to me. And you just watched, you just **let it happen***".

"What happened?" asked the therapist, turning to face the parents.

"*A few months ago*", said the father, "*after the police came to our house, Annie told Sophie she was grounded. That she couldn't go anywhere after school or on the weekends. But she found a way to get out the window and we chased her and brought her home. Then one night when I was out at a meeting, she tried to sneak out again and Peter caught her and gave her belting…*"

"*Belting*"? Sophie shouted. "*He used **his fists**. He hit me in the **face** and the **guts**. He **beat me up***", she cried, pointing at her mother "*And **you** were in the next room and you **knew** he was doing it and you **let** him do it*".

"*I didn't know then that he was hurting you badly*", said the mother.

"*You **did** so. You **wanted** him to do it*". Sophie pulled her legs up to her chest, buried her face, and sobbed. Peter had taken on a "parental" role in "*disciplining*" his sister, evidence that he was in a coalition with his mother, supporting her against Sophie. Sophie felt betrayed by her mother's failure to stop the brother's abuse. This betrayal meant that it would be difficult for the therapist to help the parents set limits for Sophie because she would reject their authority as undeserved. Sophie's sense of hurt and betrayal would block her from seeing her parents as genuinely caring about her and acting in her best interests.

Earning back Sophie's trust was an important first step in restoring the parents to an appropriate hierarchy. They had to listen to Sophie's anger and respond with empathy and remorse. In subsequent sessions, the therapist created an enactment between Sophie and her parents where Sophie sobbed out her anger and sense of betrayal at how the parents had allowed her older brother to hurt her so badly. At the end of that session, the therapist helped the mother and Sophie arrange twice weekly mother-daughter times, during which they would do an activity that they would both enjoy. Immediately following this first session, Sophie became less argumentative; she began to sleep at night, stopped waking, and stopped pacing around the house.

Next the therapists met with Peter and the parents, a session in which the parents told Peter that under no circumstances was he to hurt, restrain, or discipline his sister. From now on, they said, dealing with Sophie's behaviour was the parent's responsibility, not his.

Creating an enactment to restore the parental hierarchy

The goal for the next session was for the parents to agree upon some rules and expectations for Sophie's behaviour. The therapist gave each parent a piece of paper, asking them to write down the top ten behaviours that they would like to see Sophie change. When they had written their lists, the therapist asked them to compare their lists to see if they had three issues in common which they did: school attendance, Sophie's whereabouts after school, and speaking disrespectfully.

The therapist decided to use an enactment and instructed the parents to sit in chairs next to each other so that they were able to see each other as they spoke. Asking them to come to an agreement about the rules concerning these three issues, the therapist emphasised the importance of them working out a plan they could both agree to. She then pulled her own chair back and looked down at the floor.

The father spoke first but he addressed the therapist. She did not look up but simply gestured towards the mother. He turned back towards the mother.

"*The most important thing is that she goes to school every day*", said the mother, speaking directly to the father.

"*Of course, she should go to school every day*", he answered. "*But how are we going to make her?*"

"*If she is going to get out of bed in the morning, she has to go to bed at night on time....*"

Sophie interrupted, "*You treat me like a **little** kid. You **can't** tell me what time to go to bed anymore*".

"*.... and that means that she needs to be off the computer by 10 o'clock*", the mother continued.

"*10 o'clock – you're so stupid.........*"

"*Sophie! Don't call your mother stupid........*" said the father, turning towards Sophie.

"*I wasn't just calling her stupid. You want to cut me off from all my friends, don't you? You want me to be a loner, don't you?*"

"*Sophie, you **know** that's not true*", said the father. "*We **want** you to have friends. I know it's important at your age*".

"*Sophie*", said the mother, her voice rising, "*You **have** to go to bed on time*".

It became evident that the parents could not hold a conversation with Sophie present without her interrupting and escalating the interaction, detouring the parents in their struggle to reach an agreement. Each time, the therapist intervened to keep the parents talking to each other.

"*She's got you off track now. Ignore her*", said the therapist. "*Talk to each other. What are the rules?*"

"*So **how** do we get her off the computer by 10?*", asked the father, turning back towards the mother.

The interaction in the room between the parents and Sophie revealed the following sequence: the parents talk to each other; Sophie interrupts; the father responds to Sophie; and Sophie talks more. The father talks to Sophie. The mother talks to Sophie. This sequence repeated through the session and each time the therapist focused the parents back to their own conversation, strengthening their ability to resist Sophie's interruptions.

With the therapist's support, the parents resisted Sophie's interruptions and after a while Sophie stopped interrupting.

"*There **has** to be a rule about what time the computer and all the devices are off and lights are out and then we have to stick to it*", said the mother.

"*But **how** can we make her do that? The last time you tried she got out the window and stayed out all night*".

"*I'm **sick** of arguing with her. You **have** to get involved in following through more. You **always** leave it all up to me*".

"*I **don't** always leave it up to you*".

"*You **do**, Tony. I'm asking you to just work with me on this*".

"*So what **do you want** me to do?*"

"*I **want** you to go into her room at 10 o'clock and take away the modem, pull out the cable*".

"*I said I would back you up. But maybe we don't have to start with taking away the modem. Why can't we start with me just going in and telling her it is time?*"

Glancing over at Sophie who had been sitting quietly, listening, the father invited Sophie into the parent's conversation. "*What do you think Sophie? Are you willing to be that more cooperative? Get ready for bed when I come in and tell you it is 10 o'clock?*"

"*I **told** you. 10 o'clock is **lame**. I'm old enough to decide for myself*".

"*Sophie, why do you have to be like that?*" said the father "*Can't you see we're trying to get somewhere here?*"

This time it was the father who had reactivated the triangle giving evidence to the therapist that when the conflict between the parents intensified, the father triangulated Sophie.

Exploring successes and failures between sessions

The parents eventually reached an agreement about three basic rules and the consequences for breaking the rules. In the following session, however, they reported that Sophie had defied the rules. When the mother had tried to follow through with the consequences, the father had overruled her, allowing Sophie to evade the consequences both parents had agreed to in the previous session.

"*What happened? What happened that you went back on your agreement?*" asked the therapist.

The father threw up his hands and then ran his fingers through his hair. "*Look*", he said, his voice getting louder. "*I know I agreed when we were here. But when it happened at home, Sophie got so upset and she*", he paused, pointing to the mother, "*she was screaming at her and I can't stand it when she treats her like that. There's no point. It gets us nowhere…*"

"*…Treats her like what? You mean makes her stick to the rules?*" said the mother.

"*…She comes down on her like a ton of bricks*".

"*…Like a ton of bricks? Really? Because it is always all up to me. Because you refuse to do anything*".

The therapist expected this "setback" and welcomed the opportunity it presented to reveal the underlying conflict in the relationship between the parents. It took a few more sessions, some in which the therapist saw the parents alone to deal with a couple of issues, before both parents were able to clearly stick to their agreements and follow through in a calm, consistent, and authoritative manner in parenting Sophie. By the end of therapy,

Sophie's behaviour was no longer a concern and she enjoyed happy times with her mother who was calmer and less stressed. The father no longer undermined the mother and took on a more active role in the household and in helping to care for the grandmother.

Conclusion

This chapter has demonstrated how aspects of the Milan approach and of Structural/Strategic family therapy can be integrated providing the therapist with a view into family relationships that uses both family members' verbal descriptions of their own perceptions and therapist's direct observations of family process in the session.

The case example illustrated using the Milan questioning method to scan relationships in terms of bonds and hierarchy, revealing the underlying structure of family relationships: a coalition between the father and the daughter and an escalating complementarity between the parents – a "soft-hard" split indicative of unresolved couple conflict. The questioning process also brought to light the daughter's hurt and anger at her parents for failing to protect her. The therapist used the Structural Family Therapy technique of "enactment" with the daughter and her parents and then with both parents. An enactment allowed the daughter to give voice to her experience and receive validation and remorse from the parents. Enactments involving both parents highlighted their difficulties in working together, revealed how their daughter became involved in their conflicts, and ultimately helped them resolve differences and work together effectively. How this came about is described in more detail in the next chapter which addresses why and how the therapist meets separately with the parents in family therapy.

Notes

1 In response to criticism that therapists cannot and should not always be "neutral", Cecchin introduced "curiosity" as a more accurate depiction of the therapist's stance (Cecchin, 1987; Cecchin, Lane, & Ray, 1992).
2 This case is a compilation of several cases. Any similarity to actual families is coincidental. The transcript is continued in Chapter 9.

References

Baumrind, D. (1978). Parental disciplinary patterns and social competence in children. *Youth and Society, 9,* 238–276.

Boscolo, L., & Cecchin, G. (1982). Training in systemic therapy at the Milan centre. In R. Whiffin & J. Byng-Hall (Eds.), *Family therapy supervision: Recent developments in practice.* London, England: Academic Press.

Boscolo, L., Cecchin, G., Hoffman, L., & Penn, P. (1987). *Milan systemic family therapy.* New York, NY: Basic Books.

Brown, J. (1997a). Circular questioning: An introductory guide. *Australian and New Zealand Journal of Family Therapy, 18,* 109–144.

Brown, J. (1997b). The question cube: A model for developing question repertoire in training couple and family therapists. *Journal of Marriage and Family Therapy, 23,* 27–40.

Butler, M., Davis, S., & Seedall, R. (2008). Common pitfalls of beginning family therapists utilizing enactments. *Journal of Marital and Family Therapy, 34,* 329– 348.

Cecchin, G. (1987). Hypothesizing – circularity – neutrality revisited: An invitation to curiosity. *Family Process, 26,* 405–413.

Cecchin, G., Lane, G., & Ray, W. (1992). *Irreverence: A strategy for therapists' survival*. London, England: Karnac Books.

Davis, S., & Butler, M. (2004). Enacting relationships in marriage and family therapy: A conceptual and operational definition of an enactment. *Journal of Marital and Family Therapy, 30*, 319–333.

Diamond, G., & Liddle, H. (1999). Transforming negative parent-adolescent interactions in family therapy: From impasse to dialogue. *Family Process, 38*, 5–26.

Fletcher, A., Steinberg, L., & Sellers, E. (1999). Adolescents' well-being as a function of perceived interparental consistency. *Journal of Marriage and the Family, 61*, 599–610.

Goldenberg, H., & Goldenberg, I. (2008). *Family therapy: An overview* (7th ed.). Belmont, CA: Thompson/Brooks Cole.

Greenspan, S. (2006). Rethinking "harmonious parenting" using a three-factor discipline model. *Child Care in Practice, 12*, 5–12.

Haley, J. (1986). *Uncommon therapy: The psychiatric techniques of Milton H. Erikson*. New York, NY: W. W. Norton.

Haley, J. (1987). *Problem-solving therapy* (2nd ed.). San Francisco, CA: Jossey-Bass Pub.

Haley, J., & Richeport-Haley, M. (2003). *The art of strategic therapy*. New York, NY: Brunner-Routledge.

James, K. (1989). When twos are really threes; the triangular dance of couple conflict. *Australian and New Zealand Journal of Family Therapy, 10*, 10179–189.

James, K., & MacKinnon, L. (1986). Theory and practice of structural family therapy. *Australian and New Zealand Journal of Family Therapy, 7*, 223–233.

Jiménez, L., Hidalgo, V., Baena, S., León, A., & Lorence, B. (2019). Effectiveness of structural-strategic family therapy in the treatment of adolescents with mental health problems and their families. *International Journal of Environmental Research and Public Health, 16*, 1255. https://doi.org/10.3390/ijerph16071255

Jones, E. (1993). *Family systems therapy: Developments in the Milan systemic approach*. UK: Wiley Pub.

Levy, J. (2006). Using a meta-perspective to clarify the structural-narrative debate in family therapy. *Family Process, 45*, 55–73.

MacKinnon, L. (1983). Contrasting strategic and Milan therapies. *Family Process, 22*, 425–438.

MacKinnon, L. (1988). Openings: Using questions therapeutically. *Dulwich Center Newsletter*, Winter, 15–18.

MacKinnon, L. (1998). *Trust and betrayal in the treatment of child abuse*. New York, NY: Guilford Press.

MacKinnon, L., & Miller, D. (1987). The new epistemology and the Milan approach – Feminist and sociopolitical considerations. *Journal of Marital and Family Therapy, 13*(2), 139–155.

MacKinnon, L., Parry, A., & Black, R. (1984). Strategies of family therapy: The relationship to styles of family functioning. *Journal of Strategic and Systemic Therapy, 3*, 6–22.

MacKinnon, L. K., & James, K. (1987). The Milan systemic approach: Theory and practice. *Australian and New Zealand Journal of Family Therapy, 8*(2), 89–98. https://doi.org/10.1002/j.1467-8438.1987.tb01209.x

Marcone, R., Affuso, G., & Borrone, A. (2020). Parenting styles and children's internalizing-externalizing behavior: The mediating role of behavioral regulation. *Current Psychology: A Journal for Diverse Perspectives on Diverse Psychological Issues, 39*, 13–24. https://doi.org/10.1007/s12144-017-9757-7

Minuchin, S. (1974). *Families and family therapy*. London, England: Tavistock Pub.

Minuchin, S., & Fishman, C. (1981). *Family therapy techniques*. Cambridge, MA: Harvard University Press.

Minuchin, S., Lee, W.-Y., & Simon, G. (1996). *Mastering family therapy*. New York, NY: John Wiley and Sons.

Minuchin, S., Montalvo, B., Guerney, B., Rosman, B., & Schumer, F. (1967). *Families of the slums.* New York, NY: Basic Books.

Minuchin, S., & Nichols, M. P. (1993). *Family healing: Tales of hope and renewal from family therapy.* New York, NY: Free Press.

Minuchin, S., Rosman, B., & Baker, L. (1978). *Psychosomatic families.* Cambridge, MA: Harvard University Press.

Nichols, M., & Fellenberg, S. (2000). The effective use of enactments in family Therapy: A discovery oriented process study. *Journal of Marital and Family Therapy, 26*(2), 143–152.

Pinquart, M., & Kauser, R. (2018). Do the associations of parenting styles with behavior problems and academic achievement vary by culture? Results from a meta-analysis. *Cultural Diversity and Ethnic Minority Psychology, 24*, 75–100. doi: 10.1037/cdp0000149

Pirrotta, S. (1984). Milan revisited: A comparison of the two Milan schools. *Journal of Strategic and Systemic Therapies, 3*, 3–15.

Sells, S. (1998). *Treating the tough adolescent.* New York, NY: Guildford Press.

Selvini-Palazzoli, M., Cecchin, G., Prata, G., & Boscolo, L. (1978). *Paradox and counter paradox.* New York, NY: Jason Aronson Publishers.

Selvini-Palazzoli, M., Cecchin, G., Prata, G., & Boscolo, L. (1980). Hypothesizing –circularity – neutrality: Three guidelines for the conductor of the session. *Family Process, 19*, 3–12.

Shaw, D., Criss, M., Schonberg, M., & Beck, J. (2004). The development of family hierarchies and their relation to children's conduct problems. *Development and Psychopathology, 16*, 483–500.

Takeuchi, S., & Takeuchi, A. (2008). Authoritarian versus authoritative parenting styles: Application of the cost equalization principle. *Marriage and Family Review, 44*(4), 489–510.

Tomm, K. (1984). One perspective on the Milan approach. Part 1. Overview of development, theory, and practice. *Journal of Marital and Family Therapy, 10*, 113–125.

Tomm, K. (1987a). Interventive interviewing: Part 1. Strategizing as a fourth guideline for the therapist. *Family Process, 26*, 3–13.

Tomm, K. (1987b). Interventive interviewing: Part 2. Reflexive questioning as a means to enable self-healing. *Family Process, 26*, 167–183.

Tomm, K. (1988). Interventive interviewing: Part 3. Intending to ask lineal, circular, strategic or reflexive questions? *Family Process, 27*, 1–15.

Tsvieli, N., Lifshitz, C., & Diamond, G. M. (2022). Corrective attachment episodes in attachment-based family therapy: The power of enactment. *Psychotherapy Research 32*, 209–222. doi: 10.1080/10503307.2021.1913295

Chapter 5

Working with Abuse in Families

The Challenge of Establishing Safety While Fostering Therapeutic Relationships

Anne Welfare and Robyn Elliott

Introduction

Working with family violence involves a specific skill set. Of course, we want to address the violence/abuse, but it is our experience and contention that we must create a respectful and engaged therapeutic connection with all family members if the goal of safety and positive change for the family is to be achieved.

Many of us work with families where the abuse is the explicit and initial focus of the therapeutic work. However, there is always a possibility when working generally in family therapy that violence or abuse may be an underlying issue.[1] When we suspect violence or abuse in a family, we need to find a way to investigate our suspicions and prioritise safety issues while maintaining the positive therapeutic relationship we will hopefully have already established. In either case, working with abuse is not an easy task because it involves stepping out of the usual therapeutic frame in some significant ways.

In our experience of supervising and training family therapists and other health professionals, there is an embrace of practices such as collaboration, offering choice, being transparent, and focussing on what people are doing well: such as are consistent with the widely accepted principles of trauma informed practice.[2] When there is violence or abuse, these practices are often juggled with a more investigative or directive agenda.[3] This complexity of the therapeutic role can be confusing and daunting for a therapist. We have a duty of care issues to consider, safety of children and adults, professional registration board requirements, statutory requirements, and agency guidelines. Our fear can create inflexibility in our approach – it is safer to "go by the book". Similarly, in a parallel process, fear, anger, guilt, and shame can be evoked in our clients, thus placing any therapeutic engagement at grave risk.

Our goal in this chapter is to describe an approach to working with issues of safety and risk that proceeds on the belief that even those who abuse can often be effectively engaged in the project of redressing the harm they have done and of enhancing life for the whole family. Several significant questions are raised when working with these issues with this agenda. They include: what do I do if I suspect abuse but there has been no disclosure? Where does assessment fit in? How do I assess for abuse? Who do I see? How do I speak to family members about difficult issues without alienating them? How do I position myself to manage the seeming conflict of interests within the family? We will attempt to answer these questions in this chapter utilising multiple theoretical frameworks and considering types of family therapy approaches that fit best.

The answers to the above questions are also influenced by the circumstances under which the therapist is made aware of safety concerns. For example, working with abuse as

DOI: 10.4324/9781003490104-6

a presenting issue is different from the situation where it arises in the context of work that was initiated with a different agenda. Working with families where all members are cooperative around an established agenda for addressing safety is different from working with clients who are mandated to attend. This chapter will first address some issues and treatment recommendations that are applicable in all situations and then move on to discuss processes and practices specific to these different contexts and circumstances.

The whole issue of safety and risk is a very broad one. Early on, trauma literature (e.g., Cozolino, 2002; Rothschild, 2000) underlined the importance of safety in the therapeutic context in terms of a general expectation of support, respect, and predictability, careful management of pace and depth of difficult subject matter and also of conflictual family dynamics (Lowe, 2004). Our discussion is more narrowly focussed. What we will be addressing here are those situations where there are indications, however subtle, of the actual occurrence or the potential for *significant* harm from one family member to another, such as might require referral to a statutory body or the police. This incorporates physical, sexual, and emotional abuse and neglect. As well as abuse of children, some aspects of our discussion may be applicable to abuse between partners (partner violence), abuse from adolescents towards a parent, and abuse of the elderly by family members who are caregivers. Some reference will be made to these throughout this chapter.

However, it is important to note that while there are some commonalities, the treatment for the different populations will vary. For example, intervention with adolescent violence, which is often hidden by the parent due to their own shame and fear of the consequences for that young person, may involve intensive support for the parents to change their transactional patterns around the violence and rarely involves removing the adolescent from the home.[4] Work with the parents (e.g., Anglicarevic, n.d.) can dramatically change the trajectory for the young person showing violence. Similar dynamics to adolescent violence can also be present in the abuse of elderly parents by their children, but existing alongside complexities do not present in work with other populations (Dow et al., 2020). The treatment of an adolescent who has sexually harmed a sibling is also very different from an adult sex offender (Welfare, 2008).

Current understanding of the aetiology and treatment in these different areas can be so different to that for adult violence that we are unable to do them justice here. The focus of this chapter will be on violence perpetrated by an adult towards children and/or their adult partners.

Theoretical frameworks

In the introduction we referred to now accepted practices in family therapy not necessarily adhered to when working with issues involving risk. Collaboration, transparency, and strengths-focus from post-modern frameworks[5] which privilege empowerment of clients within the therapeutic context. When one or more family members may be harming others, however, the appropriate balance of power is already skewed, requiring us to rethink this issue. This still sits beside necessary considerations of how to maintain clients' engagement and uphold our responsibility to enable them to increase their choice and direction over their lives as much as possible. Such a complex enterprise needs, in our opinion, a firm foundation in both practice and philosophical frameworks or theories. In our work with abuse issues in families, we draw from a range of theories, including systems, attachment, social constructionism, and feminist theories. Using multiple lenses helps us to understand the impact of abuse and trauma on relationships and to facilitate healing. Space does not allow us to elaborate on each of these theories. Instead, we focus on systems theory and the feminist perspective as central to our work.

A systemic foundation

Systems theory is based on the concept that the whole entity that is a system is greater than the sum of its parts (von Bertalanffy, 1968). Regular patterns of mutually reinforcing inter-action mostly serve to retain the coherence of a system, such as a family, while allowing for some evolution over time to meet the changing internal and external needs of the whole or of its individual members. Key principles are that family interactions are circular, that is, mutually causal, and connected and that they are contextually constrained or facilitated (Goding, 1992; Nichols, 2011). Where the need for either coherence or change is not met, the family is in danger of dissolution. It is at this point that families often present for therapy. To understand a family, systems therapists consider these recurring patterns and their appropriateness to the family's circumstances (Lowe, 2004).

We view a holistic systemic approach to abuse as fundamental to how we conceptualise its occurrence, its impact, and the most effective means for ameliorating, if not healing, that impact. Early systems therapists often viewed the whole family as pathological and responsible for occurrences of abuse.[6] Thankfully the field has moved on from this position and now finds it more useful to concentrate on how the abuse has shaped the patterns of relating in the family. For instance, where a father is sexually abusing his adolescent daugh-ter, how he maintains the secrecy will often distance the daughter from her mother. This distance is then reinforced by, perhaps, angry interactions between the helpless daughter and the bewildered mother, thus maintaining the father's power over and access to the daughter. In fact, this has become, in our experience the kind of pattern that might raise our suspicions above the level of simple mother-daughter conflict. In addition, a central aspect of the work in such situations from a systems perspective would involve assessing this reciprocal interaction between daughter and mother within the context of the father's interactions, working through their understandings and feelings about their relationship, and slowly reconnecting them with roles more appropriate to their positions as parent and child (Miller & Dwyer, 1997). Unlike many individual approaches that utilise the therapeutic relationship as the vessel of recovery from trauma, a systemic approach in the field of family violence uses the therapeutic relationship to facilitate the reconnection or re-attachment of the traumatised person to their other significant relationships.

A systemic approach also has us consider the influence of ever broader levels of con-text from extended family through community, culture, nation state, and various kinds of biological, social, and cultural groupings on the occurrence and experience of abuse and on recovery from it. There has been significant research connecting broader risk factors, especially poverty, to child maltreatment (Lee, Coe, & Ryff, 2017). A systemic approach considers these contextual factors and endeavours to intervene with the wider system as well as with the family.

Finally, systems theory generally provides a clear articulation of the therapist as a co-creator of the therapist-family system and any change that is brought about for that system. The positions we take, the questions we ask, and the values by which we proceed will all impact on the shape of the system with which we are interacting. With this awareness, if we can be flexible enough in our approach, come both responsibility and opportunity for more positive outcomes with families.

Speaking more specifically of systems models, we have found the *Contextual Therapy* (CT) of Ivan Boszormenyi-Nagy (Boszormenyi-Nagy & Krasner, 1986) to fit well with our approach. Firstly, the concept of the ledger brings some clarity to situations where one or more members, because of their conduct, or by reason of their family position (e.g., as a parent), are in debt or obligation to other members of the family. While respecting the rights to fairness for *all* family members, the therapist in this situation is called on to lend his or her weight to those members who are least able to represent themselves within the family system. This is achieved in CT from a position of *multi-directed partiality*. That is, through giving due partiality to each member in turn and then especially supporting those "whose past injuries or current efforts to give to others call for … support the most at that moment" (Goldenthal, 1996, p. 11). This gives permission to actively support victims of abuse and at the same time to work towards resolution or "exoneration" of the position of the perpetrator of the abuse.

Secondly, the concept of loyalty provides validation for working with whole families, especially those who have hurt others. When offending family members do the work, take responsibility, acknowledge the harm they have created, and make reparation, they can take back some measure of self-regard. This, in turn, allows their family members, who are from the same stock, to also regard themselves more positively. Victims, frequently tied to them by blood and therefore legacy and loyalty, are relieved from carrying the burden of responsibility and from passing it on to their partners and children (Boszormenyi-Nagy & Krasner, 1986; Grunebaum, 1987; Hargraves & Sells, 1997; Sheehan, 2007; Van der Meiden, 2019).

Thirdly, CT is very clear in conceptualising the obligations that family members have towards each other, especially those of parents towards their children. This is not done by way of moralising but more by stating the consequences that flow from not fulfilling these obligations.

CT thus provides support for an approach that includes the offending family member as an integral part of family healing, and also provides therapists with a point of departure from the usual family therapy exhortation to take a "neutral" position.

A feminism perspective

In viewing interactions as reciprocal or circular, systems theory has been accused of, at best, a lack of clarity around issues of power (e.g., Penfold, 1989). From a systems perspective, no one was viewed as having unilateral power, yet each person was viewed as being able to influence the behaviour of others to some degree. This resulted in formulations that viewed women and children, and those who are marginalised by, for example, culture, sexual orientation, religion, or class, as responsible or blamed for the wrongs committed against them. It also implies that they have the power to extricate themselves from dangerous or harmful situations. Alongside the deplorability of blaming victims for their own victimisation, such a view can result in decreased sensitivity to risk on the part of service providers, including therapists. For example, it might leave a therapist in the position of assuming a woman could leave her violent husband "if she really wanted to". It also leaves us less cognisant of the ways in which patriarchal structures position women and children to be vulnerable to abuse. For example, single mothers overrepresented among those living in poverty (O'Brien, 2009) understandably may find a male "provider" very attractive, even if he is aggressive, but especially if he seems nice and loves the children. And if the child constantly gravitates to him, then it is difficult for her to believe that anything is amiss, even if the child later makes a disclosure. Even if *we* believe the child, lack of appreciation for the dynamics will interfere with the therapist being able to take the most useful position, particularly with the mother, that is, empathy, patience, and empowerment rather than incredulity.

Feminism also emphasises the role of offending family members as actors who make decisions to behave in particular ways, rather than being solely the victims of circumstance or of their own histories. In this way, it keeps our eye on issues of responsibility taking and the implications of this for victims and other family members.

Attachment theory

Attachment theory (Bowlby, 1969; Main, Hesse, & Kaplan, 2005) asserts that our inherent need to bond with a caregiver is crucial for both emotional well-being and survival. This bond serves as a "secure base" from which we venture into the world. People's actions are influenced by their early attachment experiences, which can elucidate seemingly paradoxical behaviours observed in therapy, such as individuals clinging to a family member who has hurt them. Understanding that distress, even that coming from an attachment figure, amplifies these attachment tendencies assists in risk assessment, offers insights into underlying motivations, especially of wrongdoers, and promotes a therapeutic approach grounded in compassion rather than judgement.

Attachment theory (Bowlby, 1969, 1973, 1980; Main, Hesse, & Kaplan, 2005) holds that attachment to a caregiver, usually manifested as proximity seeking, is a primary and biologically based motivating factor essential not only for the emotional well-being of the child, and later the adult, but also for his or her *actual* survival. The attachment relationship becomes the "secure base" from which the child can move out into the world. Depending on the actions of the caregiver, the child will adapt to their behaviour to maintain the connection. Thus, this theory contextualises people's behaviour within their childhood histories and helps us understand why people do what they do. For example, therapists are sometimes bewildered, or at worst misled, by the fact that family members often cling to the person in the family who is hurting them. Attachment theory makes sense of this when we realise that stress, even if it is caused by the attachment figure, elevates attachment needs. This understanding is important to the assessment of risk for people currently in the therapy room, but also for making sense of the motivations of those who are doing the hurting, and in intervening with them. Their actions frequently stem from patterns established in the context of attachment-related phenomena as well. Probably one of the most important results of this for the therapist is that it makes space for compassion and respect rather than judgement.

Neurobiology

Neurobiological findings have transformed both theory and practice in relation to working with abuse and neglect. One clear outcome of this is greater confidence in assessing, from family members' behaviours, what is and isn't possible at particular points depending on the level of emotional arousal (Griffith & Griffith, 1994). We realise that when there is high emotional arousal, it is difficult for people to think (Perry, 2006, 2010) and it is very difficult for new actions or perspectives to be entertained.[7] Individuals who have been subjected to neglect and/or abuse, especially as children, because of the adaptation of their brains to early dangerous contexts, are far more sensitive to being triggered into this arousal (Perry, 1997). Information from researchers and writers such as Rothschild (2000), Gottman et al. (1995), and van der Kolk (2015) about physical manifestations of emotional arousal has been helpful in assisting therapists to assess clients' emotional state during the therapy session. More than ever there is more scientific confirmation of our knowledge that feelings of acceptance and safety in the therapeutic context are vital (Perry, 2006; Schore, 2003; Siegel, 2003; van der Kolk, Roth, Pelcovitz, Sunday, & Spinazzola, 2005; Cozolino, 2020). This body of literature also provides us with strategies to help clients to settle, such as remaining calm ourselves, (usually) providing empathy and validation, focussing the conversation on success and strengths, maybe providing some direction, or increasing proximity to trusted caregivers. Polyvagal theory (Geller & Porges, 2014; Kain & Terrell, 2018) provides details of what makes for authentic therapeutic presence (vocal prosody, warm facial expression, tilting of the head, and so on) which in turn creates a context of safety.

The above applies equally to the work with offending family members, who are likely also to have experienced abuse and/or neglect as children (Creeden, 2006; Pithers, Gray, Cunningham, & Lane, 1993; Rich, 2006; Ryan, 1999). These findings have elevated the need for attending much more seriously to offending family members' own victimisation, where this has occurred, and to working systemically to develop and maintain a balance of support and accountability within their family or other networks (Jenkins, 2006a).

An important corollary, however, from the field of neurophysiology is that, even in the rare case where offending family members have not themselves been victims of abuse/trauma/abandonment, the creation of an authentic, caring, safe therapeutic relationship is the essential substrate to the process of challenge that will be necessary if family relationships are to be healed. Ossefort-Russell (2018) speaks of inducing feelings of shame when we approach people who are grieving from a more evaluative stance, which then invites defensive responses. How much more will this occur if we approach people who have done shameful things? In our experience, the paradox is that where we are more contextually aware and compassionate, this opens space for people to hold themselves more readily to account. See also the work of Jenkins (e.g., 2006a) for the need to balance compassion and challenge.

Social constructionism

Social constructionism posits that our understanding of reality is co-constructed within specific social contexts through language, allowing for multiple valid interpretations of experiences. Therapies like Narrative and Solution Focussed, rooted in this framework, emphasise the potent role of language in shaping perceptions and realities. They promote the exploration of positive self-aspects and empower individuals to decide which "version" of themselves to cultivate. This is important in managing blame and shame dynamics that arise when discussing issues of abuse (Jenkins, 1990, 2006a, 2006b). Techniques like externalisation make it easier to discuss sensitive issues, like abuse, by distinguishing the individual from the problem, emphasising choices and guiding values (Epston & White, 1990; White, 2007), and engaging clients as active participants in change yields better responsiveness. "Parts" methods like Internal Family Systems (Schwartz, 2021) and Schema Mode Therapy (Young, Klosko, & Weishaar, 2006) offer frameworks to understand behaviors without assigning blame, fostering introspection and facilitating transformation, especially when addressing complex issues like violence.

Social constructionism involves the idea that there is no "reality" or "truth" as such, but that what we understand to be reality is agreed on, often tacitly, between persons within a certain social context and mediated through language. This raises the possibility that there can be different versions of the one experience which are equally valid and open to difference or change within different social contexts and over time.

Narrative and Solution Focussed therapies, which have developed within a social constructionist framework, alert us to the power of languaging practices in shaping the realities people hold about themselves and each other. These can be utilised to positive ends by an approach that emphasises positive aspects of people's values, behaviour, and relationships and by inviting them to make choices about what particular "version" of themselves they want to develop. The specific processes developed within both models build resources and maintain respect. This is important in managing blame and shame dynamics that arise when discussing issues of abuse (Jenkins, 1990, 2006a, 2006b). Externalisation (Epston & White, 1990; White, 2007), a practice that separates the person from the problem, can make topics like violence, anger, and abuse much easier to talk about, without negating the importance of taking responsibility. Similarly, in rejecting the notion that we are made up of qualities or that we have an essential nature, good or bad, social constructionist notions emphasise the decisions that people make and the values that they use to guide these. Inquiring about these values and decisions can be extremely powerful in working with abuse issues (Jenkins, 2006a; White, 2007). Social constructionist theories such as Narrative and Solution Focussed therapies are also based on the premise that people are more responsive in a positive sense when they are active partners in change. This means treating them and their knowledge with respect and interest, working with their goals as much as possible, and striving to understand and help them contextualise those occasions when they have failed to live up to their own values. In our opinion, "parts" approaches such as Internal Family Systems (Schwartz, 2021) and Schema Mode Therapy (Arntz & Jacob, 2012; Young, Klosko, & Weishaar, 2006) are interesting and potentially powerful developments. Like White's externalisation, they provide a means for conceptualising and examining our behaviours, thoughts, and feelings in a way that obviates blame while setting the foundation for challenge and change. If we understand violence as rooted in strategies, i.e., "parts" that develop to manage vulnerability, it leaves the "Self" free to examine and understand the intention of these parts but to choose alternative strategies.

Reading through these frameworks reveals tensions, especially in their implications for practice. While feminism emphasises responsibility for offenders, systemic considerations, neurobiology, and attachment theory might prioritise understanding the offender's own victimisation. Social constructionism believes in multiple valid perspectives, but feminism cautions against undermining the very real impacts of abuse and neglect and how various cultural and historical interpretations might downplay its severity.

We align with Goldner, Penn, Sheinberg, and Walker (1990) in believing it's not beneficial to merge the different perspectives mentioned earlier. Instead, holding each view simultaneously offers a more effective and ethical approach. While we advocate for a multi-lensed stance, the feminist perspective takes precedence, viewing violence and abuse as tangible realities, not mere constructions or perceptions.

Like Goldner et al. (1990), we take the position that it is undesirable to try to integrate or amalgamate the different perspectives outlined above. It is the simultaneous holding of each of them, as comment and critique on the others that will provide not only a more effective approach but also a more ethical one. Nevertheless, our multi-lensed position does involve putting the feminist perspective in the foreground and conceptualising violence and abuse as inherently real, not constructions or perceptions of reality.

The model or lens that gets emphasised in each case often amounts to a clinical decision based on the specifics of each situation and the timing. The therapeutic decisions are idiosyncratic to the family that is being seen and their strengths and constraints. Having said this, we have found it useful to have in place some recommendations for practice to help the beginning therapist working in this murky area. The first of these (from feminism) is centred round the issue of how the therapist approaches the use of power in the therapeutic relationship. This is one of the more challenging aspects of this work.

Recommendations for practice

1.   The positioning of the therapist in relationship to power

Post-modern models of family therapy, especially, attempt to equalise the balance of power within the therapeutic relationship. This is done through measures such as taking a non-expert position (Anderson & Goolishian, 1988; Anderson, Goolishian, McNamee, & Gergen, 1992), greater collaboration around the therapeutic agenda, greater transparency, and even having family and therapeutic team swap sides of the one-way screen (Andersen, 1987; Perlesz, Young, Paterson, & Bridge, 1994). However, when dealing with issues of safety, it is, in our opinion, important for the therapist to be resolved about taking executive control in sessions, offering information and direction, directing the flow of information between members, and using therapeutic techniques that are not always totally transparent.

The therapist taking control of the session needs to be balanced with as much collaboration with the family as possible. However, families will often be in shock and chaos in the early stages of disclosures and may be looking to the therapist to provide some authority and assistance in managing feelings and family dynamics that they may not be capable of at that particular time. If families are not acknowledging this need, that is, when abuse that is occurring hasn't been made overt, it is the therapist's duty of care to provide as much containment and direction as the family will allow. (Most professional codes of ethics provide detailed information about this.)

The therapist may also find themselves locked into a power battle with one family member to have this control. This family member may not be the perpetrator of the abuse but the person most frightened about the loss of family integrity. A re-positioning to an alliance between the therapist and that person can be a strategic intervention.

The method of a therapist taking a management role for the family can involve direct advice giving. The establishment of executive control also positions the therapist as the one who sets the emotional tone of the session. If he or she stays calm and appropriately responsive, the family will more likely settle in their level of emotional arousal (Perry, 2010). This also provides for experience that is likely different from that which the family has at home and therefore opens the space for hope.

2.   *Holistic approach*

We recommend, if possible, engaging the whole system. Therapy is more effective if it utilises the connectedness of the family, as well as the broader system, if this can be done safely. The temptation for the therapist may be to separate the abusing family member from the family and banish them. However, if this is aimed for, without understanding the family and their relationship history (good and bad), then therapeutic engagement probably will not occur and the family along with the potential for a deep relational recovery will be lost. While in many situations we recommend the involvement of the abusing family member in the work, this requires careful screening as is outlined in more detail in the section on assessment which follows.

While we recommend working holistically with the family, this does not mean that we would work with everyone in the room at the same time. When it comes to family violence, it is critical to have separate conversations with individuals within the family to understand their truth. Again, this needs to be orchestrated in a transparent and fair manner to allow everyone to have a voice.

3.   *Safety first*

Primarily safety is a basic need and right of all people and it is our responsibility to provide for this as much as we are able. It is also crucial to the success of the work. As noted above, when we don't feel safe, our capacity to think and to take the perspective of another is compromised, and thus no work is possible. Therefore, all other therapeutic goals and agendas are subject to this one. The involvement of statutory authorities is often necessary to assist with this aspect.

4.   *Privileging the needs of victims*

The frequently taken position in systems work is one of neutrality, at least with respect to persons (Selvini, Boscolo, Cecchin, & Prata, 1980). When working with abuse issues, we take a position more in keeping with Boszormenyi-Nagy's multi-directed partiality in that the needs, wishes, and perspectives of victims are privileged over those of those who have caused the harm. Note that this is not to say that the needs and wishes of others are disregarded. A stance of respect and care for *all* is not only appropriate; it is, in our experience, what works.

5.   *Challenging secrecy*

Our practice goes outside the usual conventions governing confidentiality. Abuse is something that thrives under secrecy, so, as much as possible, we would seek to free up the flow of information. To this end, we encourage regular joint sessions and the permission from families to share information between members. Most notably, where we have the engagement of offending family members, we are clear with them that our practice is to share, where appropriate, their information with other family members, but to maintain the confidentiality of the victim. This reverses the previous power imbalance between victim and offender and prevents the therapist from becoming entangled.

Responsibility and accountability

Those who perpetrate the abuse are seen as totally responsible. A mainstay of the work is working with all members of the family to take this position. If it is appropriate to work with the perpetrator, a goal of this work is to help them become accountable for their actions and to paradoxically suffer emotional distress (Jory & Anderson, 2000) for the harm they have done to loved ones and to experience shame (Jenkins, 2006a). Systemically, the more a perpetrator experiences this emotional distress, the more the burden is lessened for the victim (Jory & Anderson, 2000). In this work, we need to be aware of practices that attempt to coerce demonstrations of remorse (Jenkins, 2006a). On the contrary, people who inflict harm on others, alongside all the other family members, should be treated with respect and compassion, with a genuine interest in their history, their functioning, and their well-being.[8]

Patience and compassion

We have become aware that families' responses to disclosure of abuse will be a complex and dynamic process. We recommend not judging people based on their initial responses. For instance, often a non-offending parent, for several reasons, may not initially believe the child's allegations (Humphreys, 1992). That parent will require time, and probably our support, to adjust and make sense of the situation.

Assessment

It is beyond the scope of this chapter to cover the vast area of risk assessment and we recommend using assessment guides published online (see endnote). However, drawing from a range of domains of information,[9] the following list has been constructed:

- Physical Presentation of Family Members
    - Observable injuries or signs of malnutrition, although these can be concealed.
    - Persistent urinary tract infections or anal bleeding that might be indicative of sexual abuse.
- Presenting Difficulties
    - Symptoms include anxiety, depression, conduct disorder, aggression, self-harm, compulsive behaviours, poor academic performance, bed-wetting, sexual acting out, nightmares, sleep issues, eating disorders, and developmental delays.
- Affective Dysregulation
    - Notable aggression and externalising behaviours.
    - Overly quiet, compliant children or those with a flat emotional affect. While these signs alone don't confirm abuse, in certain interactional contexts they should be cause for concern.
- Interactional Dynamics
    - Observable fear and hesitancy to speak or maintain eye contact in therapy sessions.

- Absence of engagement or empathy from parent to child.
- Overly harsh or blaming behaviour from parents towards children.
- Inappropriate boundaries between children and parents or other family members.
- Reluctance by parents/caregivers to permit individual sessions with other family members.

a **Physical presentation** of the family members. For example, obvious signs of injury, malnutrition, and so on, though these can be easily covered up. Other physical manifestations that might be attributable to sexual abuse would be persistent urinary tract infections or anal bleeding.

b **The presenting difficulty or difficulties**. Clues can be found in these problems. For example: anxiety, depression, conduct disorder and/or aggression, self-harm, compulsive behaviours, poor school performance, bed-wetting, sexual acting out, nightmares, difficulty sleeping, eating disorders, developmental delay, and so on.

c **Affective dysregulation.** This particularly stands out as warranting further investigation. Aggression and externalising behaviours are easily identifiable, but we should also be mindful of children who are overly quiet and compliant and/or who present with flat affect. These may be attributable to other factors and by themselves don't necessarily indicate abuse. However, alongside particular interactional dynamics, they should ring alarm bells.

d **Interactional dynamics**. These dynamics would include signs of fear demonstrated by children, or even adults, being reluctant to speak in sessions or being reluctant to make eye contact; lack of engagement and empathy from parent to child; parents being overly harsh or blaming of children; lack of appropriate boundaries between children and parents or other family members; and reluctance by parents/caregivers to allow individual sessions with other family members.

In addition to behavioural indicators in children, it is helpful to understand the heterogeneity and typologies for perpetrators of violence and sexual abuse. Therapists need to understand the role of the offending family member in the family and the aetiology of their behaviours to intervene effectively. Some types of perpetrators are less likely to benefit from therapeutic work while others will respond well.

Numerous studies differentiate between different kinds of violence, different kinds of perpetrators, and distinguishing male from female violence (Gondolf, 1988; Gottman et al., 1995; Hamberger, Lohr, Bonge, & Tolin, 1996; Holtzworth-Monroe & Stuart, 1994; Johnson, 1995; Simpson, Doss, Wheeler, & Christensen, 2008) to ascertain who would benefit from intervention and what that intervention should comprise of. For instance, in their study focussing on couple violence and seeking to synthesise the various typologies for violent men, Ross and Babcock (2009) suggest that the violence of men who use it proactively, that is, as a means the perpetrator sees as legitimate to gain/maintain control,[10] might be better addressed by "increasing punishments and/or decreasing reinforcers" (2009, p. 615). Such measures don't fall within the therapeutic domain and, more importantly, this suggestion reveals something of the poor prospects for "workability" of individuals who use violence in this way. These men have been said to be highly anger-prone and use violence outside the family as well as within (Carlson & Jones, 2010) and as such could constitute a safety risk for the therapist.

It is noteworthy that (Gottman et al., 1995) found that the men they term "cobras" had a divorce rate of zero; their partners were too afraid to separate. Many of these partners will be at risk of severe injury or even death.[11] Thus the therapist needs to assess the level of risk for all family members in the initial stage, and the first element of the therapeutic work may involve supporting and enabling the family or partner to seek a court mandated intervention order (in Australia called an Apprehended Violence Order or AVO) and/or removal of the family to a safety house. In extreme situations, this may be difficult to action as it may appear to the threatened person to further compromise their safety. In some situations, this may be true, for instance, where the violent person might have access to computer databases that reveal the whereabouts of the threatened person.

People who engage in a more reactive use of violence[12] may still constitute a danger to their partners and families, especially because they are quite unpredictable (Ross & Babcock, 2009). However, treatment recommendations include targeting hyperarousal and emotion dysregulation when there is expertise and support for this. In this situation, there might be scope to engage the offending family member in a contract to cease all violent activities while the therapy and interventions can proceed.

Many authors (e.g., Johnson & Ferraro, 2000; Stith, Rosen, & McCollum, 2003) make the point that frequently women are violent in couple relationships. Johnson and Ferraro (2000) present evidence that this falls into two types. The first is "common couple violence" (CCV): a more mutual type, arising in the context of individual instances of conflict, less likely to escalate over time or to involve severe forms. This presumably is the more reactive type of violence described above rather than the proactive kind. The second is violent resistance (VR) where women retaliate against a violent partner. Clearly, the first may be appropriate for conjoint therapy. Even if women's violence is not as lethal as that of men, research has found that in couple violence "cessation of partner violence is highly dependent on whether the other partner also stops hitting" (Stith, Rosen, & McCollum, 2003, p. 411). The second implies considerable violence by the partner and should be a red flag when thinking about conjoint therapy. Clinically we have had no experience of proactive use of violence by women either against men or children. This is not to say that women never fit the criteria for anti-social personality disorder but our perception is that their numbers are few. We also know that some women are violent towards their children (Australian Institute of Family Studies, 2014). It needs to be acknowledged and recognised here that family violence can be extreme and much more common than we would like to think. In Australia, one woman is killed every 9 days and one man every month by a current or former intimate partner (AIHW, 2019).

Sexual violence can be used for the same ends as physical violence, that is, to gain and maintain power, and it is reasonable to assume that some people use both. It is worthwhile to note here that previously sexual offending has been framed *solely* as an attempt by (usually) men to assert their control over women and children. Lane (1991) asserts that some type of power issue appears to be present in every type of sexually abusive behaviour. We have found clinically, however, that motivation can *sometimes* be more about seeking intimacy or connection, albeit in inappropriate and harmful ways. This makes a difference to the focus of treatment, the prospects for success, the way the abuser's behaviour has been internalised by the victim, and the overall response of other family members. This more individualised assessment is supported by the more recent work of Ward and Marshall (2004). Broadly speaking, however, sexual offending family members can fall into similar categories to violent offending family members in terms of their capacity to take advantage of treatment. Where there has been sadistic abuse, and where there is a total absence of remorse and empathy for the victim, we would recommend referral to other forms of treatment (Carlson & Jones, 2010; Knight & Prentky, 1990; Salter, 1988).

It is worth noting here that the greatest prevalence of sexual abuse in families is from a sibling (Caffaro & Conn-Caffaro, 2005). Similar to adolescent violence, the aetiology and treatment of young people who sexually harm is different from that of adult abuse of children, the recidivism rate for sexual harm is very low compared to adult offenders and importantly treatment should be wholistic and targeted for both the victim and the young person who sexually harmed is critical (Welfare, 2008).

We thus recommend *very* careful assessment processes to screen for current or historical use of violence and for the particular ways in which it is used before deciding whether or not to proceed with conjoint couple or family work.[13] Schacht, Dimidjian, George, and Berns (2009) summarise recommendations for the structure of such a process. Routine screening of all couples, including individual interviews with both partners[14] and written self-report measures, helps to reduce stigma and the possible interference that this can constitute in the therapeutic relationship. The domains to be covered include the type, context, function, and consequences of violence as well as the involvement of third parties (e.g., children) both inside and outside the family. If violence is disclosed, therapists should check for severity and lethality, including frequency and severity of violence, presence of weapons, use of alcohol or other drugs, perpetrator's mental health, and so on.[15]

To continue therapeutic work or re-refer?

The above are some useful indications of whether abuse or neglect is occurring. However, even if it is, our position would advocate that the therapist *may*, if the family is willing, continue with therapy, with abuse issues now firmly on the agenda. We italicise "may" here because further assessment needs to be done in relation to the offending family member and his or her capacity to engage safely and fruitfully in a therapeutic process.

Context of the referral

Much of how we respond to safety concerns and to the maintenance and development of relationships within the therapeutic context depends on how and when those concerns present themselves. In the following scenarios, we outline our responses within five different but typical contexts which are determined by the nature of the referral and/or the way in which the issue arises.

Scenario A – Currently working with the family on other issues and the therapist has suspicions that abuse might be occurring

As mentioned in the introduction, it is statistically quite possible that a family or couple who presents for general work is harbouring a violent or abusive situation. If there are indicators in the presentation of the couple or family that concern the therapist, it is critical that the therapist organises separate individual sessions in order to explore this further. The issues around maintaining secrecy and power mean that it is unlikely for disclosure to occur in family or couple sessions. The power imbalances that go with abuse and violence effectively silence victimised family members. If the family understand that individual assessment is a routine process, then this can usually be organised without undue distress. The following are some suggestions for conducting these.

Conducting separate sessions

Separate sessions, quite apart from suspicions of abuse, can be helpful for taking a more thorough assessment, for building a stronger engagement, and for doing some preparation with family members for difficult conversations with each other. These activities should be engaged with, even if there are suspicions of abuse, as they can help explore the matter further. In introducing the idea of separate sessions, it is important to recognise and defer to the current family hierarchy by speaking first, and usually separately, with those persons who are, or who one might expect to be, in a major caregiving position.[16] This is not only engaging those who have the power to return or withdraw; it is also an opportunity to clarify the flow of information and to prepare them emotionally for handling negative information. It thus reduces the potential for shame and misunderstanding. This practice, a mainstay of our work, is now widely known as "talking about the talking". The following is an example of how this might look in talking with the caregivers:

> *One of the routine things we do here is to have a session alone with children. Sometimes kids can feel a bit freer to speak about their problems when other family members aren't around. And it's then a good chance for us to report back to you on what we find. Because, in general, we prefer for information to flow freely in a family, especially to Mum and Dad. Of course, we would check with your son or daughter about that first and it's always subject to the proviso that we think that no one is at risk. How would you feel about us talking with Susie by herself? What do you think she might say about your family?*
>
> *If she told us some difficult stuff, what would that be like for you to discuss it here? I think that sometimes as parents we are in a really difficult situation, in that we want to know what is worrying our children, and we want to change what we can so things are better for them. But I also think that one of the hardest things is for someone else to start questioning how we are parenting. It can be quite hurtful. How do you think it would be if Susie didn't think things were all right at home? Is that something you think we might be able to talk about here? How do you think she would respond to that? Do you think she might be worried about how you would respond?*

We would want to underline here that caregivers saying everything is fine is not necessarily an indication that they are. What this does is put the process of talking about difficult material on the table in a way that frames it as normal and starts to establish this within the broader goals stated by the family. It is also an opportunity to observe the more telling non-verbal communication that goes with these topics. Note that one of the issues that needs to be clarified in this conversation is that of confidentiality. Engagement will be greatly compromised if parents expect to be told what their child has said and then are not told. So be clear and realistic.

If the child discloses significant abuse, we will of course follow the procedures outlined in the scenarios that follow later. However, if a child disclosed, for example, feeling that Mum or Dad didn't love them, that they got yelled at a lot, or that their older brother or sister was a bully, we would see this as an issue to be discussed in therapy, even though it may not be reportable.

Before addressing any kinds of issues with the child, the same process of talking about talking is used. This should especially include talk about what will happen to the information they might give us. We usually encourage the sharing of information, for example, to the child:

> *Do you know why you are here? What are the things that you really like about living in your family? Is there anything you would like to be different? Do you think that Mum and Dad want things to be better like that for your family too? Would you like it if I could actually help things be better in your family?*
>
> *I know that some things can be difficult to share with your family and there might be some hard things that you might want to keep to yourself, or just between us. But to help your family I am going to need to pass on some at least of what we talk about, and especially the important stuff. How will that be for you if I do that? Is there anything that you might be worried about if Mum and Dad knew? etc.*

We consider it helpful to find out the good stuff that parents or siblings have been doing too, as well as getting the context of the bad stuff. It cannot be emphasised enough that when conducting individual sessions with children where there are suspected safety issues, the therapist must not ask leading questions. Several simple tools such as drawings, sculpture, use of puppets and figurines, and so on can be useful, though these are projective in nature and again should be used with caution.[17]

When reporting back to the parents, even though they will be waiting for the difficult material, it is important to give them *the specifics* of the positives first and to give the negatives with the context attached. It may also be useful to ask the parents, either before or after the session with their child, what worries they think he or she may talk about. For example, to the caregivers:

> *John and Jane, Susie and I had a great talk and she told me some really useful things. Now I know that you are here because you are keen to make things better in your family, and Susie told me that she wants that too. I feel that it's best then if I am able to tell you as much as possible of what we talked about. (Say all the good stuff first.) This is all good but there were some things that I know you would want to hear, that are a bit more difficult to talk about. Susie and I have discussed talking with you about this and she is on board with (me) telling you. Is it all right with you if I'm straight with you about these things? You seem to be the sort of people who want to hear it like it is.*[18]

When working with couples and with families where there are older parents being cared for by their children, and violence is suspected, the situation is similar in that individual interviews help explore further. However, broader contextual information, perhaps from a GP, may also be required. For instance, some problems with ageing involve dementia and paranoia that lead unintentionally to false accusations of their adult children. Nevertheless, many abusing older children also hide their abuse under the guise of the illness of their parents.

If you conduct an individual assessment with a child or adolescent who discloses abuse of some kind, good note taking involving verbatim questions and responses is recommended. Many young people will open up to the therapist but retract or minimise when the repercussions in their family become obvious (Sorensen & Snow, 1991; Summit, 1983).

A further note about confidentiality – As family therapists we believe that while confidentiality is good under some circumstances, in general, the freeing up of information is a good thing. Secrets tend to tie people, including therapists, up in knots and are part of the general tendency towards avoidance and defensiveness that pervades individuals and systems where there is a perception of threat. As therapists we need the flexibility to be able to access and share information between family members at a pace that is helpful for their relationships. We will therefore attempt to be clear with family members that the way we work is to ask them permission to share information where we see it to be helpful, albeit with prior discussion where possible. The exception to this is, as previously stated, when we are working with offending family members in cases where their confidentiality is required to ameliorate a power imbalance and to prevent further transgression of the victim's boundaries and loyalties. This approach to confidentiality is quite a significant responsibility as it requires the therapist to continually assess the resilience of individuals and the system. It is, however, in our experience, a lighter burden than having to wonder in each interaction whether or not we can say something we have heard from other family members and fearing that a slip will irretrievably damage relationships.

What if the situation is assessed as unsafe?

If, once an assessment is made, it is decided that someone in the family is unsafe, it is time to move from a therapeutic frame to a protective frame, that is, to do whatever needs to be done to maximise the possibility of safety for everyone concerned. This may mean notifying Child Protection, or the police, or the agency manager, or the supervisor. It may also mean, during the session, thinking carefully about what information is or isn't appropriate to be shared with the caregivers in the family, and how this should be done. For example, in sitting with a family where there is a father who is very angry and unreasonable, and everyone else seems afraid of him, it would be unwise to ask to speak to other family members alone as he may not be able to tolerate the possibility of their speaking about him. This could put them at risk of later repercussions. A possibility might be to let the family go home and to contact the school, or other agencies you know to be involved, to obtain information which might help you to decide about what to do next. The therapist needs to pay very careful attention to non-verbal cues before introducing anything that might elevate risk to any family members. He or she must wait until there are signs that the family is both engaging and settling emotionally in the therapy before stepping outside what the family are prepared for.

With all people in this situation, it is important to ask them what they would like to have happen. Where the person is 17 or under, the age at which one might seriously consider a notification to statutory authorities, it is important not to make any undertakings about this. If the person who is being hurt is a teenager or an adult, capable of discussing the situation in its complexity, it is important to also talk about their perspective on the level of risk. With lower levels of abuse, some young people cannot bear to open their families to further outside intervention but will be open to offers of help with, for example, problem-solving and finding ways to connect with other safe adults in their lives. The therapist who goes further than this in this situation risks losing engagement with the parent(s) *and* with the young person. Remaining engaged holds the hope of change at some time in the future. These situations are often difficult for the therapist to hold, and supervision is important.

If the level of abuse/neglect is significant[19] and/or the person who is at risk is a young child not capable of making their own complex decision, it is important to first assess the capacities of a non-offending parent or guardian to protect, believe, and support the child. This will include the parent's history, their material and emotional resources, and as well their level of dependency on the perpetrator. If there is sufficient resource and independence, this parent may be able to be engaged in the process of a notification. *It is important to do this separately from the abuser and with due regard for any requirements of possible statutory or legal processes that may be necessary.* If the parent doesn't believe the child, it is important to not take this as a given, but to slow the process down and to work as previously described, with the issues that are underlying the reluctance (Miller & Dwyer, 1997).[20] It is possible that sometimes engagement with the family is successful enough to allow for therapy to continue after notifications have been made and formal structures are in place to ensure safety for all. How to approach the subject of making a notification is crucial to this ongoing engagement. We prefer to discuss this with the family before this takes place. This will almost inevitably be difficult, and it is important, if possible, for the family to understand the reasons. The dialogue might proceed as follows:

Therapist: So Jane, what you are telling me is that you do accept now that the fights between you and Erin have got out of control and that you can't seem to stop yourself once it gets to a certain point.

Jane: Yeah. I guess so. I don't mean to hurt her but...

Therapist: It's really hard to stop yourself at that point isn't it, with so much on your plate to deal with?

Jane: Yeah.

Therapist: Mm. This is probably one of the hardest things to talk about but I'm thinking that we need to get some outside help with this so things don't keep going down a track that you don't want them to.

Jane: What do you mean?

Therapist: I'm talking about making a call to Child Protection.

Jane: So you want them to take my kids off me?

Therapist: No, that's actually the opposite of what I'd like to have happen, but I'm thinking that that's what may end up happening if we don't do something now. You see, I know that in your heart of hearts you want the best for your children. We've talked about your values, and they are really sound. What you've been telling me, though, is that with everything going on now for you, you're finding it hard to hold to them, which must be devastating for you, and is actually dangerous to your kids. Calling Child Protection is scary, and I don't know exactly what will happen, and indeed you may never speak to me again after this. But we've talked about those values you have about parenting, and the value that you place on your children, and right now I'm being loyal to them. I'm also going to be here to help you through the process, if you want me to be.

When the notification process is handled well enough by the therapist and family, and everyone is adamant that the situation is now safe, it is important that the therapist not collude with a very understandable tendency by exhausted and overwhelmed family members to "park" the issue. In our experience, where there has been abuse, even if it has now ceased, it is unlikely that any other agenda presented by the family will not be influenced by this. We need then find ways to support the family to attend, as a matter of priority, to the personal and relational sequelae of the abuse.

Talking with the offending family member

One complexity to manage here is that, perhaps having already worked successfully towards a certain level of engagement with the offending family member, shame and/or distress may become an issue for them and may inhibit further progression in therapy. The therapist then has the task of engaging in a different way (usually less confronting). Given, as mentioned, that the material is likely to be shame triggering, it would be important, just as it is with victims, to talk first about the talking. We might start off with something like the following:

> *Hi Anna. This is the first time we've got together since Sarah told us about the things that have been happening at your house. It must be a bit strange to be meeting like this after everything that's happened. What is it like for you? Is strange the right word?*
>
> *I think it's going to be important though for us to talk about these things and to figure out where we go from here. Do you agree? Otherwise, it's going to be a bit like the elephant in the room. How do you think it will be for you to talk about the things she has said you have been doing? I don't think it's going to be easy at all.*

Where it develops from here will largely rely upon whether the abuser denies everything or admits to at least some of the things to which he or she is accused. No matter how hard we work, sometimes the constraints are too great for the abuser, and he or she, if not mandated, may decide to discontinue. However, frequently, we have found that people who hurt others are at least partly uncomfortable (sometimes horrified) at what they have done and will cooperate to some extent. Often the point of leverage is their wanting to keep the connection to their families. How we engage can make all the difference. More will be said on this in the next scenario.

Scenario B – Mandated but cooperative

The family has been referred by a statutory body, e.g., child protection, the abuse is verified and the family are cooperative

This scenario is the most straightforward in terms of engagement with the family. Safety concerns have been attended to by statutory means, and hopefully by the non-offending parents or guardians as well. The abuse allegations, and the issue of risk and safety, are on the table, as is the question of guilt and blame, and who will take responsibility. It is by no means that the offending family member will necessarily be admitting to everything he or she is accused of, or accepting full responsibility, but these are things that can be openly addressed from the beginning as part of the engagement process. The complexity that arises is often about maintaining the involvement of the statutory authority and of fostering a relationship of active collaboration. The first risk is that in cases like this the matter will seem to be settled into the hands of another agency, so overburdened protective workers are likely to see this as a low priority or to decide that there is no further risk. A second danger is that there can be a divergence or lack of clarity around goals and roles between the agency and the protective worker. It is vital that the therapist's good working relationship with the family is not at the cost of the relationship of the protective worker's relationship with either the therapist or the family. Progress will be enhanced by judicious cooperation with the statutory worker, not weakened by it. The management of the case and the issue of risk will be much more effectively held if the therapist can firmly establish the therapeutic frame from the beginning. Relevant questions here are: What are the goals from the perspective of the statutory party? And do these fit with those of the client's family?[21] What is the therapist's role? What are the reporting requirements? How long is the statutory party going to stay involved? How is the family going to get to see the therapist? How is payment going to be made, if any, and for how many sessions? How will communication happen between the statutory party and the therapist? How will all these things be negotiated with the family?

The therapy can founder on any one of these areas if they are not clear and firm, but more relevant to our discussion here is that they can interfere with both safety and therapeutic engagement. For example, if the family and therapist are not clear about what is going to be written into reports and the therapist includes something the family thought would not be included, it may be very difficult to retrieve trust. If the Department has agreed to pay a private therapist to see a family, a short-term basis is not likely to be sufficient, and the family will likely not be able to afford to pay for themselves. The therapist has the job then of closing, which is a difficult call ethically, or to enter into a fee arrangement which may not be sustainable for the therapist, and which is likely to influence the nature of the relationship.

In terms of who to see first in this situation, this decision partly depends on the age and wishes of the child or young person who has been abused. If that person is old enough to understand and wants to be seen alone or with someone other than a parent, we would usually agree.[22] If it is a younger child, we would usually see either the non-offending parent(s) or guardians with the child(ren) who have been abused. Sometimes, there may be issues that need to be discussed just between adults, and in those cases, we might see them before including the children. An example of this might be to address conflict or disruption from a bad experience with the statutory body that is now impinging on our relationship with the family or to discover and work with the parents' positioning and support for the child. These things can often be done in subsequent sessions, and it is our preference to see the child as early in the involvement as possible, *with the non-offending parent(s)*. This is to (re)establish this relationship as primary, and as central to healing, rather than to replace it with one that is therapist centric.

In the case of sibling sexual abuse, we would likewise want to see the young offending family member firstly with his or her parents rather than on his or her own because we believe their support is also crucial to engagement and progress in therapy. It is important to balance this with the parents also supporting the victim in therapy, as they are often overlooked at this time. Where the abuse has been from someone in an authority position over the child, for example, a parent, step-parent, uncle, or grandfather, we would usually see the offending person on his or her own. Couple therapy might be appropriate later but where abuse is from adult to child, the relationship between non-offending parent and child is prioritised.

Therapy with the family would then probably move to regular individual sessions with the victim by one therapist, with the abuser by another, and with the non-offending parent(s) by one or both of these therapists. The support of non-offending parents is paramount. They will be struggling with their own issues as well as having to manage those of their children. If the case is one of sibling abuse, they are frequently in a no-win situation (Welfare, 2008).

Even though the non-offending parent(s) may be believing and supportive of the child, respectful discussion about, and engagement of, the offending family member will enhance their capacity to cooperate with the process. Partly this will be because of the attachment the person has to the offending family member and all that this entails, especially if he or she is a partner, son or daughter, or parent. We have also come to understand, however, and the Contextual Therapy of Ivan Boszormenyi-Nagy is instructive here, that the issue of the offending person's shame extends to other members of the family. *Where my son is someone who has abused my daughter, what does that make me? Or where I have chosen a man who would abuse my child, what does that say about me? If my father is a monster, what does that make me?*

Shame, however, is something that can be put on the table with the offending person from the beginning of the engagement (Jenkins, 1990, 2006a). Following Lane (1991), we are open from the first session about how difficult the work is going to be, particularly how heavily the person will feel the burden of shame, and how inviting it will be to want to avoid it. We anticipate that it, perhaps accompanied by all kinds of fears, will contribute to a tendency to want to forget, to deny or minimise the events or their impacts, or to in some way shift the blame to others. We state that this is so normal and understandable that we will be expecting that whatever the person tells us can only be a partial truth. We frame the facing of shame, however, as utterly necessary for progress to be achieved. Alongside this, we also attempt to make space for the person's honour to become visible. This is part of what we would do working with anyone facing the possibility of over-whelming affect – to talk about the talking. Our conversation with the person might go something like the following:

Therapist: Hi John. It's good to meet with you. I'm not sure if you're thinking that right now. I suppose you'd probably almost prefer to be anywhere but here. I think I would be in your shoes. But it is a big thing that you are here. How do you feel about the idea of starting to talk about the stuff that Sarah has been talking with us about?

John: I don't know what to feel.

Therapist: I suppose that's true because you've probably never done this before. … I think that most people in your shoes try to find lots of ways to not think or feel about what they've done. Would you say that's right about you or are you someone who thinks about it all the time?

John: No, I suppose I try not to think about it.

Therapist: How do you think it will be for you to start talking to me about it?

John: Hard.

Therapist: Yes. I think that's right. In fact my experience with other people I've worked with around these issues is that it ends up being harder than they could even have imagined at the beginning. What are some of the things that you think might get in the way?

John: Feeling bad.

Therapist: What sorts of bad feelings?

John: I don't know.

Therapist: Well, I agree with you that bad feelings will be pretty high up there. Lots of people are afraid of all kinds of things. So, there's fear. Is that one of the things for you?

John: Mm.

Therapist: What are the sorts of things that you would be afraid of if we started to talk?

John: Well, I don't know … I suppose what people would think of me.

Therapist: Which people? Who would you be most worried about?

John: My family … Mary…

Therapist: Mary, and your family … they mean a lot to you.

John: Yeah.

Therapist: What are you worried that they would think?

John: That I'm no good.

Therapist: Because of what's happened?

John: Yeah.

Therapist: So you feel bad about what's happened?

John: Yeah.

Therapist: What would you call that? Guilt? Shame?

John: Yeah something like that.

Therapist: Well, I think those things are huge when people are dealing with this stuff. And in fact, I think they are so huge that they often make it very difficult for people to move ahead, to face up to what has gone on, to do the work that's needed. I think this is so much the case that I pretty much assume these days that when I'm talking to someone in your situation, they'll be finding it very difficult to tell me the truth, especially the whole truth. And it's understandable, because it's hard. It's also necessary though to sit with the shame if you are going to do the work. What do you think it says about you that you are prepared to be here at least talking about starting to talk? Like we said you'd probably rather be almost anywhere else.

Jenkins (2006b), in writing about his work with young sexual offenders, notes the importance of attending to fairness by acknowledging any injustices the young person may himself have been subject to. This is a matter of ethics *and* efficacy, as it is unlikely the person will be receptive to taking responsibility for his own actions without this. Jenkins' approach with young men is also slower than that demonstrated above. He gives some time and space for the usual processes of avoidance and reluctance to occur and works into challenges at a pace that the young person can tolerate. We consider this to be a clinical judgement rather than a rule of thumb. We have been quite direct with young men from the beginning and found this effective when combined with respect and empathy. We are also direct about the issue of the offending family member's fear of blame from us.

> *Of course, you are going to be afraid that I, and everyone else will blame you and see you as a terrible person. I want to put it on the table that that's not what this is about. This is mostly about you finding out about you so that the thing that you, and your family, are feeling so bad right now won't happen again.*

We agree with both Lane (1991) and Jenkins (2006a) that challenge is about leading the offending family member to "aha" moments rather than about trying to convince or manipulate him or her into seeing the error of their ways.

While the elements of respect and compassion are crucial to the engagement of the offending family member, they do however raise one of the central dilemmas in this work and that is how to hold to this without colluding with their understandable wish to avoid the pain of confronting what they have done. Aside from hindering therapeutic progress, this can be dangerous. "Cognitive distortions" is a construct in the field that describes the various ways that an offender shifts responsibility for, or minimises the seriousness or impact of, their offending (Marshall, Anderson, & Fernandez, 1999). This behaviour appears almost universally in the initial stages when people are confronted with the abusiveness of their behaviours. It is important to realise that it does not mean that they are purposefully lying, although this can and does happen. What is more frequent is that the thinking is actually and genuinely misled, sometimes because of the developmental experience of the offender and frequently as a defence against overwhelming shame. Knowing the source of the distortions is extremely useful in addressing them.

The temptation here is to, however gently, just confront the offending family member with their distortions. In our experience, unless there is a robust engagement already, this almost always evokes further defensiveness. In our opinion, there are several elements of an optimum approach. One of these can involve, as noted in Jenkins (2006a) above, a staging of the language the therapist uses to refer to the abuse, that starts out benign until the relationship is established but becomes more confronting over time. It is possible in some circumstances, however, to use elements of directness, as exemplified in the dialogue below (Young, 2023). Another element involves education about the frequently engaged behaviours of offenders, along with their explanations. For example, education about addiction cycles, the various stages leading to offending behaviour, and the nature of cognitive distortions can be helpful. The real work of straightening out the distortions, however, most effectively occurs in unpacking the minutiae of the abusive event, including the pre-planning and post-abuse stages, and within a systemic frame, so including all affected members. It is in this that empathy, which is an antidote to cognitive distortions, starts to be developed (Marshall, Anderson, & Fernandez, 1999). There is no space here to go into substantive detail about work with offenders, but the following is an example of dialogue from fairly early-stage work with a man who has been violent to his partner. This scenario provides a strategy for a therapist to establish safety in the initial stages of work with a couple where there has been violence:

Therapist: So Alan, you're saying that you think Leonie is turning a mountain into a molehill. Can you tell me from your perspective what happened?

Alan: Well, we were having an argument, and she just kept at me and at me, like she always does. I've told her before that she needs to stop before I get too riled up. Anyway, she didn't and so I just pushed her. It was no big deal. I'm not a violent person. She's more violent than I am. She hits me all the time.

Therapist: Ok, so you're saying it can get pretty heated between you two and it sounds like you place some value on not being a violent person. I'm presuming then that you would prefer that violence wasn't part of your relationship with Leonie? I don't want to just assume that though. Am I right, or do you see violence as being a legitimate part of your relationship?

Alan: Of course, I'd prefer it wasn't there. But she's just as much to blame as I am. She knows she can only push me so far.

Therapist: Ok, so there's a few issues there but for now let's just focus on that you're saying that you don't want violence in your relationship. You seem like a person who likes people to say it like it is. You're a pretty direct guy. Is that right?

Two other important issues here are Alan's blaming Leonie and the implication that he can't control his own temper. She has to do it for him. The crucial issue to pursue here is the safety of the situation, and this involves getting Alan to recognise that even though he might not intend his behaviour to be violent (dangerous), it is.

Alan:	Yeah, I'd agree with that.
Therapist:	So, is it okay for me to be pretty direct with you John?
Alan:	Yeah, I think so.
Therapist:	Well, I'm hearing you say that you don't want violence in your relationship and that you only pushed Leonie, and I would also think that you didn't really mean, in that case, for her to get hurt, but she did, didn't she?
Alan:	Yeah, she did.
Therapist:	You also seem to be saying that, in a way, you're relying on Leonie to stop you from losing your temper. Now there are lots of questions here about whether you want to have to rely on her to help you manage yourself, but probably the most important at this stage is whether or not this is a safe thing to do. I understand that Leonie has got hurt before too.
Alan:	Well, nothing like this before, and it was an accident. She just overbalanced.
Therapist:	If Leonie were here, what do you think her perspective would be?
Alan:	Well, I don't know, you'd have to ask her.

The therapist introduces an invitation to John to entertain Mary's perspective but doesn't push this as, while it is important to sow seeds, this also risks disrupting the early engagement.

Therapist:	I know this is hard to talk about, but I am hearing clearly that you have some values around what you want for your relationship. Is it okay if we keep on going so that we can bring things back to the way you want them to be?
Alan:	Okay, I suppose so.
Therapist:	Ok. That's great. So, you seemed to be saying that this is the worst it's ever got. In what ways have either of you been hurt before?
Alan:	Oh, just a bruise once or twice.
Therapist:	Okay. So, who has had the bruises? Can you tell me how it all happened?

As stated above, it is often in getting the person to talk about the detail of their interactions that the gravity of the violence becomes evident to them. It is possible to add to this by asking questions like:

> *And if the children (or Leonie's family) had witnessed this, what would they have been feeling and thinking?* or
> *Where does this happen? Has it ever happened in public? What's your thinking about that? What do you think others would think if it did?*

Especially in the early stages of treatment, it is important to engage non-offending parents, even those who are cooperative, in helpful positions with regard to the offending family member. Especially in cases of sibling abuse, parents are in an invidious position. The most helpful stance for these parents is to support the offending family member whilst strongly holding him or her accountable for the abuse. At the same time, they must privilege the safety and healing needs of the victim and validate the reality of their abuse experiences. However, this can be very difficult for parents to manage at a practical and emotional level. The tendency can be for parents to reject either the offending family member or the victim and to focus their support on the other. Parents are also having an extremely difficult time coming to terms with the occurrence of the unthinkable in their family and may blame themselves. This is natural but unhelpful to both the offending family member (as he does not become accountable) and the victim (as she is not validated by her parents' protection of their son). It may be a revelation to them, only available through the therapist, that they can, and in fact that it's best to, maintain a connection with both children (even if the children are adults when the disclosure occurs[23]). Much support from the therapist will be needed if parents are to sustain this position.

It would be easy to assume that the engagement of the victim in these circumstances is a given, but this is by no means the case. This depends on many factors. The victim may feel guilty for getting their family member into trouble, for hurting the non-offending parent, and for breaking up the family. Depending on what has been internalised from the offending behaviour, she or he may indeed feel that the abuse was her fault. The resultant shame can be just as much an impediment to talking about the abuse as it is for the one who perpetrated it (Herman, 2007). She may be locked in conflict with other family members; particularly mothers tend to be blamed by their abused children. Protracted periods of fluctuating belief or denial by the parent will likely make it difficult for her to trust anyone. Again patience, respect, predictability, and empathy are required. Productive engagement with the non-offending parent is probably the most powerful means of engagement here.[24]

Scenario C – Mandated and non-cooperative

The family has been referred by a statutory body, there has been an initial disclosure and then a retraction, and the whole family are now denying that anything has happened

This situation, particularly related to Child Protection referrals, is a difficult but not uncommon one.[25] Frequently the child's worst fears about disclosure are realised, and often under explicit or implicit pressure from their families, the child will say that they made the whole thing up. In this situation it is important, if possible, to see the child on his or her own. The therapist needs to truly appreciate what the child is up against and to convey that understanding. However, the main aim of the session needs to be to enable the child to speak of these constraints so they can be worked through both with the child and with other potentially supportive family members. One might begin by not disputing the retraction but by asking about the hypothetical, "What if it did happen?" "What would the repercussions for your family be?" We have found that if the child feels safe enough, they may give the therapist some useful information even if they don't reassert the initial disclosure, something more likely if the child has support to do so within the family. It is for this reason that it is important to see the non-offending parent next.

The non-offending parent should be seen separately from the alleged offending family member and the child. It is important to first assess the capacities of that parent or guardian to protect, believe, and support the child, and in this case, it would be safe to assume that there are significant constraints to this. Assessment will include the parent's history, material and emotional resources, and, related to these, his or her level of dependency on the perpetrator (Miller & Dwyer, 1997).[26] Denial that the abuse occurred doesn't necessarily imply that the parent doesn't believe. It may be that the parent is protecting herself or her partner from the consequences of disclosure while trying to handle the situation privately. Whether or not this is the case, it is vital to persist with joining and trying to engage the parent in working through the various issues. The person is likely to be flooded with feelings around a multitude of issues. Fear of the offending family member is one of these. Shock, grief, or fear at the multitude of potential losses of things such as income and/or housing, significant (attachment) relationships, and loss of the family ideal (Dwyer, 1999; Welfare, 2006) commonly occurs. There may also be shame at the choice of partner, betrayal by that partner, and possibly by the child, and guilt at not having been aware of the situation. It may also be that a poor relationship between the parent and child or teenager has occurred because of the sequelae of abuse or because of the positioning of the child by the offending family member. This then often makes the child less believable than the one who hurt them.

Again, we find it useful, in this circumstance, to take the position of not knowing if the abuse has occurred or not. Against a background of empathy and normalising, we explore the hypotheticals of what if it had, and what if it hadn't happened. Some examples of what we might say are:

> *I understand that Sarah initially made a disclosure about your partner and that she has since taken that back and said that she had made it up. This whole situation must have come as an enormous shock to you and now here you are talking to us? What sense do you make of it all?*
>
> *I can see how it must be incredibly difficult to know what to believe and, in your shoes, I think I might go along with what you are saying. We've seen these circumstances before, however, and we know how serious it is for everyone and so we take it very seriously. Being honest with you, it's not unusual for young people to make a disclosure and then take it back even if it is true, and there are some very good reasons for that. I'm not saying that that's the case here, but would it be all right with you if we dealt with this with the seriousness that it deserves and explore things thoroughly so that we don't end up making decisions that we'll regret in the long run?*
>
> *If it wasn't true, why do you think Sarah would say these things?*
>
> *And if it were true, what would that mean for you and your family, and for Sarah?*

It is wise to assume that the attachment relationship that likely exists between non-offending parent(s) and the offending family member is active at this point. Even if they partly believe the child and are furious at some level, they will still engage in the process of exploration far more readily if respect and concern are demonstrated for the abusing family member as well. We will sometimes say something like:

> *I'm not saying that this has happened but even if this information is true, it doesn't mean your partner (or son, or father, or uncle) is a bad person. We don't yet know the full circumstances but in our experience it's important to find out so that they can get some help as well. We have found that many times people who do these sorts of things are deeply troubled by them and, as difficult as it is, are sometimes relieved when the truth comes out.*

Real patience along with sustained respect and curiosity is sometimes required here. It can take quite a long time for families to trust the therapist enough to engage in the therapeutic process. Sometimes, in our experience, it's just a matter of time before something in the system shifts to allow this to happen.

Scenario D – Self-referral and cooperative around the issues concerning abuse

Where there is a child or adolescent involved as the victim, this can be a very difficult but not uncommon situation. A disclosure has been made, the parent or parents have confronted the offending family member, and he has admitted to it. However, everyone, while they want help for both family members, doesn't want involvement with the authorities. The crucial issue is whether there is a current risk to the child and any other children. It may be that on finding out about the abuse the parent(s) have ensured there is no contact. Some circumstances make this more achievable than others, for example, if the offending family member is a grandparent. If the offending family member is a parent who is living in the family home with the child, then this is a different story.

Respected practitioners and researchers have expressed strong opinions that families in this situation should not be seen without some kind of statutory involvement (Morrison, 2006). There are good reasons for this as it is very difficult to assess whether families are complying with the requirements to ensure the safety of children, even if they are outwardly agreeing to them. Even child protection workers in visiting the home cannot always guarantee compliance and it is rare that family therapists conduct such visits. We also know that people do extraordinary things given circumstances, especially within attachment relationships such as might pertain between an offending parent and his non-offending partner, or his non-offending daughter or parents, ambivalent about whether they believe their son or their daughter.

Thus, seeing families without statutory involvement is not something that we would recommend either. Having said this, there is the dilemma of knowing that some families will forfeit any kind of treatment if it means *any* statutory involvement. If the therapist believes that a child, any child, is at risk of abuse, regardless of whether or not they are covered by legislation mandating a notification, there is a moral obligation to notify. If the therapist does not believe there is a risk however the choice, of course, is theirs. We would strongly recommend against inexperienced workers seeing families under these circumstances. This would also apply to workers in private or public settings who do not have the support of a team, and/or management who are fully informed and supportive about this course of action. In addition, it is a decision that would need to have the full consent of all family members, and it would need to be supported by a very thorough assessment.

There are, however, situations where families might present for counselling where children are being abused by other family members at a level that is not notifiable. For example, an older brother or sister might be bullying a younger one, or a parent might be aware that they are becoming angry or irritable and saying things that they know to be unacceptable and are later regretful of. Engagement of this person is easier where they accept responsibility. We would tend to engage with *reluctant* family members in a similar way to that described above for offending family members, that is, with respect, and allowing for some avoidance while on the way to facing the full extent of their abuse and being credited for what they are doing to face up to this. And at the same time, we would work with non-offending family members on the most appropriate stance for them to take in regard to the abuse.

If the victim is an adult, the situation is clearer as there are no mandatory requirements on workers to notify authorities. This is not to say that the situation is necessarily safe. Careful assessment of risk is still necessary. Possible presentations could be couple therapy, or at the other end of the life cycle, elder abuse.

When seeing couples, even though abuse issues might be on the table, there are important considerations. In the ongoing debate in the literature about the appropriateness of couple therapy where there is violence, one of the clear reasons given for not seeing these couples conjointly is that it could increase the risk of that violence recurring (Schacht, Dimidjian, George, & Berns, 2009). This would immediately violate the highest priority, that of safety. Another reason is that couple therapy implies joint responsibility for the violence (Schacht, Dimidjian, George, & Berns, 2009). Both, aside from their ethical implications, have implications for the positioning of the therapist in regard to each partner. As noted above, it is difficult for clients to engage cognitively and to take risks where their nervous systems are activated by current or imminent threats. Where there is a risk of violence, this also means that the power differential between the partners is significant, and in this circumstance, there will either not be cooperation or the therapist will find a restriction to their therapeutic flexibility with the couple.

However, there are also very good reasons for offering conjoint therapy to couples where there has been infrequent low-level violence and/or abuse of other kinds,[27] where none of the risk factors for lethality are present, where both partners enter into the therapy willingly and are not fearful of each other, and where cessation of any violence is the primary goal (Schacht et al., 2009). A major reason is to address the interactional patterns that may be serving to maintain the violence. Another reason is that couples often stay together despite the abuse, and therapy may be a way of empowering the less powerful member (where this can be done safely), as well as providing a way to monitor the violence, at least for some time (Jory & Anderson, 2000).

With the cessation of the violence established as the primary goal and with both or all parties consenting to this, a question arises as to whether one would take a similar position to that discussed for Scenario B above. This partly depends on the level of responsibility being taken by the abusing party. Jory and Anderson (2000) describe an approach (built upon CT) that takes the same position about the abuser's accountability, and the anguish (shame) that is generated when he confronts this, as does Jenkins (2006a). That is, the abuser, and no one else, is responsible for their actions, and facing shame is absolutely necessary to the recovery of the person they have hurt – "…to the degree an individual fails to embrace the anguish of accountability for his or her own actions and attitudes, the anguish of abuse will be shifted to others in the emotional system" (Jory & Anderson, 2000, p. 330). Moreover, the reinstatement of the abusing person in his own and others' eyes is also dependent on this facing up to shame. Jory and Anderson's position with such couples is, like our model, used with families where there has been sexual abuse, and that is to privilege the perspective and the needs of the victim and to establish for that person an "environment of affirmation" (2000, p. 334). Like our model, Jory and Anderson (2000) set up a "challenging environment" for the abuser "early in the first session" (2000, p. 335). There is still an emphasis on gentle and respectful engagement and a focus on the abuser's self-discovery but more strongly the approach is infused with the conviction that his "struggle over anguish" is an integral part of the therapeutic relationship as well as of the couple relationship. Thus, in conjoint therapy the different needs of the partners are overt from the first session and the therapist uses his or her position to rebalance "the already-tipped scales of intimate justice" (2000, p. 336) by persistently affirming the less powerful member and challenging the more powerful one.

Scenario E – Currently working with an individual and a disclosure is made

This situation is similar in some respects to scenario A above, when a disclosure is made in a separate session. The main difference is that the other family members, while they may have contact with the therapist, are not including themselves in the therapy agenda. The decision then needs to be made as to whether to proceed with individual therapy or to try to involve other family members, or if the person is young enough, whether to make a notification. Our position, as stated in our general guidelines, is to try to work with as many people in the system as possible where this is safe to do so and following the fulfilment of any mandatory or duty of care obligations.

If the person is young enough to require the involvement of statutory authorities, the therapist has less manoeuvrability than when they are seeing the whole family. The therapist is not engaged with the other family members and is not able to involve them in the disclosure process. There may be a possibility to allow this to happen but generally if a disclosure occurs in this context and abuse is currently occurring, statutory authorities need to be immediately involved and they would then make the connections with the non-abusive parent.

If a person is older, they may still need police involvement and can be assisted to go through this process. This is particularly true regarding domestic violence and childhood sexual abuse (disclosed as an adult). If they are well connected to other family members, it would be useful to try and engage those persons in the process. Often the non-involved parent may be elderly at the time of the disclosure and when the perpetrator is their partner of many years, it is a difficult dilemma of whether to even tell them of the assaults.

Conclusions

This chapter has outlined the complexity of working with violence and abuse in families. There are many different types of violence and abuse but they all involve a violation from a loved one. The family therapist involved in the treatment of these victims and their families is faced with unique dilemmas that go beyond the general rules of family therapy, systems therapy, and narrative therapy. A key to the management of these abuse and violent situations involves the maintenance of the therapeutic relationship in order to progress the work but not at the expense of sacrificing safety. Awareness of the type of perpetrator involved in the abuse or violence is critical for the family and therapist's safety. Good collegial working relationships with statutory authorities and police are also critical to work effectively. Much stronger management and guidance from the therapist is required to assist families move towards recovery and an awareness of the power differentials that particularly mark these families is critical.

Notes

1 Whitzman (2008) cites the following statistics *for the general population*: 3% of Australian women in relationships will have experienced violence in the last 12 months; 36% of women abused by a male violent partner reported that the violence happened while they were pregnant; US and UK studies found the average number of violent incidents from partner violence to be three and seven times per annum, respectively; 5% of the US parents say they have hit their children with an object, kicked them, beaten them, or threatened them with a knife or gun on at least one occasion; the rate of violence towards children from parents from other cultures can be much higher, for example, 45% of Korean parents; international studies estimate child sexual abuse to be 20% for girls and 5–10% for boys; elder abuse is said to be between 4% and 6% where surveys have been conducted (Canada, USA, The Netherlands, Finland, UK). It stands to reason that with these statistics in the general population amongst clinical populations the rate of abuse will be higher.

2 Harris, M., & Fallot R. D. (2001). Envisioning a trauma-informed service system: A vital paradigm shift. *New Directions in Mental Health Services, 89*, 3–22.

3 It is important to acknowledge here that investigation is not properly the role of the therapist. Some assessment, however, is required to determine whether or not to refer the matter to those who have the legal mandate to undertake this.

4 See, for example, the work of the Meridian Program (Anglicarevic n.d).

5 These are, namely, Collaborative therapy (Anderson & Goolishian, 1988), Solution-focussed therapy (De Shazer et al., 1986), and Narrative therapy (White & Epston, 1989).

6 Early family therapy literature and practice with abuse issues viewed the whole or parts of the family (often the non-offending parent and the victim) as dysfunctional or pathological and causing the abusive behaviours (Alexander, 1992). Modern theories (informed by a feminist analysis of power, CBT addiction models, and attachment theory) now locate the aetiology of the abusive behaviours firmly within the offender (Marshall, Anderson, & Fernandez, 1999; Morrison, 2006; Ryan & Lane, 1991).

7 Cozolino 2020 (esp pp. 94–97) makes a distinction between "intelligence", which may be required, for example, in conveying information about a technical problem, and "wisdom", which tailors information to a specific situation and requires the exercise of empathy. Each depends on different parts of the brain. It is wisdom that is needed by the therapist and adult clients in particular.

8 We will expand later on some of the contributions from Jenkins (2006a), but the reader would do well to read this chapter in full to get a fairly comprehensive perspective on an invitational approach to working with shame in the therapeutic context.

9 A number of reasonable assessment guides are available on the internet, for example: Child Welfare Information Gateway (2007). Recognizing child abuse and neglect: Signs and symptoms. http://www.childwelfare.gov/pubs/factsheets/signs.cfm

10 These are Holtzworth-Monroe and Stuart's (1994) "intimate terrorist" and Gottman et al.'s (1995) "cobra". They correlate in Ross & Babcock's (2009) study with a diagnosis of anti-social personality disorder and a "dismissing" attachment style.

11 Australian statistics show that over a ten-year period (1989–1999), 20.8% of all homicides in Australia involved intimate partners (Mouzos, 1999).

12 These may include both the "family-only batterer" and the "dysphoric or borderline batterer" of Holtzworth-Monroe and Stuart (1994) and the "pit-bulls" of Gottman et al. (1995) and correlate with Ross & Babcock's (2009) borderline personality disorder diagnosis and a "preoccupied" attachment.

13 Carlson & Jones (2010) gives a reasonable summary of the research on typologies of violent men and Knight and Prentky (1990) provide a good typology with treatment recommendations for sexually abusive men.

14 Kropp's review of the violence assessment literature stresses the need for scepticism around self-report from offenders about their own violence. In contrast, they strongly support the involvement of victims in the assessment, stating that they can provide crucial information. A word of caution is added however in that victims can also "grossly minimize or underestimate the risk posed by their partners" (2008, p. 211).

15 See Schacht et al. (2009, p. 48) for a fairly comprehensive list and for other references.

16 This applies to the more powerful partner in a couple relationship too. This is not out of respect in this case but out of the wisdom that in engaging with this person one is more likely to get an assessment of whether it will be safe to see their partner individually, and/or that we may be able to engage with this person in a way that minimises their perception of threat, by engaging with them. This then minimises the risk to their partner.

17 There is a rich literature on resources for working with children, including those that relate specifically to drawings (e.g., DiLeo, 1973; Farokhi & Hashemi, 2011; Foley & Mullis 2008; Malchiodi, 1998) and those that cover a wider range of methods in less depth (e.g., Webb, 2007).

18 This approach draws on a model developed by Jeff Young, No Bullshit Therapy (2006), which emphasises directness with warmth.

19 Note, for example, that in the state of Victoria, Australia, legislation (CYFA, 2005) for Department of Human Services Child Protection involvement includes consideration not only for children safety needs but also for their stability and development. Practitioners should consult their own state or country legislation for requirements particular to their situation.

20 Miller and Dwyer (1997) hold the relationship of the non-offending parent to the perpetrator as a central influence on the non-offending parent's belief. Plummer (2006) found that mothers were most influenced in their belief of their child by a direct verbal disclosure and the child's behavioural and emotional reactions helped to confirm this. The most prevalent barrier to belief was the idea that the parent would or should have known, followed by the denial of the abuser.

21 It needs to be remembered here too that the family may not be speaking in one voice. Victim, abuser, and non-offending parents are likely to have different goals.

22 In one family the young girl wished her brother, the offender, to be present. We went along with this, although it did become apparent to her during the session that there were things she didn't wish to discuss with him present and we asked him to step out.

22 Sibling sexual abuse has the lowest rate of disclosure at the time of its occurrence. More than 80% of sibling sexual abuse is only disclosed when the siblings are adults. Consequently, parents of adult children are often faced with managing this situation (Welfare, 2008).

24 It may be helpful for non-offending parents to have therapy on perhaps long-standing issues from their own histories that may be influencing their positioning and functioning here (McIlwaine & O'Sullivan, 2015).

25 After Summit's (1983) assertion that 25% of children retract their disclosures, which was supported by Sorenson and Snow's (1991) study finding 22%, prevalence rates were disputed in the literature ranging from 3% of cases seen in a sample from Child Protection (Bradley & Wood, 1996) to 27% of children who were victims of ritual abuse (Gonzalez, Waterman, Kelly, McCord, & Oliveri, 1993). The difference may reflect 13 years of awareness and skills building on the part of workers and parents.

26 Miller and Dwyer (1997) hold the relationship of the non-offending parent to the perpetrator as a central influence on the non-offending parent's belief. Plummer (2006) found that mothers were most influenced in their belief of their child by a direct verbal disclosure and the child's behavioural and emotional reactions helped to confirm this. The most prevalent barrier to belief was the idea that the parent would or should have known, followed by the denial of the abuser.

27 See James and McKinnon (2010) for a framework for identifying different forms of non-physical abuse and their consequences.

References

AIHW (2019). *Family, domestic and sexual violence in Australia: Continuing the national story.* Canberra, Australia: AIHW.

Alexander, P. C. (1992). Application of attachment theory to the study of sexual abuse. *Journal of Consulting and Clinical Psychology, 60,* 185–195.

Andersen, T. (1987). The reflecting team: Dialogue and meta-dialogue in clinical work. *Family Process, 26,* 415–428.

Anderson, H., & Goolishian, H. (1988). Human systems as linguistic systems: Preliminary and evolving ideas about the implications for clinical theory. *Family Process, 27,* 371–393.

Anderson, H., Goolishian, H., McNamee, S., & Gergen, K. (Eds). (1992). The client is the expert: A not-knowing approach to therapy. In *Therapy as social construction* (pp. 25–39). Newbury Park, CA: Sage Publications.

Anglicarevic (n.d.). *Breaking the cycle.* https://www.anglicarevic.org.au/news/breaking-the-cycle/

Arntz, A., & Jacob, G. (2012). *Schema therapy in practice.* Wiley.

Australian Institute of Family Studies (2014). Who abuses children? Policy and practice paper. Retrieved July 5, 2023, from https://aifs.gov.au/resources/policy-and-practice-papers/who-abuses-children

Boszormenyi-Nagy, I., & Krasner, B. R. (1986). *Between give and take: A clinical guide to contextual therapy.* New York, NY: Brunner/Mazel.

Bowlby, J. (1969). *Attachment and loss.* (2nd ed., Vol 1. Attachment). New York, NY: Basic Books.

Bowlby, J. (1973). *Attachment and loss: Vol 2. Separation.* New York, NY: Basic Books.

Bowlby, J. (1980). *Attachment and loss: Vol. 3. Loss, sadness and depression.* New York, NY: Basic Books.

Bradley, A. R., & Wood, J. M. (1996). How do children tell? The disclosure process in child sexual abuse. *Child Abuse and Neglect, 20,* 881–891.

Caffaro, J., & Conn-Caffaro, A. (2005). Treating sibling abuse families. *Aggression and Violent Behavior, 10,* 604–623. 10.1016/j.avb.2004.12.001

Carlson, R. G., & Jones, K. D. (2010). Continuum of conflict and control: A conceptualisation of intimate partner violence typologies. *The Family Journal, 18,* 248–254.

Center for Sex Offender Management. (2004). Supervision of sex offenders in the community – A training curriculum.

Children, Youth and Families Act. (2008). Victorian Government. www.legislation.vic.gov.au/

Cozolino, L. (2002). *The neuroscience of psychotherapy: Building and rebuilding the human brain.* New York, NY: W. W. Norton & Co.

Cozolino, L., 2020. *The pocket guide to neuroscience for clinicians.* New York, NY: W. W. Norton & Co

Creeden, K. J. (2006). Trauma and neurobiology: Considerations for the treatment of sexual problems in children and adolescents. In R. E. Longo, & D. S. Prescott (Eds.), *Current perspectives: Working with sexually aggressive youth and youth with sexual behavior problems* (pp. 395–418). Holyoke, MA: NEARI Press.

Daversa, M., & Knight, R. (2007). A structural examination of the predictors of sexual coercion against children in adolescent sexual offenders. *Criminal Justice and Behaviour, 34*(10), 1313–1333.

DiLeo, J. H. (1973). *Children's drawings as diagnostic aids.* New York, NY: Brunner/Mazel.

Dow, B., Gahan, L., Gaffy, E., Joosten, M., Vrantsidis, F., & Jarred, M. (2020). Barriers to disclosing elder abuse and taking action in Australia. *Journal of Family Violence, 35,* 853–861.

Dwyer, J. (1999). *Loss, trauma and the familial ideal: Some Australian women's responses to the incestuous abuse of their children* (Unpublished doctoral dissertation). The University of Melbourne, Melbourne.

Epston, D., & White, M. (1990). *Narrative means to therapeutic ends.* New York, NY: W. W. Norton.

Farokhi, M., & Hashemi, M. (2011). The analysis of children's drawings: Social, emotional, physical, and psychological aspects. *Procedia-Social and Behavioral Sciences, 30,* 2219–2224.

Foley, Y. C., & Mullis, F. (2008). Interpreting children's human figure drawings: Basic guidelines for school counselors. *Georgia School Counselors Association Journal, 1*(1), 28–37.

Geller, S. M., & Porges, S. W. (2014). Therapeutic presence: Neurophysiological mechanisms mediating feeling safe in the therapeutic relationships. *Journal of Psychotherapy Integration, 24,* 178–192.

Goding, G. (1992). *The history and principles of family therapy.* Melbourne, Australia: VAFT Publications.

Goldenthal, P. (1996). *Doing contextual therapy: An integrated model for working with individuals, couples and families.* New York, NY: W. W. Norton.

Goldner, V., Penn, P., Sheinberg, M., & Walker, G. (1990). Love and violence: Gender paradoxes in volatile attachments. *Family Process, 29*, 343–364.

Gondolf, E. W. (1988). Who are these guys? Toward a behavioural typology of batterers. *Violence and Victims, 3*, 187–203.

Gonzalez, L. S., Waterman, J., Kelly, R. J., McCord, J., & Oliveri, M. K. (1993). Children's patterns of disclosures and recantations of sexual and ritualistic abuse allegations in psychotherapy. *Child Abuse and Neglect, 17*, 281–289.

Gottman, J. M., Jacobson, N. S., Rushe, R. H., Shortt, J. W., Babcock, J., La Taillade, J. J., & Waltz, J. (1995). The relationship between heart rate reactivity, emotionally aggressive behaviour, and general violence in batterers. *Journal of Family Psychology, 9*, 227–248.

Griffith, J. L., & Griffith, M. E. (1994). *The body speaks: Therapeutic dialogues for mind-body problems*. New York, NY: Basic Books.

Grunebaum, J. (1987). Multidirected partiality and the "parental imperative". *Psychotherapy, 24*(supplement 3), 646–656.

Hamberger, L. K., Lohr, J. M., Bonge, D., & Tolin, D. F. (1996). A large sample empirical typology of male spouse abusers and its relationship to dimensions of abuse. *Violence and Victims, 11*, 277–292.

Hargraves, T. D., & Sells, J. N. (1997). The development of a forgiveness scale. *Journal of Marital and Family Therapy, 23*, 41–62.

Herman, J. (2007). Shattered shame states and their repair. *The John Bowlby Memorial Lecture, Harvard Medical School, MA*. Lecture retrieved from http://www.cha.harvard.edu/vov/publications/Shattered%20Shame-JHerman.pdf

Holtzworth-Munroe, A., & Stuart, G. L. (1994). Typologies of male batterers: Three subtypes and the differences between them. *Psychological Bulletin, 116*, 476–497.

Humphreys, C. (1992). Disclosure of child sexual assault: Implications for mothers. *Australian Social Work, 45*(3), 27–36.

James, K., & McKinnon, L. (2010). The tip of the iceberg: A framework for identifying non-physical abuse in couple and family relationships. *Journal of Feminist Family Therapy, 22*, 112–129.

Jenkins, A. (1990). *Invitations to responsibility: The therapeutic engagement of men who are violent and abusive*. Adelaide, SA, Australia: Dulwich Centre Publications.

Jenkins, A. (2006a). Discovering integrity: Working with shame without shaming young people who have abused. In R. E. Longo, & D. S. Prescott (Eds.), *Current perspectives: Working with sexually aggressive youth and youth with sexual behavior problems* (pp. 419–442). Holyoke, MA: NEARI Press.

Jenkins, A. (2006b). The politics of intervention: Fairness and ethics. In R. E. Longo & D. S. Prescott (Eds.), *Current perspectives: Working with sexually aggressive youth and youth with sexual behavior problems* (pp. 143–165). Holyoke, MA: NEARI Press.

Johnson, M. P. (1995). Patriarchal terrorism and common couple violence: Two forms of violence against women. *Journal of Marriage and Family, 57*, 283–294.

Johnson, M. P., & Ferraro, K. J. (2000). Research on domestic violence in the 1990s: Making distinctions. *Journal of Marriage and the Family, 62*, 948–963.

Jory, B., & Anderson, D. (2000). Intimate justice III: Healing the anguish of abuse and embracing the anguish of accountability. *Journal of Marital and Family Therapy, 26*, 329–340.

Kain, K. L., & Terrell, S. J. (2018). *Nurturing resilience*. Berkeley, CA: North Atlantic Books.

Knight, R. A., & Prentky, R. A. (1990). Classifying sexual offenders: The development and corroboration of taxonomic models. In W. L. Marshall, D. R. Laws, & H. E. Barbaree (Eds.), *Handbook of sexual assault: Issues, theories, and treatment of the offender* (pp. 23–52). New York, NY: Plenum Press.

Kropp, P. (2008). Intimate partner violence risk assessment and management. *Violence and Victims, 23*, 202–220.

Lane, D. (1991). The sexual abuse cycle. In G. Ryan, & D. Lane (Eds.), *Juvenile sexual offending – Causes, consequences and correction* (pp. 103–141). Lexington, KY: Lexington Books.

Lee, C., Coe, C. L., & Ryff, C. D. (2017). Social disadvantage, severe child abuse, and biological profiles in adulthood. *Journal Of Health and Social Behavior, 58*, 371–386. https://doi.org/10.1177/0022146516685370

Lowe, R. (2004). *Family therapy: A constructive framework*. London, England: Sage.

Main, M., Hesse, E., & Kaplan, N. (2005). Predictability of attachment behaviour and representational processes at 1, 6, and 18 years of age. The Berkeley longitudinal study. In K. E. Grossman, K. E. Grossman, & E. Waters (Eds.), *Attachment from infancy to adulthood* (pp. 245–305). New York, NY: Guilford Press.

Malchiodi, C. A. (1998). *Understanding children's drawings*. New York, NY: Guilford Press.

Marshall, W. L., Anderson, D., & Fernandez, Y. M. (1999). *Cognitive behavioural treatment of sexual offenders*. Chichester, England: John Wiley & Son.

McIlwaine, F., & O'Sullivan, K. (2015). 'Riding the wave': Working systemically with traumatised families. *Australian and New Zealand Journal of Family Therapy, 36*(3), 310–324.

Miller, R., & Dwyer, J. (1997). Reclaiming the mother-daughter relationship after sexual abuse. *Australian and New Zealand Journal of Family Therapy, 18*(4), 194–202.

Morrison, T. (2006). Building a holistic approach to the treatment of young people who sexually offend. In R. E. Longo & D. S. Prescott (Eds.), *Current perspectives: Working with sexually aggressive youth and youth with sexual behavior problems* (pp. 349–368). Holyoke, MA: NEARI Press.

Mouzos, J. (1999). Homicidal encounters: A study of homicide in Australia 1989–1999. Australian Institute of Criminal Research and Public Policy. Series No 28. Canberra: Australian Institute of Criminology.

Nichols, M. P. (2011). *The essentials of family therapy* (5th ed.). Boston: Allyn & Bacon.

O'Brien, M. (2009). Social work, poverty and disadvantage. In M. Connolly & L. Harms (Eds.), *Social work: Contexts and practice* (2nd ed., pp. 68–80). South Melbourne, Australia: Oxford University Press.

Ossefort-Russell, C. (2018). Grief through the lens of polyvagal theory: Humanising our clinical response to loss. In S. W. Porges & D. Dana (Eds.), *Clinical applications of the polyvagal theory: The emergence of polyvagal informed therapies* (pp. 312–338). New York, NY: Norton.

Penfold, P. S. (1989). Family therapy: Critique from a feminist perspective. *Canadian Journal of Psychiatry, 34*, 311–315.

Perlesz, A., Young, J., Paterson, R., & Bridge, S. (1994). The reflecting team as a reflection of second order therapeutic ideals. *Australian and New Zealand Journal of Family Therapy, 15*, 117–127.

Perry, B. (1997). Incubated in terror: Neurodevelopmental factors in the 'Cycle of Violence'. In J. Osofsky (Ed.), *Children, youth and violence: The search for solutions* (pp. 124–148). New York, NY: Guilford Press.

Perry, B. (2010). Workshop presentation, Melbourne, 7th September.

Perry, B. D. (2006). Applying principles of neurodevelopment to clinical work with maltreated and traumatized children. In N. Boyd (Ed.), *Working with traumatized youth in child welfare* (pp. 27–52). New York, NY: Guilford Press.

Pithers, W. D., Gray, A. S., Cunningham, C., & Lane, S. (1993). *From trauma to understanding*. Brandon, VT: Safer Society.

Plummer, C. (2006). The discovery process: What mothers see and do in gaining awareness of the sexual abuse of their children. *Child Abuse and Neglect, 30*, 1227–1237.

Rich, P. (2006). *Attachment and sexual offending: Understanding and applying attachment theory to the treatment of juvenile sexual offenders*. Chichester, West Sussex, England: John Wiley and Sons, Ltd.

Ross, J. M., & Babcock, J. C. (2009a). Proactive and reactive violence among intimate partner violent men diagnosed with antisocial and borderline personality disorder. *Journal of Family Violence, 24*, 607–617.

Ross, J. M., & Babcock, J. C. (2009b). Gender differences in partner violence in context: Deconstructing Johnson's (2001) control-based typology of violent couples. *Journal of Aggression, Maltreatment and Trauma, 18,* 604–622.

Rothschild, B. (2000). *The body remembers: The psychophysiology of trauma and trauma treatment.* New York, NY: W. W. Norton.

Ryan, G. (1999). Developing a contextual matrix. In G. Ryan & Associates. (Eds.), *Web of meaning* (pp. 19–31). Brandon, Canada: The Safer Society Press.

Ryan, G., & Lane, S. (1991). Integrating theory and method. In G. Ryan & S. Lane (Eds.), *Juvenile sexual offending – Causes, consequences and correction* (pp. 255–297). Lexington, KY: Lexington Books.

Salter, A. (1988). *Treating child sex offenders and victims: A practical guide.* Newbury Park, CA: Sage.

Schacht, R., Dimidjian, S., George, W., & Berns, S. (2009). Domestic violence assessment procedures among couple therapists. *Journal of Marital and Family Therapy, 35,* 47–59.

Schore, A. N. (2003). Early relational trauma, disorganized attachment, and the development of a predisposition to violence. In M. F. Solomon & D. J. Siegel (Eds.), *Healing trauma: Attachment, mind, body and brain* (pp. 107–167). New York, NY: W. W. Norton and Company.

Schwartz, R. C. (2021). *No bad parts: Healing trauma and restoring wholeness with the internal family systems model.* Louisville, CO: Sounds True.

Selvini, M. P., Boscolo, L., Cecchin, G., & Prata, G. (1980). Hypothesising-circularity-neutrality: Three guidelines for the conductor. *Family Process, 19,* 3–12.

Sheehan, J. (2007). Forgiveness and the unforgivable: The resurrection of hope in family therapy. In C. Flaskas, I. McCarthy, & J. Sheehan (Eds.), *Hope and despair in narrative and family therapy: Adversity, forgiveness and reconciliation* (pp. 161–171). London, England and New York, NY: Routledge.

Siegel, D. J. (2003). An interpersonal neurobiology of psychotherapy: The developing mind and the resolution of trauma. In D. J. Siegel & M. F. Solomon (Eds.), *Healing trauma: Attachment, mind, body and brain* (pp. 1–56). New York, NY: W. W. Norton and Company.

Simpson, L. E., Doss, B. D., Wheeler, J., & Christensen, A. (2008). Low-level relationship aggression and couple therapy outcomes. *Journal of Family Psychology, 22,* 102–111.

Sorensen, T., & Snow, B. (1991). How children tell: The process of disclosure in child sexual abuse. *Child Welfare, 70,* 3–17.

Stith, S. M., Rosen, K. H., & McCollum, E. E. (2003). Effectiveness of couples treatment for spouse abuse. *Journal of Marital and Family Therapy, 29,* 407–426.

Summit, R. C. (1983). The child sexual abuse accommodation syndrome. *Child Abuse and Neglect, 7,* 177–193.

van der Kolk, B. A. (2015). *The body keeps the score: Mind, brain and body in the transformation of trauma.* UK: Penguin.

van der Kolk, B. A., Roth, S., Pelcovitz, D., Sunday, S., & Spinazzola, J. (2005). Disorders of extreme stress: The empirical foundation of a complex adaptation to trauma. *Journal of Traumatic Stress, 18,* 389–399.

Van der Meiden, J. (2019). *Where hope resides, a qualitative study of the contextual theory and therapy of Ivan Boszormenyi-Nagy and its applicability for therapy and social work* (Doctoral dissertation). University of Humanistic Studies, Netherlands.

von Bertalanffy, L. (1968). *General systems theory.* New York, NY: Braziller.

Ward, T., & Marshall, B. (2004). Good lives, aetiology & the rehabilitation of sex offenders: A bridging theory. *Journal of Sexual Aggression, 10,* 153–169.

Webb, N. B. (Ed.) (2007). *Play therapy with children in crisis: Individual, group and family treatment* (3rd ed.). New York, NY: Guilford Press.

Welfare, A. L. (2006). *Sibling sexual abuse: Understanding all family members' experiences in the aftermath of disclosure.* Paper presented at the 27th Annual Australian Family Therapy Conference, Melbourne.

Welfare, A. L. (2008). How qualitative research can inform clinical interventions in families recovering from sibling sexual abuse. *Australian and New Zealand Journal Family Therapy, 29,* 139–147.

White, M. (2007). *Maps to narrative practice.* New York, NY: W. W. Norton.

White, M., & Epston, D. (1989). *Literate means to therapeutic ends.* Adelaide, Australia: Dulwich Centre Publications.

Whitzman, C. (2008). *The handbook of community safety, gender and violence prevention: Practical planning tools.* London, England: Earthscan.

Young, J. (2023). *No bullshit therapy: How to engage people who don't want to work with you.* UK: Routledge.

Young, J. E., Klosko, J. S., & Weishaar, M. E. (2006). *Schema therapy: A practitioner's guide.* UK: Guilford Press.

Chapter 6

Including Children in Family Therapy

Catherine Sanders

Introduction

A family walks into a family therapist's consulting room; a father who appears uncomfortable and apprehensive, and a mother who irritably pushes two children, aged two and nine years, into the room before her. They have been referred by their general practitioner who is concerned by reports of the youngest child's hyperactivity and the older child's lying, stealing, and suspension from school. Who frightens the therapist most?

Of course, the answer is highly personal, but the literature suggests it would probably be the children. Several authors have noted the paradox that while the term family implies the presence of children, family therapists have struggled to fully include younger members in sessions. Ackerman (1970) noted that there had not been a single publication devoted to the inclusion of children in family therapy and urged the field to address this omission. Nearly 30 years later, Ruble (1999) used a systematic research synthesis of non-empirical and empirical literature on practices and beliefs of family therapists in relation to the inclusion of children. She concluded that therapists routinely excluded children from sessions with the primary reason being lack of training. Oehlers and Shortland-Jones (2013) reviewed child and family therapy texts and training in Australia to ascertain the extent to which knowledge and information about child development and emotional and psychological problems were included. They concluded it was 'limited, therefore contributing to children being unseen in the therapy process'. This is borne out by Korner and Brown's (1990) research which demonstrated that therapists whose education did not incorporate direct training in working with children were reluctant to include them as part of the therapeutic process.

Another constraint is the more complicated 'issues of privacy, confidentiality, and legal privilege due to the competing interests of parents and children and other stakeholders' identified by Sori and Hecker (2015, p. 450) who outline the need to understand law and ethical codes when working with children.

While it is tempting to exclude children from abusive or pathologising conversations, O'Reilly and Parker (2012) assert that the therapist is responsible for managing conversations that are permissible in the context of the family's social and cultural boundaries while encouraging openness and interaction. Taking responsibility and asserting authority for deciding what topics can and should be discussed with children carries risks to the therapeutic alliance. They recommend embedding strategies for managing inappropriate talk, including addressing this directly while setting up the therapeutic process. A study by Helimäki, Laitila, and Kumpulainen (2022, p. 124) with children diagnosed

DOI: 10.4324/9781003490104-7

with conduct disorder demonstrated that parent's symptom-oriented and negative talk produced a 'stagnated and unproductive interactive cycle' and that it is the therapist's task to set rules for appropriate conduct to address this. Developing these skills protects clients from abusive exchanges and therapists from unnecessary exclusion of children as a valuable resource.

The focus of this chapter will be to explore the many benefits of including children more fully in family therapy, take note of exceptional circumstances when they might best be excluded, and work flexibly and responsively with the whole family, subsystems, or the child alone while maintaining a systemic view. A wide variety of strategies and skills will also be described that can foster greater inclusion, along with a detailed case study.

The benefits of active involvement

When Sith, Rosen, McCollum, Coleman, and Herman (1996) asked children about their family therapy experience, they all, regardless of age or gender, were enthusiastic about talking in sessions and indicated a desire to be actively included. All but the youngest child of five understood the purpose of therapy and described it as helpful to themselves and their loved ones. The children did not want their difficulties to be the singular focus and were eager to learn more about the workings of their family and participate in finding solutions. While this was a limited study, with only 16 participants, it points to the desire of younger clients to be included as full and valued family members at a time when their family is experiencing difficulties. Active inclusion of children enhances their cooperation and desire for change and potentially engages them as allies in the therapeutic process. Treating all family members as important and resourceful, both in terms of understanding difficulties and discovering solutions, may change family dynamics in ways that provide invaluable resources for the future of the family. These benefits will now be explored in more detail.

Access to information

Often children can provide the therapist with a richer understanding of the family more rapidly than many adults (Gil, 1994; Zilbach, 1986). The expression 'out of the mouths of babes and sucklings' aptly describes a child's response to a skilful therapist who has established a clear and safe context for conversation. Sometimes the greater challenge for the therapist is to manage the child's candour in a way that allows both parents and child to participate openly and without risk of reprisal.

Access to the world of non-verbal communication

A related advantage is that children break our reliance on words and force us into nonverbal forms of communication (Whitaker, 1982). Drawing, role-playing, and sculpting with puppets and toys to create the current and desired shape of a family are both engaging and instructive. Moore and Seu (2011) explored how children construct their experience of therapy and noted that younger clients expressed a need for stimulation and amusement, as well as the comfort of familiar surroundings. These ways of telling the family's history and describing their situation are often experienced as more valid than words and are less likely to be swept aside in favour of more comfortable linear descriptions.

Direct observation of family interactions

Including children in the session gives the therapist the opportunity to directly observe both the process of interaction between family members and the content of discussions about the difficulties. These observations form the basis of hypotheses that can be tested and provide the opportunity to directly intervene to interrupt unhelpful patterns and support new interactions. For example, the therapist may notice that every time there is a discussion of a child's behaviour, one parent criticises the other, and the problems never get resolved. In recognising this, the therapist may choose to share their observation with the family and insist on a conversation about the child, thus disrupting a pattern that may contribute to the perpetuation of difficulties. Interviewing the parents or child alone would not have provided this vital piece of information or the opportunity to effect change.

Access to the resources of the sibling subsystem

The inclusion of all children also provides the practitioner with another powerful resource, the sibling subsystem. The sibling subsystem is a child's first peer group where its members 'support each other, enjoy, attack, scapegoat, and generally learn from each other' (Minuchin & Fishman, 1981, p. 19). The power of this group to both harm and help is often underrated, and it is important that the possibility of physical, sexual, and emotional abuse by children to each other is explored and addressed. Omer (2004) has drawn attention to this, suggesting that the failure to recognise its prevalence and potential severity is like the earlier denial of the extent of parental violence towards children.

In traditional child therapies, where primarily the mother and child attend sessions, the power of siblings is hidden, and the intimacy of therapy may weld mother and child closer and exclude others. This process may increase the isolation of the child from their siblings and further reinforce the perception that they are different. It may also burden them with a greater knowledge of and sense of responsibility for adult matters than is healthy. With all family members present, the therapist can act to strengthen bonds within the marital and parenting subsystems and return the child to their place with their siblings. In understanding the patterns which apply between the children, intervention can be actively targeted to reintegrate the child into a group where they can safely learn valuable skills. A positive sibling group can provide a place to hide when parents are in serious conflict with each other, suffer a mental or physical illness, abuse alcohol or drugs, or are generally facing stressful life events which make them sad and bad-tempered.

Exceptions to inclusion

While we may like to believe that the decision to exclude children from family therapy sessions is based on sound clinical judgement or constraints of organisations, this may not be the case. As Scott (1999) identifies, many of the reasons relate to therapists' lack of knowledge, confidence, or skill. She speaks of how time-consuming and difficult it can be to ensure the children are present and the pressure the therapist may experience from parents and other agencies to separate the identified child from the family and engage in individual therapy. A sense of protectiveness towards children or a reluctance to reconnect with one's own childhood can also increase the therapist's reticence as can a fear of the chaos children can introduce to a session. Practitioners may feel a lack of skill in translating from the world of adults to children where time, understanding, and pace are so different and be under-resourced in their knowledge of normal and disrupted child and family development. Clearly, it is important to differentiate reasons for exclusion that relate to the therapist or their agency and those that are a function of clinical judgement and active decision-making. Below are some specific occasions when a clear argument can be made for exclusion.

When managing sensitive information

The decision to exclude children varies across practitioners. However, most would agree that this is a valid clinical judgement when the adult's sexual relationship or financial concerns are the major focus or where a child is a victim of abuse by one of the parents.

Practically, it is helpful to consider boundaries between different subsystems in the family and information which should be shared with each person and group in each situation. These should be responsive to the developmental age and stage of the family and its members and their cognitive ability to apprehend complex concepts. It is also highly dependent on the focus and purpose of information sharing. Imagine a parent has become highly distressed and anxious as they begin to acknowledge their own sexual abuse in childhood. They may have become excessively protective and irritable with their children who in turn react. A child in this situation may be hugely relieved to learn that they are not the cause of their parent's distress. The provision of limited and sensitive information about the source of their parent's distress may mean the child can be more understanding and empathic and less burdened and guilty. The therapist would be wise to speak to the parents alone to fashion an explanation that is suitable for all family members and then support the adults as they speak to their children. In this case, it would be important to explain to the children that their exclusion was to discuss their parent's history.

Financial difficulties can be handled in a similar fashion, whereby the adults initially discuss their situation and identify the elements that directly affect and concern the children and should be shared. If children must move house and change schools, it is reasonable they be given some rational, accurate explanation which releases them from responsibility and does not alienate them from either parent.

By contrast, most therapists would agree that to explore the parents' current sexual difficulties with the whole family would be entirely inappropriate and that a separate interview in which the children are not invited should be arranged. The same may apply to other aspects of the adults' family of origin or personal history.

The possibility of adults meeting alone can be introduced at the beginning of therapy, where parents are told that they are welcome to decline to answer questions that they believe are inappropriate to discuss in front of their children and that the therapist will always be willing to privately explore such matters. This does not mean the therapist will necessarily agree or that absolute confidentiality from the children will always be appropriate. The same right should be extended to children, especially as they get older, with the clear understanding that if they disclose information that suggests they or others are being hurt, this cannot be kept confidential. At times, a child may not wish their private concerns shared with siblings for fear of embarrassment or bullying. However, whenever a decision is made to break the family into smaller units, the therapist should be alert to the drift towards individual explanations and the expectation that therapy is best conducted with the child alone.

To reinforce the parental hierarchy

A different form of exclusion of a child may be decided by the therapist to draw a boundary and reinforce the adult hierarchy. Asking a child to leave the room while the adults talk may be a way of empowering parents and restoring a defiant and irresponsible child to a more cooperative role in the family. However, rude and difficult behaviour may be a child's only way to express anxiety and distress, which is better explored and addressed with all family members present.

When children are too disruptive to allow for an effective session

The suggestion by some authors (for example, Lund, Schindler-Zimmerman, & Haddock, 2002) that children should be excluded if they have an organic disorder or are highly disturbed or psychotic should also be questioned, as this may reflect therapists' discomfort and lack of skill rather than an objective decision. Highly disruptive and uncooperative children can be managed in the context of a family session and their difficult behaviour becomes an opportunity for the therapist to use enactment techniques (Minuchin & Fishman, 1981) to support the parents to challenge problematic family patterns. The inclusion of children with severe developmental disorders is also important as they are key family members and should be recognised as such. The presence of these children provides the practitioner with the opportunity to observe interactional patterns first-hand and intervene in a more informed way.

Working with subsystems or individuals

The hallmark of effective therapy is the practitioner's capacity to respond flexibly to the needs of the child and family as they present. This may require different groupings at different times. For example, inviting a mother or father and a highly disengaged child may provide an opportunity to create closeness with one another and a more appropriate distance from an overinvolved sibling. Working with the sibling subsystem can draw a boundary with parents and allow children to develop a supportive bond, while an individual session with a child gives the practitioner an opportunity to connect with them and better understand their perspective. Equally, a session with an individual adult or the parents may be indicated.

Specific skills to support the inclusion of children

A wide variety of skills are available to the therapist wishing to be more inclusive of children, from the regular modification of the standard means for interviewing to the use of creative tools for assessment and intervention. These include the use of books, drawings, and art, in unstructured or more structured formats, the use of specially designed pictorial resources, behavioural techniques, and reframing. The aim here is not to provide an exhaustive summary but to provide examples of strategies to support the inclusion of children in family therapy.

Modification of standard interviewing skills

Interviewing children successfully requires a good understanding of expected language and cognitive development and the tailoring of questions to suit the receptive and expressive language skills of the individual child. Here is an example of how to adapt a standard relationship question to the needs of a six-year-old child, Sue, and her ten-year-old brother, Tom. The adult version of the question might be, 'Are you closer to Mum or Dad now, compared to before you started school and when Dad was working away all week?' This is a complex question and one that Sue at six would find impossible to answer. Instead, she could be asked to show how close she is, first to her mother and then to her father, by using toys to demonstrate. The therapist would need to explain the concept of closeness using toys of her choice to represent each family member. The child could then be asked to reflect on when she was 'a little girl and went to kindergarten and Daddy used to go away for work'. Checking that she could remember this time, the therapist could then ask her once again to position the toys to reflect relationships at this time. Rather than asking the question as one, the answer is built up from a series of simpler questions. Sue's ten-year-old brother, Tom, may find toys 'too babyish', yet he too would have difficulty with the complete question. He is now capable of understanding relational terms like closer, happier, and sadder, unlike his sister, who would understand the concept of 'closer' in absolute rather than relational terms. She would be unable to place family members in relation to each other using this idea. Tom can now answer the question 'Is Sue closer to Mum or Dad?' However, to complete the response, he will need a second question, 'Was Sue closer to Dad or Mum the year when Dad was away for work all week?'

Sanders (1985) suggests modifications to more complex difference questions which make them accessible to children, combining verbal and non-verbal elements, including the use of scales, and physical demonstrations to compare each person's experience and changes in the system over time. Benson, Schindler-Zimmerman, and Martin (1991) also address the issue of adapting circular questioning to children, making specific suggestions for modifying relationship difference questions, degree differences, behavioural sequences, hypothetical/future questions, and now/then differences. They warn that work with children requires a careful selection of questions which are integrated into play, art, and drama. Wilson (1998) devotes a chapter of his book 'Child Focused Practice' to adapting adult style circular and reflexive questions to encourage children's voices into the dialogue. He recommends the use of multiple-choice questions, where a child is very diffident or unable to answer open questions. However, the therapist must be vigilant that they retain neutrality and that the session does not deteriorate into an inquisition. Successful use of such questions also requires a good understanding of experiences of children in families and familiarity with the literature in relation to children's issues.

The same requirements apply to the use of 'playful mindreading', a technique suggested by Wilson (1998), for children who are particularly withdrawn and uncommunicative. Here the therapist asks the child for permission to be his or her mind and answers on their behalf. The therapist asks the child to correct them if they are wrong. This is perhaps a more successful strategy when the therapist's hypothesis fits the circumstances but should be used judiciously and respectfully. It is like a more direct approach, where the therapist asks the child about their hypothesis. This may be done by asking: '*I was wondering if*' or more indirectly '*I have spoken to other children in situations a bit like your and they told me … I wonder if this is more the same or different for you*'.

Children's literature

Other people's circumstances and solutions can be introduced using books, either read out directly to the child and family in the session or for older children lent for reading between sessions. Talking about the character's experience and how it is similar to and different from that of the child can be a gentle way of opening a conversation that is painful and therefore avoided. 'The Worry Tree' by Marianne Musgrove is a good example of a book that is ideal for therapists. The story revolves around Juliete whose idiosyncratic family, irritating younger sister, and demanding friends all contribute to overburdening worry. The story explores her positive and empowering response to unchangeable circumstances and is an excellent resource for children who experience fear and anxiety in contexts which will allow for little external change. Wilson (1992, 1994, 1996, 2000), an English author, has also written several novels for young adolescents which touch on common and painful situations, including parental separation and divorce, moving house, friendships, bullying, school difficulties, falling in love, and peer and relationship difficulties. While these are not books written by therapists or specifically for use in therapy, they are popular with young clients and can be a vehicle to open conversations that have been difficult to broach more directly. Books with a humorous twist, like those of Cole (1995, 1996, 1997, 2000), combine quirky illustrations with amusing text and are often more successful with both adults and children than many formal texts written for therapeutic purposes. These are particularly appealing to younger children and can be read in the session to introduce a different perspective to both parents and children.

For over 30 years, the Australian Association of Family Therapy has presented an award to a children's novel and younger readers' or picture book which depicts a challenge in family life and positive steps towards resolution. A list of these books is available on the website and ranges from parental mental illness, refugees, disability, dementia, foster care and adoption, substance abuse, and friendship. These can be used in the session to raise and discuss difficult topics or suggested as reading by parents and children at home.

Family sculpting

Family sculpture, where family members are asked to physically create the 'shape' of the family, was initially developed by Kantor and Lehr (1975) and used extensively by Satir (1972). Asking a child to help arrange for family members to demonstrate interaction can be very empowering and serves as a platform for a wide variety of conversations. These can include a comparison of each person's view, an exploration of how and when the family came to operate in this way, a mapping of how each would like the family to look, and a discussion of each person's potential role in effecting change. A similar process can be conducted using toys, where the child or children are asked to pick different toys to represent family members and arrange them to illustrate the family's processes. This can be done in a family session or with a child alone. The toys can be asked to enact scenes from family life as a way of mapping a sequence, telling a painful story, or imagining a different set of relationships. A similar way of doing this is by using puppets, who can comment upon conversations or stories and, with the therapist's help, suggest different possibilities.

Drawings

Drawing the family genogram is used extensively by family therapists and is easily adapted to engage children. One can bring family members together around a large sheet of paper, give each their own marker, and ask them to work together to draw the family genogram. This can be adapted for engagement and serves as a platform for the assessment of family interactions or the collaborative exploration of change. Dumont (2008) draws a family map where each person is given a different colour pen and asked to represent their view of the family within circles drawn on the paper. Each person is asked to represent the relationship between people using yellow double lines to denote closeness and brown zigzags for conflict. This forms the basis for dialogue about the child's perception of their family and allows discussion of their wish for the future.

A whiteboard can support the inclusion of children in family therapy in a variety of ways. It enables the therapist to draw diagrams of repetitive patterns of interaction, to work with children to depict pie-graphs of the percentages of time or energy that is expended by family troubles, or to develop other more idiosyncratic visual representations of the child's experience. Sometimes, however, the children's best drawings occur spontaneously as adults talk and can then be incorporated into the adult conversations. This was the case with seven-year-old Millie whose parents had separated. Millie's mother had begun a relationship with a mutual friend and was describing their plans to live together. Both Millie's parents were overtly relaxed and 'civilized' about the situation and spoke calmly and kindly to each other. Millie followed their lead saying how much she loved 'Uncle Ben' and how happy she was with the plan. However, she then jumped to her feet and frantically drew on the whiteboard. She explained that her drawing depicted a bushfire approaching a ravine. At the bottom of the ravine was a person in a wheelchair with a bucket trying to put out the approaching fires. Using her picture as a cue, it was then possible to explore the dangerous and burning feelings which Millie experienced as encroaching from all sides and her sense of responsibility to 'put them out' with cooperation and silence.

Bower place protocols

The protocols developed at Bower Place (Robinson & Sanders, 2023) to manage inequality incorporate many of these approaches and are particularly useful in working with children. These authors assume that wherever possible both word and image are used in both enquiry and intervention. All sessions are conducted according to these protocols. In setting the agenda, the practitioner explains the format of the session and puts the paper in full view so that everyone can see each item as it is addressed. The agenda includes the drawing of an ecogram, an extended family tree inclusive of non-family, friends, professionals, and other support systems, as well as family members' pets and toys. While constructing the ecogram, a timeline is drawn, detailing key positive and negative events in the life of the family with good events recorded in green above the line and negative events below in red. Wherever possible, children are engaged in the creation of the ecogram and the timeline with the goal of putting the pen in the hands of the child wherever possible. Even the most disengaged child finds this hard to resist and when asked to take responsibility for the timeline by writing events onto the line, unexpected and important information may appear. Notes are also printed in bright colours, so that they are easily readable, and all family members are invited to check them as the session unfolds and during the break. At the conclusion of the session, notes are scanned and the original is given to the client.

Structured art

Kozlowska and Hanney (1999) detail a more structured approach to art. Their interactive art exercise, designed for children from two to eight years, requires a family to plan and execute an art task and allows the observing therapist to note how each person and the group respond. The authors describe a variety of tasks designed to span the developmental requirements of family members using drawing materials, clay, or magazine cuttings with simple instructions to create a portrait, object, or collage together. Once the exercise is complete, the therapist returns to discuss the artwork with the family and explore the similarity between the exercise done in the session and life at home. From these, therapeutic goals are set. Kozlowska and Hanney (2001, 2003) have applied these techniques to traumatised children for whom words may not be a preferred or accessible modality while Klop (2017) directly integrates art therapy into working with families.

St Luke's resources

Another valuable set of resources designed for children are produced by St Luke's Innovative Resources. Strength Cards, each representing one strength as demonstrated by a cartoon animal, can be invaluable in supporting the deviation amplification process as described in Chapter 3, providing a concrete method of affirming progress and ensuring that it is recognised by the child and caregivers alike. Bear Cards are also useful, consisting of a host of bears, each representing one emotion. These cards allow children to express emotions non-verbally in a cartoon format and can also be used to build empathy between children and parents in the context of circular questions. These are just two examples of over 50 types of cards, designed for children across the age range.

Reframing

Reframing a problem to change the understanding of its context is a technique from the strategic school (Watzlawick, Weakland, & Fisch, 1974). It is ideally suited to work with children as it can be playful, engaging, and non-blaming of the child and contains within it implicit alternative responses to the situation from other family members. A charming example applied to a child's difficult behaviour by Coppersmith (1981) is developmental reframing. Following a thorough assessment, the therapist declares 'He's not bad, he's not mad, he's just young' which carries the message of hope that the child can grow up and the expectation that parents may need to set firmer limits for them to do so. Externalisation, a practice from narrative therapy, may be viewed as a form of reframing. Problems can be separated from the child, personified as tricksters or bullies, thus removing guilt and making room for personal agency. This practice originated in White's (1984) approach to encopresis or 'sneaky-poo' but has been adapted for a host of other difficulties, including obsessive compulsive disorder (March & Mulle, 1994), night-time fears (Epston, 1986), aggression (Epston, 1989), and challenging behaviours in children with an ASD diagnosis (Chimpen-Lopez, Andres-Garrizand, & Pretel-Luque, 2022).

The 'Sit-In'

Omer (2000, 2001, 2004; Omer, Schorr-Sapir & Weinblatt, 2008; Omer, Steinmetz, Cathy & Von Schlippe, 2013; Omer & Dolberger, 2015) employs the principles of non-violent resistance and the concept of parental presence in the management of violent, aggressive, and self-destructive children. Whereas many of the tools described so far have been designed for the exploration of relationships and the development of solutions in the therapy room, this technique is designed for active intervention with children in the home.

The 'sit-in' is a strategy designed to empower parents and foster responsibility in the child while avoiding expressed emotion. Parents are instructed, at a time of their choosing and not in the context of conflict, to inform their child that they are no longer willing to accept the behaviour which is causing them concern. They then sit at the child's bedroom door, blocking the child's exit, and state that they will sit there until a reasonable suggestion is made for addressing the problem. The parent is instructed not to respond to the child's efforts to engage them in debate and to accept any reasonable suggestion. The sit-in continues for up to an hour and is repeated daily until the child provides a solution. In between sit-ins, the parent is instructed to engage in gestures of reconciliation to enhance the relationship. The theory and strategy have been further developed and refined by Omar and others to address sibling violence (Omer et al., 2008), threats of suicide (Omer & Dolberger, 2015), violent behaviour by children in foster care (Van Holen, Vanderfaeillie, & Omer, 2015), and multi-stressed families within their wider system (Jacob, 2018).

Online therapy

Working online brings unique challenges but is crucial in a country as big and remote as Australia and became essential to the ongoing provision of services during the 2020 pandemic and resultant lockdowns. Vermeire and Van den Berg (2021) recommend encouraging playfulness 'as an atmosphere' to create new interactions between family members and therapists and propose strategies to engage and manage confidentiality and safety while maintaining a broad systemic scope. Children can be encouraged to 'invite' toys and pets to a session who can then be interviewed about their perspective on the child and family's situation and asked for their advice. Ensuring children bring drawing materials allows non-verbal exploration and expression, even at this distance.

Open dialogue practices

The principles of dialogisity and open dialogue form the basis for a model of systemic social work assessments developed by Clement and McKenny (2019) who describe an adaptation for work with children and their families where there are safeguarding and child protection concerns. This work was developed in the context of an assessment service for children and families referred to Children's Social Care Services with concerns about abuse or neglect. They report that parents felt respected and heard and were more likely to listen to concerns expressed by professionals and make positive changes.

Case study

The case study below demonstrates the value of including children in family therapy. Two sessions are described, the first with only the mother and father and the second with the whole family. In the second session, the frankness, perspective, and insights of the children caused the parents to question unhelpful familial interactions.

Gemma was seven years old when her parents decided 'something was wrong' and they needed to seek help. She had always been an anxious child, like her mother, reluctant to try new things, nervous of strangers, and 'a homebody'. However, when she refused to participate in her first school sleepover and became extremely distressed at attempts to persuade her, they began to worry.

Gemma and her younger brother Alex, four, were the children of Geoff and Maria who were both in their early forties. The couple had met through an environmental action group which they had joined in their teens and had married at 21. They described each other as 'best friends'. After ten years of marriage, they had encountered a difficult issue. Geoff was eager to have children but Maria, who had come from a neglectful and abusive family, believed she was unable to be a good mother. They had struggled to the point where Geoff announced he would leave if they could not have children and Maria had decided she was unwilling to lose the relationship. Within months Maria was pregnant with Gemma, but the relationship had changed. Geoff appeared more interested in the baby than his wife and while he had always been available to help her resolve her anxieties and fears, he now appeared irritated by them. Gemma was hard to settle to sleep and breast-feeding was painful for Maria and frustrating for Gemma. Within three months, Geoff suggested weaning Gemma so he could get up to her at night and Maria was relieved. Gemma's difficulties sleeping and Geoff's willingness to help her continued into childhood.

Other things changed too. Geoff's mother, with whom both he and Maria had been very close, became ill and died just before Alex was born, and six months later Geoff's father moved into the household. Alex was an easy baby who fed contentedly and slept without assistance and was blessed with a sunny and sociable disposition. Everyone loved Alex.

Geoff and Maria attended the first session alone, explaining that they did not want Gemma to believe there was anything wrong with her or that she was to blame for the difficulties. They said they had been shocked at the strength of her refusal to attend the sleepover as she was normally cooperative, if anxious. However, it was also clear that she had rarely been challenged in this way before. While her friends had been sleeping at each other's homes for at least a year, Maria had been reluctant to accept invitations as she could not be sure of her safety and the thought of being responsible for other people's children made her too anxious, so no invitations were issued. Gemma had been reluctant to attend kindergarten, but her teachers and father had worked hard to support and encourage her, and she now attended school regularly, if reluctantly. Until this year, Maria and Geoff had been happy with Gemma's teachers but they felt her current teacher was unsympathetic to her anxieties and too 'robust'. There had been days when Gemma expressed a reluctance to attend, and Maria had given her the occasional day off to rest and these were becoming more frequent.

In exploring their history, the couple explained that except for Geoff's father, they had little contact with either family. Maria had disconnected herself from her parents when she became pregnant with Gemma, fearing the possible risks for her children given her abusive childhood. She had a sister who she had been close to in childhood, but she had moved to another city, had little in common with Maria, and they rarely spoke. Geoff was an only child. Both Geoff and Maria were employed outside the home and enjoyed their work. Geoff reported good relationships with his colleagues, but these did not extend to social contact outside work. Maria said she did not socialise with workmates. Where once they had close friends from their early years together, these bonds had loosened when they had children and they no longer spent time together.

In exploring the couple's relationship, Geoff reported that he was 'fed-up' with his wife's anxiety and attempts to control him and the children. In turn, she spoke of feeling a failure as both a wife and mother and clearly not as good a parent as her husband.

At the conclusion of the first session, it was suggested that Gemma and Alex be invited to attend to provide them the opportunity to express their views which could prove helpful. Initially reluctant, Maria agreed on the understanding that if she believed Gemma was becoming 'too stressed', the session would end.

A week later, the family arrived. Gemma was small for her age and immediately sat between her parents. While reticent she was polite and willing to respond to ordinary questions about her name and age. Alex appeared much less constrained and immediately began rummaging in the toy box. After explaining the process of the session and the limits to confidentiality, the therapist asked the parent's permission to speak directly to Gemma.

Therapist: So, Gemma, who told you about coming to talk to me today?
Gemma: Mum.
Therapist: And what did Mum say about this?

Gemma hesitated and looked directly at her mother who nodded encouragingly.

Gemma: She said we needed to come and talk to you so we could be a happier family.
Therapist: A happier family, I see … so, could you show me how much happiness there is in this family right now? Is it this much? (therapist holding her hands close together in front of her) Or this much? (therapist holding her hands further apart) Or this much? (therapist holding her arms fully extended) Can you show me?

Once again, Gemma hesitated, seeking both her parent's expressions, and then slowly moved her hands forward, leaving a gap of about 15 centimetres.

Therapist: I see … and how much happiness would you like to be in this family?

Once again, the therapist demonstrated with her hands and Gemma responded indicating that she would like a much larger amount. Questioning then explored the differences between family members by asking Gemma to demonstrate how happy she perceived each one to be and how happy they wanted to be. Attention then turned to Alex who, while apparently absorbed with the toys, had clearly been listening.

Therapist: Hey, Alex, can you show me what you think about happiness in this family?

Alex turned to respond and as he did so, Gemma interrupted saying '*he doesn't know he's too little*' and Alex picked up the toys again. Here was a challenge with Gemma indicating that Alex was not to be troubled by the family difficulties.

Therapist: I see. So, Alex, perhaps you can help me understand more about your family? (Alex nodded and Gemma watched warily) What I want you to do is to pick a toy that we can pretend is Dad. (Alex selected a monkey) Excellent, just bring him over here and sit him on the floor. (Alex placed the monkey between the therapist and his parents sitting opposite) Good. Now can you pick a Mum? Where does she go, is she close to the Dad or more far away?

With both his parents and sister watching, Alex selected toys to represent each family member and placed them in relation to each other. The toys were arranged with Mum and Dad close, Alex a short distance in front of them, and Gemma wedged between. The grandfather was behind Alex. The therapist then turned to Gemma.

Therapist:	So, Gemma, do you think it looks a bit like this or would you make it differently? (Gemma nodded in agreement) So what would have to happen to make this family happier?
Gemma:	The fighting would have to stop.
Therapist:	Who would have to stop fighting?
Gemma:	Mum and Dad.
Therapist:	Is this fighting with words or fighting with fists?
Gemma:	With words ... and Mum cries.
Therapist:	Mum cries and what does Dad do?
Gemma:	Dad yells.
Alex:	(interrupting) and stomps off!
Therapist:	So, Alex, when Mum cries and Dad yells, what does Gemma do?
Alex:	She goes up to them and says, 'Stop fighting, stop fighting!' or tells me to tell them to stop and I say, 'Stop fighting, stop fighting!'
Therapist:	Does that stop them?
Alex and Gemma:	NO!
Therapist:	So, what happens next?
Alex:	Gemma tells grandpa.
Therapist:	What does Grandpa do?
Gemma:	He says 'Don't worry' but sometimes he tells them to stop.

This introduced a new person to the system and the opportunity to explore grandfather's role. All agreed that although he seemed able to stop individual instances of conflict, this did not prevent another episode. The session proceeded with an exploration of the impact of the conflict on Gemma and her anxiety for her family. She spoke of feeling very sad when her parents fought and when asked to rate her sadness out of 10, she said it was 'big, 10 out of 10'. She also spoke of her worry for her family, 'That Dad might go and never come home'. Gemma's anxiety and sadness had been directly connected to the parental conflict, but the relationship to the school sleepover had not been established.

Therapist:	So, Gemma when you are away from Mum and Dad, are you more worried about the fights or less?
Gemma:	More.
Therapist:	And would you be more worried to be away during the day or at night?
Gemma:	At night, cause they fight when they think we are asleep in bed but we hear them!

Throughout the session, both Geoff and Maria had listened intently and with increasing distress as their children spoke. They then began to clarify the conflict. Maria explained that because Geoff was a better parent, he would spend time with the children after dinner, bathing, reading stories, and settling them for sleep while she cleaned up the meal. However, he would take so long that she would go and remind him that it was past the children's bedtime. This would annoy Geoff who would become angry, feeling she did not trust him. He would then withdraw and eventually lose his temper, resulting in a fight. Maria felt she was left with the role of policing the rules while Geoff maintained she was rigid and controlling of both him and the children. When questioned directly, Maria was clear that she did not believe Geoff was inappropriate with his children. Throughout the session, the therapist observed the interaction between parents and the children and noticed that they interacted freely and confidently, approaching them equally and being warmly and appropriately received by both. The therapist then took a break and returned with the following message.

Therapist: I think it has been very important that both Gemma and Alex came today as they have helped me understand this family much better. Gemma, you asked that I help your family become happier and I think this is exactly what needs to happen. I have watched you, Geoff and Maria, with your children and it is clear that you have been excellent parents who have raised capable children who love you both. However, it is also clear that the fighting is hurting you all and needs to stop. (Turning to the children) I know both your parents believe it is important to be fair and you are all telling me that it is unfairness which seems to cause the fighting. Geoff, you tell me Maria's monitoring of you with your children feels unfair and Maria, you tell me that your exclusion from the night routine with the children feels unfair.

Both children say they experience the fighting and its impact on this family as unfair. So, this is what I am suggesting. Geoff, just until the next appointment, you are to be in charge of managing the fairness balance in this family. For one week you are to plan the evenings so there is a fair balance between you and Maria in terms of both household chores and parenting tasks. Maria, next week it will be your turn.

Everyone accepted the task. When they returned next session, Gemma and Alex reported that their father had taken responsibility for the 'fairness balance' in the family and there had been no more fighting. Maria also endorsed Geoff's role and was eager to take her turn. The parents noted that Gemma had been eager to go to school and had even conceded that she would 'think about' the sleepover. At the conclusion of the session, it was agreed that couple therapy was now the most useful direction.

Conclusion

The temptation for family therapists to exclude children from sessions is understandable. Children are noisy and disruptive and do not participate in therapy like adults. They have the potential to touch the heart of the practitioner in ways that are disconcerting and painful and can render us powerless and uncertain with their directness. Effective work with children in their families requires a thorough knowledge of child and family development and a comprehensive understanding of the impact of both expected and unexpected events on children.

Despite this, there is a powerful argument to include children, both for the family and the therapist. Children provide information quickly and clearly in ways that cannot be ignored. They allow us to see the whole system at work and to harness the power of their attachments to their parents and each other. Equipped with an array of techniques, both verbal and non-verbal, the therapist can engage in a process that reveals the basis of a child's distress and then act to address it.

References

Ackerman, N. (1970). Child participation in family therapy. *Family Process, 9,* 403–410.

Benson, M., Schindler-Zimmerman, T., & Martin, D. (1991). Accessing children's perception of their family: Circular questioning revisited. *Journal of Marital and Family Therapy, 17,* 363–372.

Chimpen-Lopez, C., Andres-Garrizand, C., & Pretel-Luque, T. (2022). Narrative practices for children with ASD: Hey! My therapist has an imaginary friend and other anti-tantrum practices. *Australian and New Zealand Journal of Family Therapy, 43,* 210–222.

Clement, M., & McKenny, R. (2019). Developing an open dialogue inspired model of systemic social work assessment in a local authority children's social care department. *Journal of Family Therapy, 41,* 421–446.

Cole, B. (1995). *Mummy laid an egg.* London: Random House.

Cole, B. (1996). *Princess smarty pants.* London, England: Harper Collins.

Cole, B. (1997). *Dr dog.* London, England: Random House.

Cole, B. (2000). *Two of everything.* London, England: Random House.

Coppersmith, E. (1981). "Developmental" reframing: He's not bad, He's not mad, He's just young. *Journal of Strategic and Systemic Therapies, 1,* 1–8.

Dumont, R. (2008). Drawing a family map: An experiential tool for engaging children in family therapy. *Journal of Family Therapy, 30,* 247–259.

Epston, D. (1986). Nightwatching: An approach to night fears. *Dulwich Centre Review,* 28–39.

Epston, D. (1989). Temper tantrum parties: Saving face, losing face, or going off your face! *Dulwich Centre Newsletter,* 12–26.

Gil, E. (1994). *Play in family therapy.* New York, NY: Guilford.

Helimäki, M., Laitila, A., & Kumpulainen, K. (2022). Why am I the only one you're talking to, talk to them, they haven't said a word? *The American Journal of Family Therapy, 50*(2), 113–130. doi: 10.1080/01926187.2020.1870582.

Jacob, P. (2018). Multi-stressed families, child violence and the larger system: An adaptation of the nonviolent model. *Journal of Family Therapy, 40,* 25–44.

Kantor, D., & Lehr, W. (1975). *Inside the family system.* CA: Jossey-Bass.

Klop, S. (2017). Sometimes words just ain't enough – Enhancing the contribution of children in therapy through creative expression. *Australian and New Zealand Journal of Family Therapy, 38,* 283–294.

Korner, S., & Brown, G. (1990). Exclusion of children from family psychotherapy: Family therapists beliefs and practices. *Journal of Family Psychology, 3,* 420–430.

Kozlowska, K., & Hanney, L. (1999). Family assessment and intervention using an interactive art exercise. *Australian and New Zealand Journal of Family Therapy, 20,* 61–69.

Kozlowska, K., & Hanney, L. (2001). An art therapy group for children traumatized by parental violence and separation. *Clinical Child Psychology and Psychiatry, 6,* 49–78.

Kozlowska, K., & Hanney, L. (2003). Maltreated children: A systems approach to treatment planning in clinical settings. *Australian and New Zealand Journal of Family Therapy, 24,* 75–87.

Lund, K., Schindler-Zimmerman, T., & Haddock, S. (2002). The theory, structure and techniques for the inclusion of children in family therapy: A literature review. *Journal of Marital and Family Therapy, 28,* 445–454.

March, J., & Mulle, K. (1994). *How I ran OCD off my land: A guide to cognitive-behavioral psychotherapy for children and adolescents with obsessive-compulsive disorder.* Toronto, Canada: Multi-Health Systems.

Minuchin, S., & Fishman, H. C. (1981). *Family therapy techniques.* Cambridge, MA: Harvard University Press.

Moore, L., & Seu, I. (2011). Giving children a voice: Children's positioning in family therapy. *Journal of Family Therapy, 33,* 279–301.

O'Reilly, M., & Parker, N. (2014). 'She needs a smack in the gob': Negotiating what is appropriate talk in front of children in family therapy. *Journal of Family Therapy, 36,* 287–307.

Oehlers, K., & Shortland-Jones, R. (2013). Is family therapy including children? *Australian and New Zealand Journal of Family Therapy, 34,* 215–231.

Omer, H. (2000). *Parental presence.* Phoenix, AZ: Zeig, Tucker and Co.

Omer, H. (2001). Helping parents deal with children's acute disciplinary problems without escalation. *Family Process, 40,* 53–66.

Omer, H. (2004). *Nonviolent resistance.* Cambridge, UK: Cambridge University Press.

Omer, H., & Dolberger, D. (2015). Helping parents cope with suicide threats: An approach based on nonviolent resistance. *Family Process, 54,* 559–575.

Omer, H., Schorr-Sapir, I., & Weinblatt, U. (2008). Non-violent resistance and violence against siblings. *Journal of Family Therapy, 30,* 450–464.

Omer, H., Steinmetz, S., Carthy, T., & Von Schlippe, A. (2013). The anchoring function: parental authority and the parent-child bond. *Family Process, 52,* 193–206.

Robinson, M., & Sanders, C. (2023). https://bowerplace.com.au/bower-knowledge/

Ruble, N. (1999). The voices of therapists and children regarding the inclusion of children in family therapy: A systematic research synthesis. *Contemporary Family Therapy, 21,* 485–503.

Sanders, C. (1985). Now I see the difference – The use of visual news of difference in clinical practice. *Australian and New Zealand Journal of Family Therapy, 6,* 23–29.

Satir, V. (1972). *Peoplemaking.* CA: Science and Behaviour Books.

Scott, E. (1999). Are the children playing quietly? *Australian and New Zealand Journal of Family Therapy, 22,* 88–93.

Sith, S., Rosen, K., McCollum, E., Coleman, J., & Herman, S. (1996). The voices of children: Preadolescent children's experiences in family therapy. *Journal of Marital and Family Therapy, 22,* 69–86.

Sori, C., & Hecker, L. (2015). Ethical and legal considerations when counselling children and families. *Australian and New Zealand Journal of Family Therapy, 36,* 450–464.

Van Holen, Vanderfaeillie, J., & Omer, H. (2015). Adaptation and evaluation of a nonviolent resistance intervention for foster parents: A progress report. *Journal of Marital and Family Therapy, 42,* 256–271.

Vermeire, S., & Van den Berge, L. (2021). Widening the screen: Playful responses to challenges in online therapy with children and families. *Journal of Family Therapy, 43,* 329–345.

Watzlawick, P., Weakland, J., & Fisch, R. (1974). *Change:Principles of problem formation and problem resolution.* New York, NY: W.W. Norton & Company.

Whitaker, C. A. (1982). The ongoing training of the psychotherapist. In J. R. Neill, & D. P. Kniskern (Eds.), *From psyche to system: The evolving therapy of Carl Whitaker* (pp. 121–138). New York, NY: Guilford.

White, M. (1984). Pseudo-encopresis: From avalanche to victory, from vicious to virtuous cycles. *Family Systems Medicine, 2,* 150–160.

Wilson, J. (1992). *The suitcase kid.* London, England: Random House Children's Books.

Wilson, J. (1994). *The bed and breakfast star.* London, England: Random House Children's Books.

Wilson, J. (1996). *Bad girls.* London, England: Random House Children's Books.

Wilson, J. (1998). *Child-focused practice: A collaborative systemic approach.* London, England: Karnac Books.

Wilson, J. (2000). *Vicki angel.* London, England: Random House Children's Books.

Zilbach, J. J. (1986). *Young children in family therapy.* New York, NY: Brunner/Mazel.

Chapter 7

Improving Relationship Security for Distressed Adolescents

Suzanne Levy, Torrey A. Creed, and Guy Diamond

Introduction

Our culture perpetuates the myth that adolescent development is predicated on separation and individuation. While important, we now know that continuity in connection and attachment to parents is essential (Steinberg, 1990). Therefore, the central task of adolescence is transforming parent-child relationships to support an appropriate balance of attachment and autonomy. Adolescents who present in therapy have typically fallen off this healthy developmental trajectory. Thus, therapy could aim to refurbish or repair this developmental cocoon by promoting secure base family relationships. To accomplish this, parents must be more emotionally sensitive and available (secure base) and support autonomy and competency (safe haven). In this context, adolescents can learn to better express themselves, tolerate difficult emotions, and learn more effective problem-solving skills. Attachment Based Family Therapy (ABFT) provides a road map to accomplish these goals in an organized and systemic manner. This chapter provides an overview of that map and a case study to help the therapist better understand its application.

Rationale

ABFT theory base

The quality of interpersonal relationships, social experience, and life events can cause, maintain, or buffer against suicide and/or depression (Diamond, Diamond, & Levy, 2021). This view is best articulated in interpersonal theories of depression (Coyne, 1976; Gotlib & Hammen, 1992; Joiner & Coyne, 1999). In this framework, factors such as parental depression (Weissman & Paykel, 1974), marital conflict, ineffective parenting practices (Cummings & Davies, 1994), unmet attachment needs (Greenberg, 1999), loss (Harris, Brown, & Bifulco, 1986), and negative parent-child interactions (Asarnow, Goldstein, Tompson, & Guthrie, 1993) are viewed as etiological and reinforcing factors of depression. This orientation to understanding and treating depression is particularly relevant for children and adolescents, for whom the family context has a more potent and inescapable impact than for adults (Maccoby & Martin, 1983; Rutter, 1984).

Adolescent attachment theory and research serve as the primary conceptual framework of ABFT (Allen, Moore, Kuperminc, & Bell, 1998; Kobak & Sceery, 1988; Lynch & Cicchetti, 1991; Rosenstein & Horowitz, 1996). The importance of appropriate attachment during adolescence has been well documented (Grotevant & Cooper, 1993; Steinberg, 1990). Healthy adolescent development depends, in part, on the presence of at least one

DOI: 10.4324/9781003490104-8

parent (caregiver) as a stable attachment figure. Secure attachment leads to more direct communication, which fosters perspective taking and problem-solving skills (Ewing, Diamond, & Levy, 2015; Kobak & Duemmler, 1994), essential abilities for the suicidal adolescent. In contrast, a caretaker's unavailability and unresponsiveness, particularly at critical moments (e.g., suicide attempt), lead to insecure attachment. Insecure attachment has repeatedly been associated with depression in infants, children, adolescents, and adults (Ainsworth, 1989; Greenberg, Siegel, & Leitch, 1983; Kobak & Sceery, 1988; Sund & Wichsgtrom, 2002).

Application

Based on the rationale above, we have developed ABFT, an empirically informed brief psychotherapy. The efficacy of ABFT has been demonstrated with adolescents who are depressed, suicidal, anxious, have high family conflict, and have experienced trauma. Several clinical trials have demonstrated that ABFT is better than usual care found in the community for treating both adolescent depression and suicide ideation (Diamond, Reis, Diamond, Siqueland, & Isaacs, 2002, 2003, 2010, 2019, 2021).

Rather than a primary focus on cognitions, ABFT aims to re-establish or strengthen the family's capacity to offer (parents) and receive (adolescents) a secure base of love and protection. To accomplish this, the therapist guides families through a series of in-session tasks or episodes that prepare for and facilitate corrective attachment experiences. ABFT rests on the notion that interpersonal problems within the family such as abandonment, betrayal, neglect, distrust, abuse, over control, and high criticism must be addressed initially and directly, as these themes often underlie many of the behavioural problems that bring families to therapy. Without a strong foundation of trust and safety, problem-solving interventions will be undermined. Therefore, a focus on interpersonal functioning between family members is the first order of therapeutic business in the treatment. As interpersonal themes are resolved, parents begin to adopt a more caring, non-critical, authoritative parenting style. This helps adolescents revise their internal working model of their parents. Adolescents once again begin to perceive and interact with their parents as caring, safe, protective attachment figures. As the secure base is strengthened, adolescents increasingly turn to their parents for support to manage the stressors that can exacerbate depression or suicidal thoughts.

The ABFT manual (Diamond, Diamond, & Levy, 2021) offers a set of guiding principles, processes, strategies, and goals to repair these interpersonal attachment ruptures. It is a road map through and across the treatment tasks but requires clinical judgement and decision-making. Certainly, families come to treatment with their own list of goals and problems. But their concerns usually focus on behavioural management issues. Do they get up on time? Do they go to school? Do they cooperate at home and have good friends? These are important problems to solve. In ABFT, psychological science guides our treatment goals. We know that repairing attachment, developing more trust-based relationships, teaching affectively attuned parenting skills, and improving adolescent affect regulation and conflict resolution skills will rebuild a new relational foundation. Therefore, we initially focus our treatment on these goals on this more fundamental aspect of family life. Rather than talk about behavior change, we first focus the conversation on trust, safety, and relational disappointments that we believe drive many behavioural problems.

Theory into practice

Important influences on ABFT

The model stands on the shoulders of five clinical giants. ABFT is firmly based on the tradition of *Structural Family Therapy* (Minuchin, 1974). We use enactment (e.g., in vivo family conversations) to practice new interpersonal skills with each other. ABFT also has a strong connection to *Multi-Dimensional Family Therapy* (MDFT; Liddle, 2002). From MDFT, we have learned how to use psychological science to inform treatment development and a general sensibility of how to approach family work with adolescents. The *Emotion Focused Therapy* work of Greenberg and Johnson (Greenberg & Johnson, 1988) has helped us understand the importance of emotional processing as a therapeutic facilitator and mechanism of change. *Contextual family therapy* (Boszormenyi-Nagy & Spark, 1973) has led to our focus on "trust" as a primary organizing clinical topic and on intergenerational legacies that impact parents' current parenting practices. Finally, we have used Bowlby's *attachment theory* (1969) to redirect our clinical focus from behavioural management to focus more clearly on issues of safety, protection, felt security, and love.

Implementation

ABFT clinical model

The model can be understood as three distinct, yet overlapping, phases. In phase one, treatment focuses on helping the adolescent identify past and present family conflicts that have strained the attachment bond and damaged trust. Adolescents and parents are taught new communication and affect regulation skills in preparation for reparative conversations in phase two. This phase of treatment involves adolescents and parents discussing these past and present conflicts using their new communication skills. The final phase of treatment focuses on promoting adolescent autonomy (i.e., improving school productivity, finding a job, developing, or returning to social activities, etc.). For the suicidal/depressed adolescent, this can decrease isolation and increase exposure to positive experiences. To accomplish these goals, there are five ABFT treatment tasks. Each task may take one or several sessions.

Phase 1: Preparing for the relationship repair

Relational reframe task

Although reframing is discussed in several systemic and cognitive models of therapy, ABFT has a specific slant on this principle. Our reframe aims to shift the family's focus of treatment from "viewing the adolescents as the problem" to "enhancement of family relationships as the solution". In this regard, the reframing task frames the focus of the therapy on attachment, rather than symptom reduction. To accomplish this, the session usually begins with joining and history taking. About midway through the session, if possible, the therapist shifts his or her focus away from fact-finding and towards interpersonal problems that have damaged trust and ruptured the attachment fabric of family life. The session (and much of the therapy) revolves around the question: "When you feel so depressed or suicidal, why don't you go to your parents for help?" Ideally, the conversation remains focused on this topic long enough to soften the emotional mood of the session. The goal is not to blame anyone, but to uncover and amplify the biologically wired desire for love and protection. The session ends with a clear commitment from the family to let therapy focus on attachment ruptures and repair for the first phase of therapy.

Adolescent alliance building task

With the adolescent alone, the session initially focuses on developing client-therapist trust by exploring strengths and concerns that are important to the adolescent. The session then turns to understanding the depression narrative. We want the adolescent to express the pain or despair that he or she feels. This is our way of getting them motivated to engage in the therapy. We then turn to the attachment narrative. Here we aim to help the adolescent better understand the attachment failures with the parents. We aim to help them have a more coherent understanding of these disappointments and more easily access the vulnerable emotions that result from them. With this story developed, we link the attachment narrative to the depression narrative. "Your depression partially results from these family conflicts" or "these family conflicts exacerbate your depression". If they accept either of these assumptions, then we have leverage to motivate them to work out problems with their parents, to reduce depression. This is never a simple conversation but when they agree, we prepare them for that conversation.

Parent alliance building task

The Alliance Building Task with the parent focuses on reducing parental distress and improving parenting practices. There are three areas that could be explored in this task. First, we are concerned about how current stressors affect parenting. This could include work, other children, or psychiatric distress. Second, when we have a two-parent family, we always explore parental teamwork. Do they work well together and how we can improve this? Often, marital problems lurk behind parental conflict, and this must at least be identified and often referred for couples' therapy. Finally, we might have conversations about parents' own attachment experiences when they were a child. These "ghosts in the nursery" often linger and enter our lives when we have our own children. We are not trying to solve or resolve these past issues, but rather use parent's empathy for their own disappointment to better understand how their child feels. In this softened state, they become more receptive to learning parenting skills that focus on affective attunement and emotional facilitation (Gottman, Katz, & Hooven, 1996). The essential goal of this task is to increase parents' ability to empathically appreciate the challenges that the adolescent struggles with. This sets the foundation for a more productive conversation in Task IV.

Phase 2: Reparative discussions

Repairing attachment task

The Repairing Attachment Task is the culmination of the work from the previous three tasks and provides the in vivo context for experientially practicing new interpersonal skills. These in-session adolescent-parent conversations focus on the adolescent disclosing, often for the first time, past and present experiences, thoughts, and feelings which have violated the attachment bond and damaged trust. These attachment ruptures may be associated with perceived parental criticism, over control, parental rejection, abandonment, or abuse. When parents respond to their adolescent's pain, accusations, anger, and hurt in a supportive, understanding, and non-defensive manner, adolescents are more likely to acknowledge their contribution to past problems and move towards forgiveness of their parents. At one level, these conversations aim to work out past and often avoid difficult topics. At another level, family members are practicing new more productive interpersonal problem-solving skills. At the third level, this conversation becomes a corrective attachment experience, where parents are available and sensitive and adolescents use parents as a secure base to talk about difficult and painful experiences.

Phase 3: After the reparative conversation

Autonomy promoting task

The Autonomy Promoting Task is designed to facilitate the adolescent's re-involvement and success in extrafamilial, pro-social contexts (e.g., school, employment, peer relations, sports, etc.). Many depressed adolescents have withdrawn from these activities during the depressive episode and need help to rebuild this part of their lives. As family hostility or conflict decreases, depression usually decreases as well. Adolescents become less preoccupied with anger at their parents and more willing to turn to them for help.

While attachment repairing work is not over, more attention can be given to building opportunities for autonomy and competency. Parents are taught to encourage, support, and advocate for their children without being negative, over controlling, or overprotective. Adolescents are encouraged to use parents as emotional resources in trying to sort out these challenges. In this way, competency promotion is coupled with maintaining and appropriately using the secure base of family life.

The self of the therapist

Although this is a semi-structured treatment manual, ABFT is fundamentally a depth psychotherapy. This therapy requires respect and admiration for all family members and a therapist who is comfortable with deep, raw emotion, arousal, and conflict and will push people to go deeper. The self of the therapist is critical. The work goes to the deepest places in family life, sometimes ugly and sometimes blissful. The therapist must believe in people even considering this ugliness. The therapist is flexible; being both soft and empathic, yet challenging and directive. The therapist must have a willingness and ability to take control and keep everyone safe when necessary. This is not an approach for the faint-at-heart therapist. This is a process-oriented therapy, where sustained, explorative therapeutic conversations are viewed as the curative agent.

To some extent, the therapist's role, tone, and disposition change over the course of the three phases. During the preparation phase (Tasks I–III), the therapist must be authoritative and confident about his or her skill level and treatment plan. Shifting the family's focus from symptom reduction to attachment repair often takes a leap of faith for families. The family has to believe in the expertise of the therapist and trust in the "medicine" being proposed. In the alliance building tasks, the therapist serves as the transitional attachment object, fostering trust, safety, protection, and comfort. The therapist/patient relationship is used to resuscitate or activate these feelings, but the action of these alliance tasks occurs between the patient/parent and the therapists. The therapist is gently directive, eliciting family members' agreement to the treatment task and working with the family to explore the content of the attachment rupture and then preparing them for the reparative conversation. During the *reparative phase* (Task IV), the therapist transfers the attachment relationship back to the parents and adolescent. The therapist aims to orchestrate an attachment promoting conversation between parents and adolescent serving as the conductor who provides guidance, tempo, intensity, and focus, while the family members provide the emotion and content. These conversations are also more process than outcome oriented. The therapist helps restrain the family members from rushing to solutions and encourages more open-ended exploration. The process is the goal. In phase three, *after the reparative discussion* (Task V), the therapist becomes less directive, and the therapy becomes more client centered. The therapist continues to guide the family, but parents increasingly resume their leadership role in helping the adolescent rebuild autonomy and competency. Ideally, the adolescent, who has resumed some leadership of their own life, identifies goals and tasks to accomplish. The parents provide a supportive yet challenging secure base to promote success. The therapist's goal is to be as minimally involved as needed.

Summary of a case

In this chapter, we will illustrate each task with excerpts from transcripts from a family seen in therapy by Suzanne Levy, Ph.D. A vignette of the case is presented, followed by the description of each task and illustrative samples of transcripts from the case.

> Jane[1] is a 15-year-old African American girl who resides with her mother, Tina, step father, and half-sister. Tina and her husband are both employed, and Tina is also in school studying to get her nursing degree. Jane's biological father has had an inconsistent presence in her life. When Jane sees her father, he often lets her down and breaks promises. Jane is currently a freshman in high school and is struggling academically. She has some interest/hobbies such as fashion, hair, and poetry, but her depression has reduced her interests in these activities. Jane reports that she has felt isolated from her family her whole life. In her teenage years, Jane has become physically aggressive when upset. In these moments of crisis, Tina sends Jane to her biological grandmother's house to live for lengthy periods of time. Jane was referred for treatment by her primary care doctor for depression and suicidal ideation. Therapy sessions focused on the relationship between Tina and Jane, because Jane indicated her issues were with her mother and she had a good relationship with her step-father. Additionally, Jane's step-father was unable to attend therapy sessions due to his work schedule.

Phase I: Preparing for the relationship repair

Task I: The relational reframe

The first 30 minutes of this task are spent orienting the family to the therapy, joining with the family, and defining the problem. This is usually done in the first session because it lays the contractual foundation of the entire therapy: a focus on relational development. The session begins with a focus on the strengths of the adolescent and parents. This conversation conveys to the adolescent and parents that depression is just one component of their lives and that all aspects are important. Focusing on strengths also gives the therapist valuable information for the future Autonomy Promoting Task (Task V). The therapist asks about the general context of the family: who lives in the home, who is employed and where, whether extended family or social services are involved, religious involvement, etc.

The conversation then turns to the mental health issue. The family is asked to describe the adolescent's depression, what they think is causing the depression, and the impact it has on the family. The therapist gathers enough information to understand and punctuate the problem, but not so much detail that the session is overly focused on the patient's failures and history taking. There will be more time for that. The session should have some therapeutic value so that the family will feel hopeful and engaged in the process.

About halfway through the session, the therapist begins the reframe. The conversation shifts from history and behaviours to attachment relationships and emotions. The therapist helps the family examine why the adolescent has not used the parents for support by asking the adolescent, "*Why don't you go to your parents when you are feeling depressed or suicidal?*" or asking the parent questions such as, "*Why doesn't your adolescent come to you when he or she is upset?*" The therapist begins to explore themes of trust and protection, comfort and love, abuse, and abandonment, and how attachment ruptures get in the way of the family being a resource for the adolescent. Throughout the discussion, the therapist deepens vulnerable emotions through the use of empathy, reflection, and use of words that provoke primary emotions such as loss, love, trust, abandonment, etc. We do not aim to "resolve" these issues at this time. Rather, we highlight them enough to activate emotions of sadness and disappointment that might give us access to feelings of longing for connection.

Once the therapist has laid the groundwork above, he or she proposes to focus the therapy on repairing or strengthening attachment. A rationale is given: increased trust will help the parent to protect the adolescent from harm and make problem-solving easier. The therapist tries to get each family member "on record" saying that they desire a change, wish to be closer, and will work towards repairing ruptures and strengthening trust. Resistance to this goal should be explored. If needed, the therapist may also scale back and just ask that the hesitant adolescent or parent at least return to the next session. Below are some excerpts from Task I, beginning with the therapist starting the actual reframing task.

Therapist: Is that [feeling like you don't have a dad] something you ever talked to your mom about?
(Daughter shakes head "no".)
Therapist: (to mother) Did you know that she felt that way about her dad?
Mother: I knew, to a certain extent, I knew.
Therapist: (to adolescent) How come you never talked to your mom about that?
Daughter: Um … because … I don't even know. I feel weird – I don't know if I want to talk about it.
Therapist: What do you mean?
Daughter: When I try to tell her stuff sometimes, and I think about how she's gonna react…
Therapist: So you're worried about the way she reacts. How did she react to you before that made you feel unsafe?

Daughter: Sometimes … yelling…
Therapist: And what was that like for you when that happened?
Daughter: Just said I won't never tell her nothing no more.
Mother: I disagree with that. She … she never really tells me anything. It's to the point where I'll find out about something, then I poke and prod until I find out what it is, and then she'll tell me, and that's why I'm so angry. She never really comes to me, never, never, never, never, never.

The therapist used words such as "safe" to tap into the attachment instinct of the parent, but the mother still became defensive. Instead of challenging the mother's defensiveness directly, the therapist took a different tactic.

Therapist: Was there ever a time in the past when you guys talked about these challenges, missing dad or being in a blended family?
Mother: We never talked about that, but we have talked about things that were of concern. You know, so we have had times where I have asked her to say why she does not come to me, why won't she talk to me? And she says the same thing, because you're gonna holler and I told her at that point, I said, who cares about that, I get over it … just give me a chance to calm down and soak it through.
Therapist: Well, it sounds like for Jane, she is a pretty sensitive person and that the yelling is what kind of gets in the way. That for you [talking to mother] your first reaction is to yell, even though that is not how you feel deep down. But for Jane, that yelling is probably the hardest part.
Daughter: Yeah.
Therapist: (to Jane) So, part of you really wants to be able to go to mom and talk about things. Right? (turns to mother). Tina, did you know your daughter wants to come to you for help?
Mother: And I want her to come talk to me.
Therapist: That is great. I can see how much you love each other … I also think this would be very helpful for both of you. And provide some protection for your daughter … you know … so she can turn to you to help solve problems. Would the two of you be willing to work on this in therapy with me?

When the therapist switched the focus to whether the family had ever been able to discuss issues, the mother softened and refocused on providing safety for the daughter. The therapist reframed the mother's aggressive style of communication for the daughter as coming from a place of love, while acknowledging that this was not the optimal style for the adolescent. The therapist did not try to resolve or fix these poor communication skills in this session but rather focused on the part of each family member that wanted to connect with each other. By the end of the session, Tina and Jane acknowledged that they longed to be closer to each other and were committed to making that the initial focus of treatment. As the session progressed, the therapist also discovered other core ruptures, particularly that the adolescent is sent to the grandmother's house whenever she "acts up".

Task II: Adolescent alliance building

The Adolescent Alliance Building Task is the second task of treatment and usually begins in the second session. However, it can be interchanged with the Parent Alliance Building

Task if needed. Task II usually takes two to four sessions to complete but can last longer if the adolescent is resistant. Meeting alone with the adolescent has many purposes. First, the therapist continues bonding with the adolescent, transforming suspicion into comfort and trust. Second, the therapist helps the adolescent develop a more coherent depression narrative. Understanding their own mental health distress can help move the adolescent from a victim to an agent of change in their own life. Next, the therapist helps the adolescent better understand their attachment narrative with their parents. This may include specific experiences of abandonment or abuse, or more general dynamics such as parents who are overly critical or controlling. The therapist gets at these negative processes by asking questions such as: "*When you are upset, why don't you go to your parents? What has happened in the past when you've tried?*" Once the negative processes are determined, the therapist helps the adolescent explore the impact these dynamics have had on them. Then the therapist amplifies the adolescent's right to tell his or her parents about these concerns and helps them to understand how important it would be to get this off of his or her chest.

Whether these concerns are accurate or exacerbated by the depression, convincing the adolescent to discuss these things with the parents is critical. Getting signed on to this task is not always easy. The therapist must engage the adolescent in a dialogue regarding the adolescent's willingness to talk to their parents about the "attachment rupture". The therapist may begin by asking the adolescent, "*Have you ever told your parents these things?*" If the adolescent says yes, the therapist and the adolescent might explore the adolescent's past attempts to have these discussions with their parents or how they think their parents might feel hearing these things. If the adolescent has not tried, the therapist will ask, "*Why not?*" If the adolescent is concerned about burdening their parent, the therapist can ask, "*Why don't you deserve to have these things addressed?*" If the adolescent is concerned his/her parent won't listen, the therapist may say, "*You've never tried it with me. I can make it different. I can make her listen. I will protect you.*" All resistance or fears should be explored so that the commitment to enter into this conversation can be as solid as possible.

In the last part of Task II, the therapist attempts to prepare the adolescent for the Repairing Attachment Task. As part of this, the therapist helps the adolescent recognize and take responsibility for old behaviours and emotional reactions that have contributed to non-productive conversations. The therapist also assures the adolescent that the therapist will protect the adolescent through the process (e.g., prepare the parent, or stop the conversation if it gets too negative). The therapist then helps the adolescent to plan what to say, explore potential emotional reactions, discuss effective ways to communicate in session, explore feared parental reactions, and plan for how to handle these challenges. Finally, the therapist helps the adolescent understand why it is important to engage in the Repairing Attachment Task, even if the parents cannot do it well. This process is about the adolescent finding a voice, and not about the adolescent changing the parents.

Below is an excerpt from Task II with Jane by herself. The transcript begins with the therapist punctuating the attachment ruptures Jane has noted throughout the session. Some affect focused questions then help deepen the emotional intensity.

Therapist: So, it sounds like a couple of things have gotten in the way of going to your mom. One is that you don't really trust her and that she will not keep your information private. Another is that initially when you tell her something, she yells. And, maybe most important, you feel like she's abandoned you several times.

Daughter: Yes, that's true.

Therapist: Tell me how you really feel inside.
Daughter: Hurt.
Therapist: How else do you feel inside?
Daughter: Neglected. Like I don't belong.
Therapist: That must have been awful for you. I get the sense that you feel neglected now too, though. (Daughter nods her head "yes".)

At this point, the therapist would explore the impact these experiences have had on the adolescent's sense of worthiness of love and protection. The therapist may also explore how these experiences impact the adolescent's other relationships. Once the therapist has helped the adolescent understand and connect to their experience, the therapist can feel more confident that the patient will be motivated to make a change. Then the conversation moves more towards talk about change. The next phase of the conversation introduces the desired tasks (talk directly with the mother) and deals with the resistance that inevitably arises.

Therapist: And these are things you haven't told your mom before? (Daughter nods her head, confirming.)
Therapist: Are you willing to tell her things? Daughter: I want to – but I'm worried.
Therapist: What are your concerns?
Daughter: That she not gonna listen. She's gonna keep on doing the same thing she always does … (Silent Pause) … She will never understand, so what's the use?
Therapist: So you feel pretty hopeless.
Daughter: The last time we were in therapy with someone else, she didn't get it.
Therapist: What do you mean?
Daughter: Because it got worse. She neglected me even more.
Therapist: Neglected you?
Daughter: She just gave up on me. She always says stuff is my fault and it's not.
Therapist: That must be painful and frustrating. … (pause…) But you know, I think your mom really needs to hear these things. I know she loves you and I wonder … I wonder if she knew how you felt, she might understand you differently. Can I help you tell your mom those things? (Daughter nods head "yes".)

At this point, the therapist moves from an affect focus to a bit more focus on preparation, planning, and setting up the conversation.

Therapist: I'm so glad to hear you want to do this. I'm going to meet with your mom on Thursday. I'm gonna talk to her about what's going on with her and what she wants to say to you. And then I will prepare her for having a talk with you … I'm gonna step in if there's blame and too much anger. But I need you to do something for me. I need you to stick in there with it because your mom's not gonna be perfect – it's gonna take some practice, and I'm here to help guide both of you guys through that process. Do you think you can stick with it?
Daughter: Yes – but what if I get angry?
Therapist: If I see you getting angry, I'm gonna help you calm down. I want you to be honest and strong, but not attack her. I am going to help you. How does that sound to you?
Daughter: I'm willing to try.

In this session, the therapist intentionally punctuated the adolescent's identified attachment ruptures to focus the adolescent on those experiences and assess her willingness to engage in a conversation with her mother about these felt injustices. When the adolescent noted possible resistance to having this conversation, the therapist helped the adolescent explore these concerns and deepen the affect related to her past experiences. The therapist also highlighted why it was important for the adolescent to share these things with her mother. Once the adolescent agreed, the therapist then offered herself as a "secure base" for this conversation by describing how she would protect and help everyone during the conversation. The therapist also set realistic expectations for the mother's behavior and made clear what was expected of the adolescent. In this context, the adolescent was able to discuss her own feared reactions, thus allowing the therapist and the adolescent to plan to manage those reactions. At the conclusion of this session, Jane was prepared for the Repairing Attachment Task. She knew what she wanted to say to her mother, had practiced discussing her emotions related to this topic during the course of the session, had processed her resistance, and had planned for her own feared reactions.

Task III: Parent alliance building

The Parent Alliance Building task should be completed parallel to Task II adolescent sessions. It typically takes between two to four sessions to complete this task. The purpose of these sessions is to bond with the parent to lower defensiveness, help the parent increase empathy for themselves and their child, and build their skills in responding to emotionally charged conversations.

At the beginning of the first parent-alone session, the therapist typically describes the goals and tasks of the session to parents and briefly assesses parents' initial reactions to the goals and tasks. Parents will likely be more receptive to parent-alone sessions when they understand that having these sessions allows the therapist to better help the parents to parent more effectively. Then the therapist asks about current stressors in the parents' lives (e.g., couples' conflict, financial, etc.) and how these stressors impact them. The goal is to reduce parent blame and guilt by putting parent-adolescent conflicts into context. The therapist explores and deepens the linkage between parental stressors and their parenting by asking questions such as *"How do you think these things have impacted your parenting?"* or *"It must be hard raising an adolescent, let alone a depressed one, when you have so many other stressors in your life"*. The parents' support system is also explored. For instance, the therapist may ask, *"Who do you talk to when things are tough?"* For parents with few supports and many stressors (sometimes including their own mental health problems), it may be necessary to refer them for individual or marital counselling.

The therapist may also explore intergenerational themes related to attachment ruptures that the parents may have experienced as children. Usually, this involves the parents' own caregivers, but it might also involve relatives, peers, or other significant figures from the parents' childhood or adolescence. To gather this information, therapists ask parents to describe what their relationships were like with their primary caregivers. The critical questions to explore here are, *"Were you close to your parents growing up? Could you go to them when you were having problems? What got in the way? How did that impact you?"* Instead of asking for these stories in detail, the therapist asks parents to remember and feel the emotions that accompanied them. Once enough detail is gathered and vulnerable emotion is elicited, the therapist links these affectively charged memories to how their own child might be feeling now. For instance, "*So, you know what it is like to not be protected … I wonder if that is how your child is feeling now?*" This strategy aims to amplify parental empathy for the child and increase the parent's understanding of the child's need for secure attachment. The therapist then offers the parent the opportunity to spare their child the pain and suffering that they (the parents) experienced as a youth. If the parent did not experience attachment ruptures as a child, then we offer to help the parents provide his or her child with the good things the parent had as a child: "*You were close to your parents. It must be hard that you and your child are not close. I could help you with that*".

The therapist works with any resistance on the part of the parent until they agree to the task. Then psychoeducation and preparation begin. The therapist begins preparing the parent by asking questions such as, "*How do conversations usually go for the two of you? What would be some of the challenges for you in having this conversation? What might go wrong? What if your daughter makes you angry or hurts your feelings?*" Once these issues are explored, the therapist engages the parents in a conversation about their comfort with emotions and teaches them emotion coaching skills (Gottman, Katz, & Hooven, 1996) to be used in the Repairing Attachment Task. Teaching, discussion, and handouts help flesh out these skills. Essentially, the therapist encourages the parents to be curious, ask questions, not get defensive, and be interested in the adolescent's emotions. It is not expected that parents will be experts in emotion coaching skills by the time they engage in the next task. Rather, they will deepen their understanding of the skills by using them in the Repairing Attachment Task with coaching from the therapist. Orienting the parents to emotion coaching skills provides a shared language between the therapist and parents that will help facilitate communication in Task IV.

The transcript below begins with the therapist exploring the mother's intergenerational legacy of attachment ruptures. Tina indicated that her life was good until age 11, when her mother, father, and she moved out of her grandparents' home. Soon after that, her father abandoned the family, the family had much less money, and Tina was forced to take on a parental role with her brother. When Tina became a teenager, her mother remarried and Tina's new stepfather sexually assaulted her. Tina's mother threw her out of the house, and Tina was forced to spend the remainder of her adolescence in orphanages and group homes. Throughout Tina's narrative of her past, the therapist punctuated the theme of abandonment and the vulnerable emotions that it generated. The transcript begins when the therapist is helping Tina to see the connection between her own life and her daughter's experiences.

Therapist: How do you see yourself in Jane?
Mother: When I listen to some of the things she says, I feel like … I'm – I'm lookin' at a re-run of me – that's like, she's just replayin' everything I said or anything I did when I was younger and it's like, it's quite scary cause it's like I'm lookin' at myself and I didn't wanna deal with myself back then, so how am I gonna deal with myself right now? So how do I deal with it? I just get away from it. Just leave it alone. Just try to make the problem go away.
Therapist: But you know what it is like to be abandoned. Do you think she feels you are doing that to her?
Mother: Yeah, that's so true.
Therapist: When you were a kid, did you wish that someone was gonna step in and protect you?

Mother: I needed my grandfather and he died. And I needed him because he was the only one.

Therapist: You have an opportunity here, to do for Jane what you never had yourself – You can step in and protect her. Would you like that opportunity to do that for her?

Mother: Definitely, I wanna be able to, just sit down with her and enjoy being with her. I wanna enjoy being around her. I don't wanna make her sit and watch a movie with me or, go to the mall, or anything like that. I want her to be able to come up and say, "Oh, well, you wanna know what happened today?" And, you know? I can't – I never get that.

Therapist: I think if we show her you can be understanding and protective, she will feel more safe with you and then come to you more often.

The transcript demonstrates how the therapist used the parent's own past to motivate her to want to help her daughter, and to save her daughter from the years of pain and struggle she went through. Tina had a longing to help her daughter, but admittedly did not know how. Her attachment instinct had clearly been activated and she needed new skills to be there for her daughter. In the following session, the therapist explored the mother's history of emotions in her own family and then taught the parent emotional coaching skills for her to use with her daughter.

Phase II: Relationship repair session(s)

Task IV: Repairing attachment task

By the end of the two Alliance Building sessions, both parents and the adolescent are prepared for the conversation to take place during the Repairing Attachment Task. Important content areas have been identified, and all parties have accessed vulnerable emotional states that will be important to express and discuss. Additionally, everyone has agreed to partake in the conversation. The therapist has assured both the adolescent and parents that the therapist will be there to support them through the conversation by saying, "*I'll be there to help. I will keep us focused*". The Repairing Attachment Task concerning the core attachment ruptures may be completed in one or many sessions. The purpose of this task is to have parents and the adolescent discuss the core attachment ruptures in a new affectively regulated, emotionally sensitive manner. For parents, this is an opportunity to practice new affectively attuned parenting skills. For the adolescent, this is an opportunity to practice new affect regulation and interpersonal problem-solving skills.

During this task, the therapist should guide the adolescent and parents through this conversation rather than leading it. The therapist monitors *content* (i.e., sharing of core interpersonal or attachment rupture), *affect* (i.e., vulnerable emotions that are part of the fear structure – hurt, sadness, appropriate anger, disappointment), and *process* (i.e., the work is between the parent and the child rather than through the therapist, and the parent is listening in this phase and offering empathy). The therapist offers protection as needed and attempts to strike a balance between shaping the conversation and letting it take its own shape.

Initially, the therapist guides the adolescent to share vulnerable feelings directly with the parents and coaches the parents to respond empathically to the adolescent. For instance, the therapist will say, "*Adolescent, tell your parent(s) what gets in the way of you coming to them for comfort and support*". Ideally, the family members will do most of the talking. The therapist guides the interaction, helps the family sustain the conversation, and helps the family access deeper, more vulnerable emotions (i.e., sadness, loneliness) while blocking defensive behavior. The parents should provide protection, validation, and soothing. It is important that the parent acknowledge the adolescent's perception, so the adolescent feels heard. In this safe environment, adolescents are less defended, more reflective, and more open to new input.

At times, parental acknowledgement evolves into an apology when relevant (case dependent). This can only happen after every aspect of the adolescent's felt experience is explored. If appropriate, the therapist makes an intentional shift to have the parents explain their side of things and apologize. The therapist modulates the parental dialogue, so it does not take over the session or become the center of the work, and so that the adolescent is not put in the position of protecting or comforting the parents. The therapist helps the adolescent engage in a discussion about the parental disclosure and perspective take. During the conversation, the therapist assesses the adolescent's reaction to the parents' disclosure by asking, "*Do you believe your parents?*" In many ways, these conversations can be thought of as a forgiveness process for resolving past trauma, wherein an apology from a perpetrator expedites the victim's ability to resolve the past traumas (Herman, 1992). The therapist assesses the adolescent's level of forgiveness for the parents by asking "*What does it feel like to hear your parents say these things? How does it change things? What is the effect of this?*" It is not expected that these issues will be resolved by the end of this discussion, but rather that this is a starting point for rebuilding trust between the adolescent and parents. There are plenty of opportunities in future sessions to continue discussing the core attachment rupture or other problems between the parents and the adolescent.

Jane and Tina attended the session knowing that they would partake in the Repairing Attachment Task. After brief hellos and a few words on the importance of everyone listening and being respectful, the therapist asked Jane to turn to her mother and talk about the things that get in her way of going to her mother for help and support. Jane began by talking about how her mother listens to her stepfather over her. The therapist redirected the conversation to the core attachment rupture – the mother sending Jane away to her grandmother's house when they had a fight.

Therapist:	Ask her if she cares about how you feel.
Daughter:	Do you care about how I feel?
Mother:	I care about how you feel. I care about you and what I want is for you to just understand how I'm—how I think about things sometimes when it comes to you. The only thing I want is the best for you. So, I don't say things just to be mean—
Therapist:	I'm gonna just stop you for a minute. There's no need to justify right now. The message of "I care how you feel" is the important one here. Jane, do you believe your mom when she says she cares about you?
Daughter:	Umm … sometimes.
Therapist:	How do you know when someone cares about you?
Daughter:	They show it.
Therapist:	How do they show it?

Daughter:	Uhh … different ways … They are there for you. They work with you when things are hard. They don't give up.
Therapist:	Do you feel like your mom's given up on you before?
Daughter:	(nods head "yes")
Therapist:	When?
Daughter:	All the time. (Begins crying.)
Therapist:	(to the mother) Maybe you could ask her what made her feel that way?
Mother:	What's made you feel that way?
Daughter:	How you just take me to grandma's, even when you don't know what's going on. You just go by what you see.
Mother:	How should I find out the whole story?
Daughter:	Ask me.
Mother:	And then if I ask you? After I ask you and you won't answer me, then what am I supposed to do? How do I find out?
Daughter:	Wait for a second.
Therapist:	So I'm gonna stop you for a minute … In these situations, things escalate, but Jane you're someone who needs some time to de-escalate, to calm down. And it sounds like you're feeling unheard, like you aren't getting to tell your side of the story. You don't get to tell her, and that it just results in you being taken to grandma's. How does it feel when you are taken to grandma's house?
Daughter:	It makes me feel alone.
Therapist:	Like you've been abandoned?
Daughter:	(nods "yes")
Therapist:	So, the result of you being taken to grandma's is that you feel lonely, abandoned … is there any anger in there? Are you also angry at mom?
Daughter:	(nods "yes")
Therapist:	Can you tell her?
Daughter:	(there is a long pause and the adolescent wipes her face with a tissue).
Therapist:	Is it difficult to tell your mom that you're angry?
Daughter:	(nods "yes")
Therapist:	Tina, is it okay if she told you that she's angry at you?
Mother:	(nods "yes")
Therapist:	Let her know.
Mother:	It's okay.
Daughter:	When you take me there, I feel angry because … I'm all by myself. (Begins crying into hands.)
Therapist:	Go ahead, you're doing a great job.
Daughter:	And I don't belong there. (Adolescent is continuing to cry.)
	(The therapist motions for Mother to comfort and put an arm around Jane. Mom moves over and comforts her daughter. Jane begins crying even harder. Tina holds her daughter for about 1–2 minutes where no one is talking.)
Therapist:	Jane, is there anything you'd like to say to your mom?
Daughter:	(shakes head "no")
Therapist:	So going to your grandmother's house has made you feel alone, abandoned, and angry. (To Tina) What is it like knowing that this is what it results in?
Mother:	It's sad. I don't think it is bad though because she has family. That's something I never had when I was her age.

Therapist: I know this is different from your experience and you didn't have anyone at all, but the feelings are the same. She still feels alone even though she's with her grandmother. Remember what it felt like for you when you were alone when you were her age? Remember – what did you need then? Can you turn to Jane and give her the support you talked about wanting to give her, the kind you wish your grandfather was able to give you?

Mother: Jane, I care for you and love you. I don't want you to feel that way. I want to hear what you have to say.

We see here how the therapist helped guide this difficult conversation between the adolescent and her mother. When Tina became defensive, the therapist interrupted and helped reframe Tina's statement, pulling out the positive aspect of what she said so that Jane could hear the important message. It was clear that Tina had difficulty exploring Jane's emotions, so the therapist helped keep the mood soft and provided Tina with the words to do so. The therapist helped Jane access more vulnerable emotions (i.e., loneliness, anger) and created a safe environment in which Jane could express her feelings and thoughts to her mother. The therapist used enactment to help deepen the emotion between Jane and her mother further and assisted in engineering a tender moment between the two (e.g., Tina comforting Jane). Ideally, Tina would have done this without the therapist's help, but this was the first time had Tina tried a more empathic approach to communicating with her daughter, so the therapist felt the need to provide more guidance. As family members become more competent and comfortable with these intense emotional conversations, they assume more responsibility for them.

Phase III: After the relationship repair

Task V: Autonomy promoting

The Autonomy Promoting Task, the last of the tasks, may occur after all four other tasks have been completed or it may at times be interspersed among the other tasks. This task comprises the majority of sessions once Tasks I through IV have been completed. The purpose of this task is to have parents help adolescents re-engage in their social world and activities that have often been ignored in the face of their depression. Now that parents are viewed as a secure base, they are in a better position to promote their adolescent's autonomy while providing love and support. Re-engaging in the social world can help adolescents increase their self-esteem and sense of competency, which has been shown to buffer against further hopelessness, depression, and, ideally, suicidal ideation (Cole, 1990; Dumont & Provost, 1999). Additionally, re-engaging in activities or engaging in activities for the first time has been known to be an effective intervention for those suffering from depression. Finally, this phase of treatment helps adolescents and parents practice their newly acquired communication skills, thereby increasing their competency in their use. With these skills, parents can help adolescents identify problems, discuss their feelings, and effectively problem-solve.

Returning to our case study

After the Repairing Attachment Task, the family missed a few sessions. The next session was with Jane alone due to Tina's schedule. Jane discussed how things had been different with her mother and how much better she had been feeling. Jane indicated that her mother had been yelling less and listening more. She stated that she felt like she fit in better with the family and had started putting herself and family before her friends. Jane indicated that her mother was more affectionate with her and that while it had taken some time getting used to, she was enjoying it. She noted that she still had a fear of being sent to her grandmother's house but recognized that it would take time to start feeling more secure about that. Jane also noted that she wanted her mother's help with starting a hair braiding business. The therapist helped Jane think about how she could talk to her mother about her fear of being sent back to the grandmother's house, as well as getting her mother's help in starting the business.

The following week, Jane and her mother both attended the session. Their change in comfort and affect with each other was very apparent. They made significantly more eye contact and physical contact and were able to laugh with each other. Jane was able to talk to her mother about her fear of being sent back to her grandmother's house. Tina listened to Jane and validated her feelings. Tina indicated that sending Jane to her grandmother's house was no longer an option because they were finally communicating. Additionally, Tina told Jane that there would be other consequences for misbehavior, rather than going to her grandmother's house. Once Jane indicated that she was feeling reassured and was satisfied with the discussion, the discussion shifted to Jane's desire to start a hair braiding business. Jane asked her mother for help in starting the business. Tina noted that she was proud of Jane for wanting to do hair and supported her in eventually going to trade school, but she also felt it was important for Jane to go to college to learn how to manage a business. Jane listened to her mother but did not commit to going to college during the conversation. Tina and Jane talked about how Tina could be helpful in assisting Jane in starting her hair business by making business cards and teaching her to become organized and maintain a budget.

Given the foundation of repaired trust from the Repairing Attachment Task, Jane and Tina were able to engage in these important conversations without any of their previous non-productive communication patterns. Jane was able to share her concerns with her mother, and Tina was able to empathically listen and respond. Additionally, Tina was able to help Jane start her own business, as well as express her desire for Jane to attend college. Tina was able to tolerate Jane's ambivalence about college without yelling or becoming argumentative. Both Tina and Jane attributed their new ability to communicate to having discussed the hard topics during the Repairing Attachment Task. Jane's ability to express what she needed from her mother, and Tina's desire to offer protection to her daughter, allowed for this new communication and rebuilding of trust. They both now possess the necessary skills to handle challenging events in the future.

Note

1 Names and identifying information have been changed to protect the identity of clients.

Further reading

Diamond, G. S, Diamond, G. M, & Levy, S. A. (2014). *Attachment-based family therapy for depressed adolescents*. Washington, DC: American Psychological Association Press.

References

Ainsworth, M. D. S. (1989). Attachment beyond infancy. *American Psychologist, 44,* 709–716.

Allen, J. P., Moore, C., Kuperminc, G., & Bell, K. (1998). Attachment and adolescent psychosocial functioning. *Child Development, 69*(5), 1406–1419.

Asarnow, J. R., Goldstein, M. J., Tompson, M., & Guthrie, D. (1993). One-year outcomes of depressive disorders in child psychiatric in-patients: Evaluation of the prognostic power of a brief measure of expressed emotion. *Journal of Child Psychology and Psychiatry, and Allied Disciplines, 34*(2), 129–137.

Boszormenyi-Nagy, I., & Spark, G. M. (1973). *Invisible loyalties: Reciprocity in intergenerational family therapy.* Oxford, England: Harper & Row.

Bowlby, J. (1969). Disruption of affectional bonds and its effects on behavior. *Canada's Mental Health Supplement, 59,* 12.

Cole, D. A. (1990). Relation of social and academic competence to depressive symptoms in childhood. *Journal of Abnormal Psychology, 99*(4), 422–429.

Coyne, J. C. (1976). Toward an interactional description of depression. *Psychiatry, 39*(1), 28–40.

Cummings, E. M., & Davies, P. (1994). *Children and marital conflict: The impact of family dispute and Resolution.* New York, NY: Guilford Press.

Diamond, G., Kodish, T., Ewing, E. S. K., Hunt, Q. A., & Russon, J. M. (2022). Family processes: Risk, protective and treatment factors for youth at risk for suicide. *Aggression and Violent Behavior, 64,* 101586. doi: 10.1016/j.avb.2021.101586

Diamond, G. S., Diamond, G., & Levy, S. (2021). Attachment-based family therapy: Theory, clinical model, outcomes, and process research. *Journal of Affective Disorders, 294,* 286–295. https://doi.org/10.1016/j.jad.2021.07.005

Diamond, G. S., Kobak, R. R., Krauthamer Ewing, E. S., Levy, S. A., Herres, J. L., Russon, J. M., & Gallop, R. J. (2019). A randomized controlled trial: Attachment-based family and nondirective supportive treatments for youth who are suicidal. *Journal of the American Academy of Child and Adolescent Psychiatry, 58*(7), 721–731.

Diamond, G. S., Reis, B. F., Diamond, G. M., Siqueland, L., & Isaacs, L. (2002). Attachment-based family therapy for depressed adolescents: A treatment development study. *Journal of the American Academy of Child and Adolescent Psychiatry, 41*(10), 1190–1196.

Diamond, G. S., Siqueland, S., & Diamond, G. M. (2003). Attachment-based family therapy for depressed adolescents: Programmatic treatment development. *Clinical Child and Family Psychology Review, 6*(2), 107–127.

Diamond, G. S., Wintersteen, M. B., Brown, G. K., Diamond, G. M., Gallop, R., Shelef, K., & Levy, S. (2010). Attachment-based family therapy for adolescents with suicidal ideation: A randomized controlled trial. *Journal of the American Academy of Child & Adolescent Psychiatry, 49*(2), 122–131.

Dumont, M., & Provost, M. A. (1999). Resilience in adolescents: Protective role of social support, coping strategies, self-esteem, and social activities on experience of stress and depression. *Journal of Youth and Adolescence, 28*(3), 343–363.

Ewing, E. S. K., Diamond, G., & Levy, S. (2015). Attachment-based family therapy for depressed and suicidal adolescents: Theory, clinical model and empirical support. *Attachment & Human Development, 17*(2), 136–156.

Gotlib, I. H., & Hammen, C. L. (1992). *Psychological aspects of depression: Toward a cognitive interpersonal integration.* Chichester, England; New York, NY: Wiley.

Gottman, J. M., Katz, L. F., & Hooven, C. (1996). Parental meta-emotion philosophy and the emotional life of families: Theoretical models and preliminary data. *Journal of Family Psychology, 10*(3), 243–268.

Greenberg, L. S. (1999). Attachment and psychopathology in childhood. In J. Cassidy, & P. R. Shaver (Eds.), *Handbook of attachment: Theory, research, and clinical applications* (pp. 469–496). New York, NY: Guilford Press.

Greenberg, L. S., & Johnson, S. M. (1988). *Emotionally focused therapy for couples.* New York, NY: Guilford Press.

Greenberg, M. T., Siegel, J. M., & Leitch, C. J. (1983). The nature and importance of attachment relationships to parents and peers during adolescence. *Journal of Youth and Adolescence, 12*(5), 373–386.

Grotevant, H. D., & Cooper, C. R. (Eds.). (1993). *Adolescent development in the family.* San Francisco, CA: Jossey-Bass.

Harris, T., Brown, G. W., & Bifulco, A. (1986). Loss of parent in childhood and adult psychiatric disorder: The role of lack of adequate parental care. *Psychological Medicine, 16*(3), 641–659.

Herman, J. L. (1992). *Trauma and recovery.* New York, NY: Basic Books, Inc.

Israel, P., & Diamond, G. S. (2013). Feasibility of Attachment Based Family Therapy for depressed clinic-referred Norwegian adolescents. *Clin Child Psychol Psychiatry. 18*(3), 334–350. doi: 10.1177/1359104512455811

Joiner, T. E., & Coyne, J. C. (1999). *The interactional nature of depression: Advances in interpersonal approaches.* Washington, DC: American Psychological Association.

Kobak, R., & Duemmler, S. (1994). Attachment and conversation: Toward a discourse analysis of adolescent and adult security. In D. Perlman & K. Bartholomew (Eds.), *Attachment processes in adulthood: Advances in personal relationships* (Vol. 5, pp. 121–149). Bristol, PA: Jessica Kingsley Publishers, Ltd.

Kobak, R., & Sceery, A. (1988). Attachment in late adolescence: Working models, affect regulation, and representations of self and others. *Child Development, 59,* 135–146.

Liddle, H. A. (2002). Multidimensional family therapy for adolescent cannabis users. *Cannabis youth treatment series, 5.* Rockville, MD: Center for Substance Abuse Treatment, Substance Abuse and Mental Health Services Administration.

Lynch, M., & Cicchetti, D. (1991). Patterns of relatedness in maltreated and nonmaltreated children: Connections among multiple representational models. *Development and Psychopathology, 3*(2), 207–226.

Maccoby, E., & Martin, J. (1983). Socialization in the context of the family: Parent-child interaction. In E. M. Hetherington & P. H. Musen (Eds.), *Handbook of child psychology: Vol. 4. Socialization, personality, and social development* (pp. 1–101). New York, NY: Wiley.

Minuchin, S. (1974). *Families & family therapy.* Oxford, England: Harvard University Press.

Rosenstein, D. S., & Horowitz, H. A. (1996). Adolescent attachment and psychopathology. *Journal of Consulting and Clinical Psychology, 64*(2), 244–253.

Rutter, M. (1984). Psychopathology and development: II. Childhood experiences and personality development. *Australian and New Zealand Journal of Psychiatry, 18*(4), 314–327.

Steinberg, L. (1990). Autonomy, conflict and harmony in the family relationships. In S. S. Feldman & G. R. Elliot (Eds.), *At the threshold: The developing adolescent* (pp. 255–276). Cambridge, MA: Harvard University Press.

Sund, A. M., & Wichsgtrom, L. (2002). Insecure attachment as a risk factor for future depressive symptoms in early adolescence. *Journal of the American Academy of Child & Adolescent Psychiatry, 41*(12), 1478–1485.

Weissman, M. M., & Paykel, E. S. (1974). *The depressed woman: A study of social relationships.* Chicago, IL: University of Chicago Press.

Chapter 8

Family Therapy with Adolescents

Key Ideas and Their Application

David Allan and Lyndal Power

Introduction

It is a common misconception that adolescence is a time of separation from parents. Certainly, it is a time when an adolescent's developmental tasks involve individuation and identity formation – a time when the self is transformed – but this does not mean separating from the family. While pushing away from adults is common, maintaining connection is crucial for navigating these years well (Siegel, 2014). Indeed, as adolescents develop into individuals, they need their parents more than ever to help them with this process. Family-based therapies may be effective interventions for many of the typical clinical problems adolescents experience, such as running away; depression and self-harm; school attendance; substance abuse; adolescent violence; and other anti-social behaviours (Bickerton, Hense, Benstock, Ward, & Wallace, 2007; Carey & Oxman, 2007; Carr, 2009, 2000; Cottrell & Boston, 2002; David-Ferdon & Kaslow, 2008; Diamond & Josephson, 2005; Henggeler & Schaeffer, 2010; Henggeler, Schoenwald, Borduin, Rowland, & Cunningham, 2009; Hogue & Liddle, 2009; Larner, 2009; Lebow, 2014; Liddle, 2010; Robinson & Pryor, 2006; Robinson, Power, & Allan, 2010).

Much of the material in this chapter was developed at RAPS Adolescent Family Therapy and Mediation Service, an Australian government funded program, located at Parramatta in Western Sydney. The program saw families with adolescents where there were problems that ranged from ordinary parent–teenager developmental conflict to more serious complex situations where young people were at risk of homelessness. Over the years, the authors found there are some general principles which seem relevant for all families and these are: maintaining connection; limit setting; and parental hierarchy; and, at the same time, there can be particular social circumstances needing to be taken into account such as: culture; family composition and gender identity.

This chapter discusses the reasons why family therapy is a useful vehicle for addressing adolescent problems. First, it considers the developmental requirements of adolescents and how these can be met optimally within the context of family. Second, attention is given to three practical problems unique to family therapy with adolescents: engaging adolescents in therapy; convening sessions with both adolescents and parents together; and dealing with dilemmas around confidentiality. Third, two areas are highlighted as particularly important to address: connection and limit setting. Many of the difficulties for adolescents originate here, and this chapter looks at how to remedy problems with these and ways of working with parents. Fourth, the chapter concludes with the application of these ideas to six common adolescent problems: adolescent aggression; substance abuse; school problems; depression and self-harm; and misuse of social media devices.

DOI: 10.4324/9781003490104-9

Developmental needs of adolescents

Why do adolescents still need their parents?

The onset of adolescence is marked by dramatic hormonal and synaptic changes for the brain, and changes caused by these take over a decade to complete (Gillespie, 2019). This allows more time to optimise adaptability; however, it also means that the capacities for impulse control and good decision-making take time to mature.

Adolescents begin to think differently from children. This is the result of dramatic rewiring in the brain where synaptic connections being used are strengthened, and those not being used are 'pruned'. The brain becomes more interconnected and specialised, and so it is optimised for its environment. However, different regions mature at different rates. The process starts at the back of the brain and rolls forward finishing with the prefrontal cortex (where cognition happens); and, at the same time, deep within the brain, change happens with the limbic system (where emotions originate). Significantly, the structures in the prefrontal cortex which are involved with judgement and emotional regulation mature slower than the structures in the limbic system which are involved with generating emotion – there is a developmental mismatch and the potential for problems managing behaviour.

Until a teenager's cognitive capabilities crystallise into the stable and flexible thinking of early adulthood, an adolescent's new sense of self is fragile. It is accompanied by a range of new and intense feeling states that are destabilising, and it is very difficult for adolescents to manage these changes by themselves. First, they need help with processing their new experience of the world. They need help with recognising and managing their new emotional states. Second, in the face of all the changes, adolescents need to feel that there is someone bigger and stronger than they are who can guide them through the process of growing up; and, if this happens, they will eventually internalise the capacity for emotional regulation in harmony with good decision-making and develop the capacity for self-regulation.

During adolescence, a teenager needs someone who can reliably meet these needs, who knows the teenager, and who can tolerate the sudden shifts that occur. While meeting these needs does not depend on the person's gender (Silverstein & Rashbaum, 1994), it is hard to replace the role of parents in this.[1]

The role of the person who is endeavouring to meet the developmental needs of an adolescent can be difficult. In order for an autonomous self to develop, an adolescent needs someone to push against: a benignly opposing other (Wolf, 1994). Parents of adolescents face a challenging situation. They must try to meet the needs of their teenagers who have limited control over their emotions and who, because of their emerging cognitive capacity, often think they know more than their parents. On top of this, parents need to continue reaching out to their adolescents, who may be actively pushing against them.

Does gender make a difference?

There can be significant differences in the brains of boys and girls but the structure does not seem to be as predetermined biologically as commonly thought (Rippon, 2019). Yes, there are differences, but socialisation around gender[2] can amplify small differences at birth into troublesome gaps through childhood and adolescence (Eliot, 2009). Socialisation amplifies gender differences and so interventions for behavioural problems may need to be different.

At birth there are small, but significant differences in the brains of girls and boys particularly around communication and affect.[3] In terms of communication, development of infant girls is a month ahead of boys and, with girls, Broca's area (the brain's motor area for speech) is more active. In terms of affect, with boys, the amygdala is larger, and in infancy, this makes boys more emotionally fragile and harder to settle. Small differences such as these can lead to different parenting responses whereby communication with girls can be easier and dealing with boys can be trickier. Positive feedback loops are created reinforced by social expectations around gender.

With the onset of adolescence, these differences magnify. Girls usually enter puberty a couple of years sooner than boys, so girls' brains mature before those of boys. On top of this, because brain regions mature at different rates, the developmental mismatch between emotion and thinking further amplifies differences (Blakemore, 2018). Into this mix are added hormones which initiate sexual behaviour and teenagers' increased preoccupation with their bodies which is 'a booster shot to gender intensification' (Eliot, 2009, p. 293).

In adolescence, maturing of the limbic system has different trajectories for boys and girls. For boys, in their brains, the amygdala continues to grow bigger compared with girls. Aside from activating fight-flight responses, the amygdala is an important area for sexual arousal and the hormones of puberty have a greater impact on males than females. As boys develop a new, intense interest in sex, their bodies grow bigger which gives them a new sense of power. This is commonly associated with increased self-esteem reinforced by gender stereotypes about masculinity. The growth of the amygdala also increases the appetite for sensation seeking and risk-taking (McKay, 2018). There is a positive bias towards emphasising the 'pros' of risks while de-emphasising the 'cons' (Siegel, 2014, p. 109). Decreased fear, interest in novelty, and impulsivity breathe new life into ways of doing things and this enables adolescents to challenge their brains with the kind of skills with which they may want to excel as an adult (Giedd, 2015). The developmental mismatch between hyperactivity of the amygdala of boys and the slower development of the prefrontal cortex results in heightened risk-taking without the capacity to evaluate consequences, and this can often be the basis of problems for adolescent boys.

For girls, earlier maturing of their physiology results in a further enhancement of emotional intelligence which means they can be better at perceiving what is happening for others – a good thing. However, this comes at the cost of lower assertiveness and discomfort with competition. A greater grasp of the interior space of others (viz., mentalising[4]) is accompanied by a greater sensitivity to how others perceive them. Recognition of the state of mind of others increases vulnerability to embarrassment and shame, and relationships assume greater importance (particularly to those in their cohort). The developmental mismatch between the hyperactivity of the limbic system of girls and the slower development of the prefrontal cortex results in heightened emotionality without the capacity to manage emotions (McKay, 2018), and this can often be the basis of problems for adolescent girls.

As girls and boys enter adolescence, carers need to take account of their different developmental trajectories where their needs and the capacity to relate are different. Girls are more likely to seek support from relationships, and they are often more likely to think things through by talking. Boys, by contrast, are more likely to become aggressive or withdraw and this is likely to inhibit relationship formation. Boys are more at risk of becoming isolated. Often the parent of the opposite sex to the teenager withdraws at the onset of puberty. Fathers may withdraw from their teenage daughters and can become more controlling as a reaction to their girls maturing physically. Mothers may pull back from their sons at adolescence out of fear of making them soft and may even guard against emotional expressiveness (Kindlon & Thompson, 2000; Silverstein & Rashbaum, 1994). The situation can be more fraught for boys than girls because the mother is often the primary attachment figure, and the father may be less able to compensate for the mother's withdrawal. If a father pulls back from his daughter, the mother is likely to be available, but there is more at stake with loss of connection for boys. Adolescent males' relationships with their parents are harder to sustain and the emotional realm is more difficult to access. Paradoxically, because adolescent females have greater acuity with relationships, they are likely to be more sensitive to breaches in connection with their parents.

Why is family therapy useful to help adolescents?

Adolescents need their parent(s) in two ways. First, they need someone who is attuned to them (someone who can help them process their new experience of the world); second, they need someone to be in control (someone who can guide them until they can internalise self-regulation). If a parent is not available to provide these two functions, then adolescents must seek other ways of managing developmental processes by themselves such as by forming inappropriate relationships, acting out,[5] substance abuse, or self-harm. Remedial work with adolescents usually falls into two broad areas: building connection and limit setting. Family therapy is an ideal vehicle for this, and the work usually involves either gaining an understanding of the adolescent–parent relationship and then working to repair disconnection, or else gaining an understanding of any difficulties parents may have setting limits and then helping them with this. Sometimes, therapy may involve addressing both areas.

In determining whether it is distress or limit testing that is underlying behaviour, it can be useful to ask family members for their perspectives. For example, if the young person has started running away, the therapist could ask, '*How much do you think your teenager's running away is about factors at home and feeling unhappy, and how much is it about factors outside home, such as wanting to be with friends?*' Whether it is because of loss of connection or because of a problem with limit setting, parents need to be encouraged to pursue their teenager, and family therapy may focus on obstacles to this and what needs to happen to be successful. For instance, pursuing an out-of-home teenager may mean physically looking for the young person even by driving around and turning up at places where their teenager usually visits. With problems with adolescents, parents need to be supported to remain persistent and to signal that they are not going to give up.

A further consideration is how individual dyads can be affected by the network of relationships in which they are embedded. A particular 'parent–adolescent' dyad may be influenced by the relationships a parent may have with other children, as well as the relationships an adolescent may have with other siblings, grandparents, and so forth. For example, it is not possible to get a full understanding of a mother–teenage daughter relationship without considering the effect that the birth of a new baby will have. The mother and daughter may draw closer as the daughter is enlisted as the mother's helper, or else the mother and daughter may drift apart as the mother becomes more focused on the infant. Either scenario may develop, and to get an adequate understanding of the mother–daughter relationship, it is important to explore the impact that this other relationship has. Parent–adolescent dyads exist in a web of family relationships that affect each other, and a family-based approach enables this to be considered.

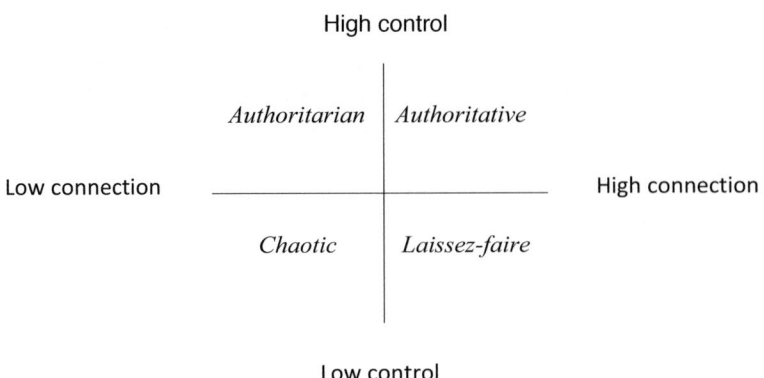

Figure 8.1 Baumrind's four types of parenting.

Within the web of family relationships, styles can be assessed in terms of 'connection' and 'control'. These dimensions are outlined in Figure 8.1. Therapy commonly involves helping each parent to work with the other as a united team to enhance one of these dimensions that may be underdeveloped. This may also involve helping parents understand how the legacy from their own past of their own experience of being parented may now be affecting the way they are parenting their children, and how the dynamics of other family relationships may be affecting their capacity to parent. Change is likely to be more enduring if parents are the ones who are positioned to meet their adolescents' needs, so therapists should take care to empower parents and be cautious of undermining or usurping their position.

Any form of relationship therapy needs to be able to conceptualise difficulties in relational terms and then disrupt dysfunctional relational patterns (Sprenkle, Davis, & Lebow, 2009). Effective family therapy with adolescents helps family members gain insight into what is happening in their relationships. This can be done by considering interactional behaviour patterns, and internal structures (such as coalitions and hierarchy), as well as understanding each person's experiences and beliefs, and the whole enterprise needs to be underpinned by a sound therapeutic alliance. The therapist has a clear goal: to move the parenting executive into the 'authoritative' quadrant of Baumrind's diagram, where a good balance is struck between connection and control (Baumrind cited in Henggeler, Schoenwald, Borduin, Rowland, & Cunningham, 2009, pp. 56–57; Baumrind, 1991).

This is a normative approach, where some family structures are viewed as better than others for adolescent development. So, therapeutic lenses that can conceptualise families in this way are particularly helpful. The structural model of family therapy is an especially useful way of seeing these families since it can take account of the dimensions of both connection and control. It provides a means of theorising about the family organisation, and its concepts of coalitions, triangles, boundaries, and hierarchies can help the therapist map the way the web of relationships operates. Also, simple behaviourist techniques that use rewards and consequences can be incorporated within the more sophisticated systemic framework that takes account of interactional patterns. These methods allow the therapist to view families in terms of underlying patterns and consequently see ways forward through what can often be chaotic and unsafe situations.

These approaches are useful in cross-cultural contexts, too. However, therapists need to be mindful of the drawback that cultural material can often lie outside the realm of awareness: things may seem to be a natural 'given', and stepping outside of conventional cultural situations involves engaging with what is outside awareness (Codrington, Iqbal, & Segal, 2012; Segal, 2010). For instance, a common problem pattern with migrant families occurs when adolescents from migrant families quickly embrace Western values of the new country to which they usually have more exposure than their parents; their parents in turn may cling to different (and often less liberal) values of their home country as a way of maintaining a sense of identity within the upheaval of migration. The scene is then set for harsh, critical interactions around beliefs and values. In situations like these, where parent–adolescent relationships are overlain by cross-cultural issues, a useful starting point can be to help the parties soften to more curious and more accepting positions by helping them gain greater understanding of the different experiences each has had. For example, the therapist could say, '*How do you think your experience of growing up in this country is different from that of your parents?*' Parents can then be asked to talk about how parenting in the new country is different from the way it was done in their homeland. Helping parents and adolescents talk about their different experiences, of which they may be unaware, can be a useful first step in fostering greater compassion towards each other, before then deploying more conventional strategies for addressing parent–adolescent issues.

Who should attend

Many therapists are understandably apprehensive about seeing adolescents and parents together in the same room. Therapists can fear that they will lose control of the session, resulting in a teenager and parents yelling at each other. Parents, on the other hand, find it hard to understand why they need to attend, because they see the problem as located in their teenager. Nevertheless, to understand an adolescent's behaviour in terms of the family system and the web of relationships, it is useful to get as many family members from the household as possible to attend the first session. It can be helpful to give parents the rationale that it is important to understand how everyone experiences the problem. However, if the adolescent who is the source of concern fails to attend, then it is still possible to proceed with just the parents, because they are likely to be the most important site for promoting change.

Therapists' fears that they will lose control of a session are well founded, and the first goal is to create a secure, containing environment by establishing structure around the session. For example, the therapist could say, '*I want to understand how each of you sees things, so it is going to be important that we speak one at a time*' or '*One at a time … I want to finish hearing your mum; I'll come to you*'. In families with adolescents, bickering can quickly escalate to more serious emotionally charged conflict. Ensuring that family members talk to the therapist rather than to each other can short-circuit this. For example, the therapist could say, '*Speak to me; tell me what you are most upset about*'. If someone is becoming uncontained, another strategy is to ask other family members about that person. For example, the therapist could say, '*What do you think your mum is most worried about?*' This shifts the conversation to another family member while still acknowledging the material of the uncontained person, and it creates a more reflective, but still empathic discussion.

Confidentiality

Before therapy starts, it is prudent to inform family members about the limits of confidentiality without unnecessarily alarming them. There are three areas to keep in mind. First, there are statutory responsibilities that the therapist needs to consider. Then there is the general effect of any secrets within the family that the therapist is being asked to hold. Finally, there are ethical considerations around parents' right to know about their children.

Like other therapists, family therapists have a statutory obligation to report children who are at risk of abuse to child protection agencies. From an ethical perspective, parents have a right to know the consequences of any disclosures during therapy; from a practical point of view, this reduces the damage to the therapeutic alliance if it turns out that a report needs to be made but parents were ignorant of this possibility. On the other hand, giving undue prominence to this makes families guarded in what they say, and it should not overshadow an assurance that, with this one exception, the usual ethical framework of confidentiality operates. For example, the therapist could say, '*Everything you say is confidential. Of course, if there are concerns someone is at risk of harm, we may need to get other services involved to help families be safe*'.

In general, any secrets within families need to be examined from the perspective of how they function. They can be powerful ways of forming coalitions, and therapists need to ask themselves what purpose a particular secret serves. In some cases, it may be important to preserve the secret, but in others it may be part of the problem. Therapists need to be especially cautious around being invited into a secret themselves. To be sworn to secrecy places the therapist in a covert alliance. The therapist needs to consider how this will affect the progress of therapy and may reserve the right not to be bound by it. For example, the therapist could say, '*Before you tell me, I think you can understand that, without my knowing beforehand what the secret is, I can't automatically guarantee that I can keep your confidence. First, let's talk about how you think it would affect other family members if they knew*'.

Since parents have the responsibility for the care and development of their children, they have the right to know about things that, from their perspective, affect the performance of this responsibility, especially when it comes to protecting their adolescent from harm. This principle should not be followed mindlessly, and it needs to be tempered by other considerations, such as the age of the adolescent and the consequences of the parents knowing or not knowing. If a therapist decides in an individual session with an adolescent that there is information the parents should know about their teenager, then the therapist needs to take the position of exploring with the teenager how the parents can be told. For example, the therapist could say, '*How are we going to tell your parents that you are smoking marijuana?*' Then the various options for telling the parents and also their anticipated responses can be explored. If the outcome seems uncertain, the therapist may decide to have a session separately with the parents to prepare them for what their adolescent is going to try to tell them and coach them about the best way to react. The process can then become an opportunity to enhance communication and trust.

Considerations for a family session with an adolescent

Therapy with families of adolescents follows the usual generic format which is set out in detail in Chapter 2. But how to join with adolescents? They are often more self-conscious than children, and less socially adept than adults, and they are usually suspicious of what is going to happen in therapy because they have been identified as the reason the family has come. Joining first with the parents, then each child in birth order, helps to take the spotlight off the adolescent. Just as with other family members, joining with adolescents involves looking for entry points into their subjective world. Open, neutral questions allow adolescents to define their own experience, so they are more useful than closed questions for which the answer is circumscribed. For example, the therapist could say, '*What is your school like?*' which is an open question that allows for a range of responses, and it is better than using a leading question such as, 'What do you like about school?' It is also useful to use the teenager's language. Thus, if an adolescent said, 'School sucks', the therapist could say, 'What 'sucks' about school?' All the while, the therapist is seeking areas where adolescents come alive and where there is energy, which is when adolescents are likely to become involved in a session in spite of their inhibitions.

If, after several attempts, an adolescent is still not responsive, it is better not to persist with something that could result in the activity of talking itself becoming an area of contention. Instead, in order to appear undaunted by what the adolescent does, the therapist could ask other members about the adolescent and then move on. For example, the therapist could say, '*What would you say your son enjoys doing most?*' And sometimes, if the conversation is about them, teenagers cannot resist interjecting in spite of themselves. However, if the therapist has not been successful in joining with an adolescent, he or she should remain alert for future opportunities to get the adolescent talking and involved in the process.

After joining with the family, the therapist asks about the problem by asking each person in turn to say what his or her concerns are. Often adolescents find it hard to respond to this and, if this happens, a useful strategy can be to ask them, '*If you were worried, would you be worried about something at home or school?*' The therapist needs to unpack the teenager's response by asking further questions. If an answer is not forthcoming, then the therapist could ask, '*Who in your family most knows what you are worried about?*', and then the therapist asks that person. No matter what adolescent problem is presented, getting a detailed, interactional, behavioural sequence is the best way to get a clear picture of what happens and who are the participants. So, after getting each person's concerns, the therapist asks family members to describe a recent upset in order to get a typical sequence.

Essential tasks for adolescent family therapy

Enhancing relationships through connection and attunement

Behaviour problems may mask a breach in relationships because adolescents are often unable to put into words what they are experiencing, so they express themselves by 'acting out', and families may become focused on problem behaviours when what is really required is that the adolescent be helped to formulate her or his experience (Stern, 2019) especially in terms of emotional regulation.[6] Typically, there can be a disjunction that escalates as an adolescent reacts to a relationship rupture by acting out her or his distress through problem behaviours, and then retaliatory actions by parents amplify an already fraught situation. On top of this, failure to respond to an adolescent's strong emotions can activate feelings of shame – 'the core affect of early adolescence' (Schave & Schave, 1989), and this is an isolating emotion that can lead to the withdrawal of adolescents or increased aggression at a time when they may most need connection and help making sense of what they are feeling. Therapists can assess in which sector to locate parents on Baumrind's four types of parenting grid (Figure 8.1) by getting an interactional sequence. If the parenting is situated towards the 'authoritarian' or 'chaotic' areas, then it is likely that the parent–adolescent relationship may need attention. Rebuilding connection involves, first, helping parents accept that disconnection is a problem and, second, providing ways to rebuild the connection.

In the first step of helping parents accept that disconnection may be the source of a problem, three useful techniques are: (a) the establishment of a relationship discourse; (b) the use of circular questions; and (c) the tracking of the evolution of problems over time in terms of relationships.

The establishment of a relationship discourse[7] means locating presenting problems in a relationship context. This means exploring the network of relationships in a family so that family members begin to see problems in terms of relationships. Discussion of relationships gives a new context and hence a new meaning to presenting problems. For instance, running-away behaviour commonly occurs after an argument, so parents usually focus on behaviours that led to the argument; however, the argument is often the consequence of an adolescent not feeling important or not close. If parents can be helped to understand this, then their adolescent is no longer seen as unmanageable but, instead, as 'on the outer': the teenager is no longer seen as bad but, instead, as sad. It is then a logical step for parents to see that change does not hinge on punitive action but on reconnection.

Circular questions can be powerful tools for establishing the link between behaviours and what is happening in relationships. There is a crucial shift in conceptualisation that makes it 'circular' which is that a circular question is aimed at discovering previously unrecognised patterns between various aspects of the system so that family members gain a new understanding of the circular nature of things; that is to say, how A affects B, and the output of B then circles back to affect A. To do this, it is usually more useful to start broadly with open questions, and then make these more concrete by seeking more exact information using closed (forced choice) questions, and even scaling questions. For example, in establishing a link between the state of a parent–adolescent relationship and an adolescent's behaviour, a therapist could ask a parent, '*How would you describe your partner's relationship with your teenager?*' The therapist could then encourage the parent to expand on this answer to get a fuller description. Then the therapist could ask a scaling question, '*On a scale of 1 to 10 (with 10 meaning close and with 1 meaning distant), where would you put your partner's relationship with your teenager?*' Having elicited this exact information, it is then possible to draw a link, that is to say, reveal a circular pattern between what is happening in the parent–adolescent relationship and other features of the system, such as, in this instance, 'behaviour', by asking a question such as, '*If your partner were to spend more time with your teenager, what difference do you think that would make to their relationship?*' followed by, '*What effect do you think that would have on your teenager's behaviour?*' In this way, a previously unrecognised link can be made between the adolescent's behaviour and the parent–adolescent relationship.

Tracking the history of how problems evolved over time in terms of relationships can also be helpful. Lynn Hoffman (1982) used the metaphor of a thick cable to imagine this history. The longitudinal dimension (lengthwise part) of the cable represents the flow of time from the past to the present. A cross section at any point along the cable reveals the web of relationships at those particular points in time. Different patterns of relationships occur at different slices along the length of the cable as they evolve over time from the past to the present. The therapist looks out for so-called nodal points, where the pattern of relationships may have altered noticeably.

Life cycle events, such as births, deaths, or children leaving home, are predictable nodal points where the pattern of relationships is likely to change, and there are also contingent ones such as accidents, changes in jobs, and so forth. Obviously, nodal points that correspond with the onset of a presenting problem are of particular interest. Nodal points can be detected by simple, open questions. For example, the therapist can ask, '*Can you remember a time when things were different?*' or '*What was it like then?*' Locating nodal points helps family members gain a new understanding of the way problems have developed in terms of how events have affected relationships, and then also how new behaviours (and perhaps new problems) have evolved because of these realignments in relationships.

Once the first step is accomplished of helping parents accept that disconnection may be an issue that needs to be addressed, the next step is to equip them with ways to rebuild connection with their teenager. To do this, three useful techniques are: (a) one-to-one time; (b) coaching parents with communication and attunement; and (c) physical contact.

Prescribing one-to-one time between an adolescent and a parent can be surprisingly effective in defrosting relationships, particularly if an adolescent is feeling on the outer. However, it is easy to underestimate the difficulties for both parents and adolescents with undertaking this when it is set as a task. Both are likely to feel bruised from past hurts, and the therapist needs to explore possible restraints and anticipate problems. To do this, the therapist can ask, '*How do you think your adolescent will react to this?*' Typically, parents may feel awkward and fear rejection, while adolescents may feel suspicious and fear their parents' withdrawal. Parents need to take the first step, and they may need to be coached about how they will cope if their adolescent is rejecting. They need to be encouraged to find ways of reaching out again (and again, if necessary). It can help the therapist to predict possible rejection and frame it as the adolescent's way of testing a parent's commitment. The task of having one-to-one time is better if it is short and frequent. For example, asking teenagers about their day is better than the one-to-one time that is of long duration, but happens only intermittently. One-to-one time should not involve other family members, and it is better if it is set up to fit with the teenager's interests. Just as with any between-session task, even if the task has not been completed, subsequent exploration of what happened can be an opportunity to get a better understanding of what restraints might be operating.

A second technique for rebuilding relationships is to coach parents around communication and attunement and undertake enactments.[8] Coaching can be set up between parents and adolescents; or between teenagers and siblings; or between parents. Enacting this in session can bring about changes in parent–adolescent relationships, not only by improving the communication process but also by allowing significant new material to be discussed. The therapist asks the participants to talk together about a particular topic or an area of disagreement, and the therapist observes the process and looks for blocks to good communication and attunement.

One useful typology of unhelpful communication patterns has been outlined by John Gottman (Gottman, 1999; Gottman & Silver, 1997), who has detected four especially harmful behaviours that predict relationship breakdown: the so-called 'four horsemen of the apocalypse'. Outlined in Table 8.1, they are criticism, defensiveness, contempt, and stonewalling. A format for an enactment around communication is the following. The therapist explains the 'four horsemen', and then asks the participants to write down how

Table 8.1 John Gottman's 'four horsemen'

Behaviour	Definition	Example	Antidote
Criticism	Any statement that attacks the character or personality of the other	Phrases that begin with 'You never ...' or 'You always ...' are indicators of criticism	Raise a complaint by making a specific statement about behaviour rather than the person
Defensiveness	Attempts to defend oneself from a perceived attack by denying responsibility, making excuses, or meeting one complaint with another	Phrases that begin with 'It wasn't my fault' or 'It was your fault' or 'Well, you don't listen to me either' or 'I couldn't help it' are indicators of defensiveness	Take responsibility: make space to hear and acknowledge what the other person is saying
Contempt	Verbal or nonverbal expression of superiority: a step up from criticising; it involves tearing down or insulting the other person	Rolling one's eyes or calling names or tearing down the other person with sarcastic humour are indicators of contempt	Develop a culture of respect
Stonewalling	Refusing to communicate when conflict arises	Not responding or leaving the conversation are indicators of stonewalling	Calm down, self-soothe, and later come back to the conversation

they would rate themselves out of 10 with respect to how much they think they use each of the four horsemen in disagreements, then also rate how the other person uses them. Each person then listens to what the other wrote, and the therapist gives information about what to do instead of these behaviours: the so-called 'antidotes'. After asking family members for permission to pull them up if any of the four horsemen appear, the therapist directs the participants to talk together about a particular issue and monitors the communication. For example, the therapist could say, 'You're coming across as a bit critical; is that your intention?' and the participants resume talking, trying to use the antidote.

Another exercise that assists communication when the emphasis is on the expression of feelings is an adaptation of the Imago dialogue developed by Harville Hendrix (1988). This variation facilitates the expression of feelings and empathic responsiveness so it can be particularly helpful in coaching parents to help their teenager formulate and regulate feelings. It can be useful to have the steps written down, and usually the person who has the most distressing issue goes first as the speaker (often the teenager). The teenager is directed to talk to the parent about an issue that is distressing. The therapist waits until the teenager has said about a paragraph's worth of content, then the parent is asked to paraphrase what the teenager said. If the parent starts replying to the teenager, the therapist reminds the parent that there will be an opportunity to be the speaker once the teenager has finished. The therapist also needs to monitor carefully that listeners do not start interpreting what was said rather than paraphrasing. If this happens, the therapist can say something like,

'*I don't think your teenager said that. Try again. Use your teenager's words*'. The next step is that the parent validates the teenager by saying, '*I can understand that*', and then the parent responds empathically by saying, '*You must be feeling …*', and the therapist encourages the parent to use one or two words to identify what the teenager might be feeling, after which the parent checks, '*Is this right?*' If not, the therapist encourages the parent to have another attempt. Once the parent has captured what the teenager is feeling, the parent then resumes by saying, '*Tell me more*', and the teenager says another paragraph about the same issue. When the teenager has exhausted what needs to be said, the teenager and parent swap roles. This exercise is particularly useful where there are strong, unexpressed emotions and, since the process makes both parties vulnerable, it is also likely to enhance intimacy and increase attachment security (James, 2007).

Intense emotional surges are a hallmark feature of adolescence but, because of the different rates of development of parts of adolescent brains, emotional regulation is difficult. In adolescents, emotions arise rapidly without the capacity to make sense of them. Adolescents need help managing intense emotional upwellings and parents can provide this. Dealing with sudden, intense emotions of an adolescent can be a daunting prospect for parents; however, these moments are valuable opportunities to help adolescents learn how to regulate themselves. When intense emotions erupt, adolescents need to learn to recognise them and manage them; just like strengthening a muscle group, it takes time and practice to develop the faculty of self-regulation.

The challenge for adolescents is to learn how to make sense of the new ways their brains apprehend the world and then manage this. They need to learn how to formulate experience and then learn how to 'respond' instead of mindlessly 'reacting' – in other words, they need to recognise how they think and feel about thinking and feeling (Allen & Fonagy in Hill, 2015, pp. 106–109).

Because of the different trajectories of development of girls' and boys' brains, adolescent girls are more likely to need help managing their emotions and help with cultivating assertiveness, while adolescent boys are more likely to need help recognising emotions and cultivating empathy. Parents are more likely to need support helping their daughter with strategies for managing emotions, while with adolescent boys, parents are more likely to need support helping their son around the recognition of emotional states.

A third technique for rebuilding relationships is physical contact. Adolescents often receive less physical contact with their parents than younger children, but touch remains an important way of connecting (Biddulph & Biddulph, 2003). Therapists need to point this out and encourage parents to explore ways of maintaining physical contact with their adolescent. It is difficult to underestimate the beneficial impact of a caring touch from a parent when an adolescent is feeling upset and isolated. It means that, notwithstanding whatever upset has happened, a parent still wants to keep connected – literally.

Setting limits for adolescents

Parents have a crucial role in setting limits for their teenagers because, although teenagers may appear to be physically mature, their brains are still immature and developing. They are not yet able to make good decisions such as, 'I should get off the couch and work on my assignment before seeing friends'. Adolescents still need an adult to guide them until they are able to internalise this and self-regulate. Furthermore, adolescents have lower motivation than adults, they take shortcuts and look for highly stimulating activities (Siegel,

2014), and it is unrealistic to expect teenagers to do uninteresting activities such as chores and homework of their own volition. Therapists can use brain research to explain to parents why teenagers are not motivated to do these activities, and why parents need to assist teenagers with such tasks.

During the dramatic changes of adolescence, limits provide a sense of structure and create a feeling of stability and predictability – they provide security. When adolescents' lives are organised into a good structure, many problems fall away. If families are encountering problems with structure, therapists can help by mapping the family's daily routine on a whiteboard, and these details can then be used to detect any problems with structure. For example, problems getting teenagers up in the morning are often linked to teenagers staying up late the previous night, so getting teenagers up in the morning depends on the effort made to get them to bed the night before.[9]

As a way of setting up good routines, the maxim 'work first then reward' can be a useful guide for parents. Thus, before computer time a teenager needs to finish homework, or before watching television a teenager needs to complete chores. Getting a teenager to do homework or chores involves work on the parents' part. In fact, getting a teenager to do a chore is usually more work for parents than doing the chore themselves. In order to see this activity as worthwhile, the therapist may need to locate it within the bigger scheme of things, which is that parents are teaching their adolescents important life skills to help them become responsible adults.

When coaching parents around setting limits, the following principles apply. Parents should show teenagers that they are setting limits out of caring for their teenagers rather than trying to be punitive. Unreasonable consequences can damage the parent–adolescent relationship, so any consequences should be in proportion to the misbehaviour. Consequences of long duration can be counterproductive: the link to the misbehaviour becomes attenuated and time breeds damaging resentment. Limits need to be developmentally appropriate; for example, with parties, parents of younger adolescents should check whether there will be parental supervision, whereas parents of older adolescents should have conversations with their teenagers about how they will keep safe. Compliance can be an opportunity for a teenager to earn trust, so taking care with setting limits can be an opportunity to enhance parent–adolescent relationships.

Developing an effective parenting team

From a developmental perspective, if adolescents still need their parents to guide them, then the best arrangement is when parents can work together as a team. This is more straightforward when parents have shared goals for their teenagers and there is goodwill between the parents. If the parenting team is not working well, this may need to be one of the first areas to address in family therapy with adolescents. 'Not working well as a parenting team' can range from minor issues, such as a parent saying yes to his or her teenager without thinking to check with the other parent, through to more serious problems, such as a parent deliberately undermining the other parent. Parents who are disaffected with their partner may side with the teenager rather than uniting with the other parent. Such cross-generational coalitions are particularly harmful; teenagers can become symptomatic,[10] and it can be very difficult to get teenagers on track. These more extreme situations may require couple therapy delivered under the guise of helping the two adults form a more effective parenting team.[11]

To ascertain the nature of the parenting team, in family sessions children and teenagers can be asked questions about how they see their parents working as a team. It is usually better to ask children before asking parents, as this may reveal new information to the parents and be an intervention in itself. For example, a therapist could ask each child, starting with the oldest, '*How would you rate your parents working as a parenting team, if 10 means working well as a team and 0 means not working well as a team (that is, they pull in different directions)?*' Therapists then ask further questions to unpack their answers. For example, the therapist could say, '*You said, they are a 4/10 as a parenting team, what do they do that tells you this?*' Asking children to comment on their parents' behaviour can be confronting for parents, and parents need also to be asked their points of view so that engagement is maintained. When there are difficulties with limit setting, another way of asking about the parenting team is to ask children how they rate the firmness or softness of each of their parents in terms of discipline. For example, the therapist could say, '*If 10 means firm (what they say they mean) and 0 means soft (you can get them to back down), how firm is your father?*' Once each child has answered, this same question can then be asked about the other parent. Parents are also given the opportunity to comment on how firm or soft they see each other and themselves. If there is a discrepancy, therapy involves understanding the restraints that may be operating with each parent before coaching each to become more aligned.

To help parents work better as a team, one useful strategy can be to meet with the parent subsystem in a separate strategy session. This becomes a brainstorming session, where parents are asked to list the problem behaviours of their adolescent and prioritise which one they want to tackle first. Once parents have agreed on the behaviour they want to tackle, the therapist asks the parents to talk to each other to come up with a plan for how they will address this behaviour. At this point, there is a risk that the parents may talk to the therapist rather than with each other, and the therapist should direct them back to each other. After a while, any problems with the couple's communication patterns are likely to become apparent.

Three typical problems are: one parent dominates the discussion; or both parents do not express their points of view in order to avoid conflict; or both parents argue and are not able to reach an agreement. In the first case, if a parent is dominating the discussion, the therapist can ask this parent to check if the other parent agrees, and then the therapist can ask the parent who is dominating to find out the other's opinion. On the other hand, if both seem to be not expressing what they really think in order to avoid conflict, the therapist keeps the parents in the process long enough for differences to emerge. In the third situation, if parents become embroiled in an escalating conflict, the therapist may focus on the common ground upon which they do agree even if the details differ. In general, with these sorts of discussions, the actual agreement that parents develop is of less importance than the fact that a united position is reached.

Not all families fit neatly within the traditional Western mould of a nuclear family. An adolescent may be in a family with a single parent; or be in a blended family with a step-parent; or in a family with a parent in a same-sex relationship; or a family where children were adopted; or in some other kinship arrangement with adults who have a parent role. Each configuration introduces unique challenges to more standard family therapy approaches.

Single parent families have the advantage of not having to consider two parents' perspectives; however, a disadvantage is that a single parent is a scarce resource where juggling being a parent with other commitments can be exhausting and there is a vulnerability around letting things slide. Aside from figuring out how to manage being a scarce resource, considering mobilising who may be available to form a support network (extended family, friends, etc.) can be helpful although this may bring with it wider system complexities (Imber-Black, 1988).

With a blended family where there is a stepparent, depending on when the stepparent came into the adolescent's life, there may be problematic dynamics. If it was early, then the young person may give authority to the stepparent as if to a parent. However, if the stepparent is a recent arrival in the family, care needs to be taken assessing changes in relationships around the nodal point of the stepparent's arrival. For instance, the young person may have formed a companionable relationship with the biological parent which the stepparent may be disrupting and the young person may feel resentful about being displaced. Alternatively, the biological parent's attention may be captured by the new partner and the parenting framework may be destabilised. Typically, the adolescent will be presented as the identified problem when what the young person is doing is an artifact of changes in family structure.

With a family where there is a parent in a same-sex relationship, as a young person enters puberty the young person can think differently,[12] and depending on when the non-biological parent enters the young person's life, there are similar dynamics to those that operate with a blended family, but any problematic dynamics may be compounded by cultural attitudes to same-sex relationships.

With a family where the young person was adopted, once again, the time in a young person's life when the young person was adopted makes a difference, and if the young person was adopted as an infant, the young person is more likely to relate to the adoptive parents as parents. However, with adoptive parents and adoptees the importance of belonging colours everything. At adolescence, a young person may challenge parents by saying things like, 'You're not my real parents' and a family therapist may be able to coach parents to respond positively to this in ways that reinforce a young person's sense of belonging. For adoptees, there can sometimes be an underlying doubt about feeling worthwhile[13] and adoptive parents may try to compensate for an unusual background by being soft. Being aware of this sort of dynamic and creating a space in which to discuss this in a family therapy session can take account of this.

Abuse by a parent

Abuse by parents can vary from overt physical behaviour, such as hitting, slapping, and pushing, to more subtle forms of abuse that are non-physical. The causes may range from conflict that has not been managed well to parents being abusive because of their own experiences in their family of origin.

In the case of physical abuse (rather than non-physical abuse), sometimes parents speak openly about using physical abuse, and at other times it is more hidden. It is important to get a sequence of an incident of conflict, and therapists need to be alert to when the description becomes vague because family members may be uncomfortable talking about this; the therapist may need to persist with seeking details and even ask straight out, 'Did things get physical?' In general, it is better to ask one person about another's behaviour because this is likely to produce more accurate information than if someone tries to give an objective account of her or his own behaviour. However, in situations where family members may feel intimidated, the therapist needs to be mindful of the possibility of reprisals after the session. To avoid this, the therapist should directly ask the person who has used abusive behaviour to describe it.

It is less easy to recognise non-physical abuse. It can sometimes be hard to discriminate between heated conflicts and when situations have become abusive. One way of distinguishing if the behaviour is abusive is to consider the frequency of the behaviour, the intention, and the effect. If the behaviour is perceived as intending to cause emotional hurt by diminishing the dignity of a person, it can be classed as verbal abuse. If this occurs over a lengthy period of time within an attachment relationship (that is, a relationship that involves dependence), then a person's emotional development can be affected, and this is better conceptualised as emotional abuse. Where the non-physical abuse results in an erosion of the target person's sense of self, then this has caused psychological injury and, as such, it is categorised psychological abuse (James & MacKinnon, 2010). The effects of non-physical abuse on the fragile, emerging self of an adolescent can be catastrophic. The effects can be long-lasting, erode self-esteem, cause depression, and lead to self-harming behaviours and a diminished sense of self.

Therapists are more likely to become aware of non-physical abuse by attending to the interaction between people in the session and staying alert to the following: hostility in tone; criticism; verbal and nonverbal signs of contempt; threats of abandonment; invalidation of the other's feelings, thoughts, and perspectives; the symptomatic person's withdrawal, confusion, and submission to the other's implicit or explicit put-downs; and finally, the differential effects of the upsetting or conflictual episode on the functioning of those involved (James & MacKinnon, 2010).

The goal in addressing all forms of abuse (be it physical or non-physical) is to gain a commitment from parents not to use these behaviours. Parents often reach for physically and verbally abusive behaviours with teenagers when they feel most powerless. Because these behaviours usually do not gain the cooperation they seek, parents often end up feeling even more powerless. The therapist looks for what motivates parents to change their behaviour; in other words, the therapist looks for leverage. One of the most effective ways of doing this is to draw a distinction between the intention and the actual effect of the abusive behaviour. This can be done when getting the sequence. For example, the therapist could say, '*When you hit your teenager, what were you hoping would happen?*' Frequently, parents say that they hit to stop their adolescents from being disrespectful.

Therapists can then explore the actual effect of the parent's abusive behaviour on the parent–adolescent relationship, and this is usually different from what they had intended. For example, the therapist could ask, '*What effect has hitting your teenager had on your relationship?*' If other family members are also asked, there is usually a confirmation of the negative effects. Releasing information about the effect of the parents' abusive behaviour can often motivate parents to change.

To confront parents around any behaviour, it is usually best for the therapist to meet with the parents without their children present since this is likely to be less embarrassing for them and so improves the chances of maintaining engagement. The therapist begins by empathising with the parent's frustration, while reiterating how the behaviour has not achieved the effect that was sought, and highlighting the unintended, negative effects on the parent–adolescent relationship. The therapist then asks the parent to make a commitment not to use these behaviours again. If this occurs, the children are then asked to come back into the session to hear the parent's commitment.

In a small minority of cases, the abusive behaviour may be quite ingrained and may be difficult to change without undertaking long-term individual therapy that addresses this behaviour. In these cases, the time frame for this may be too long given the urgency for repairing the parent–adolescent relationship. These teenagers often end up residing with the other parent or attached to other families. In this particular area of work, if things feel intractable, it is crucial to have good supervision from someone who can cast an experienced eye over the family interactions through live supervision or recordings, and who is able to recognise what change is (or is not) possible.

Strategies for serious adolescent problems

Adolescent aggression

Understanding adolescent aggression and addressing it is a priority for therapists because parents will not be able to set limits and change other adolescent behaviours if they feel frightened. In doing this, a distinction needs to be drawn between aggression that is expressive and aggression that is instrumental, as the interventions for each are different. Adolescent aggression can be regarded as expressive when the behaviour is a vehicle for the release of pent-up emotions; for example, if an adolescent were to throw down a school bag after a bad day. On the other hand, aggressive behaviour is seen as instrumental when the behaviour is used as a means to an end; for example, if an adolescent were to say, 'Give me ten dollars or I'll slash the tyres of your car'. Expressive and instrumental aggression can be either verbal or physical.

An effective way of assessing the nature of aggressive behaviour is to obtain an interactional, behavioural sequence using the techniques outlined in previous chapters. By asking about participants' thoughts and feelings associated with particular behaviours in the sequence, the therapist can determine whether the adolescent's aggression is expressive or instrumental. It is also important to recognise if what may have been expressive behaviour in the past is starting to shift to become instrumental as an adolescent becomes bigger during the growth spurt of puberty and has the potential to become intimidating.

In the case of expressive aggression, parents have a crucial role to play in helping their teenagers learn to manage difficult emotions and helping them to develop better ways of expressing feelings. To do this, parents need to know how to mirror, validate, and label the emotions of their adolescent (Gottman & DeClaire, 1997; Hendrix & LaKelly Hunt, 1997), and useful frameworks for doing this are the coaching techniques used in enactments and the Imago dialogue. The whole project of parents helping their adolescent regulate emotions can become an opportunity for parents to ally with their adolescent and build greater connection.

Parents also need to model to their teenagers how to deal with anger by demonstrating how they manage their own angry feelings. This is through parents using an appropriate tone of voice, taking a break from the teenager to calm down, and apologising to him or her if their own behaviour has been unacceptable. Work with parents may also involve helping parents identify the buttons that their teenager pushes and coaching him or her not to be reactive when this happens (Sells, 2004).[14] Rather than parents lecturing teenagers about this, it is usually more effective to ask parents to reflect on their behaviours and then offer ideas. For example, the therapist could say, '*What do you want to teach your teenager about managing angry feelings?*'

With instrumental aggression, it is important for parents not to reinforce these behaviours by allowing them to work for the adolescent. Parents need to affirm their teenagers' appropriate attempts to get what they want through asking rather than demanding. If teenagers have used aggression on parents or siblings, parents can set consequences such as removal of a phone, television, or computer time or withholding pocket money. Parents may also need to show teenagers that there are relationship consequences to their abusive behaviour by, for instance, withdrawing things they would normally do for their teenager, such as cooking or giving lifts.

It is important to establish a strong therapeutic alliance with the parent subsystem, and parents need to be able to draw confidence from the therapist. This can be fostered by the therapist helping parents to anticipate their adolescent's reactions to limit setting, and brainstorming with parents on how they can react to their adolescent's reactions, even to the point of calling the police. Many parents are understandably reluctant to take this last course of action, and it is important to take the time to explore the restraints that might be operating around this. These may range from fear that the parent–adolescent relationship might be damaged to worries that the adolescent may get a criminal record.[15] It can often be helpful to frame calling the police as a caring act. Once parents feel they can draw on this ultimate sanction, they are likely to act more confidently and decisively with their adolescent. With parents who are particularly disempowered – for instance, some sole mothers – the therapist may need to bolster them by setting up a meeting with the police and then accompany the parent(s) to this.

Parents' beliefs often restrain them from setting limits on their teenagers. To set limits on a teenager, parents need to be able to tolerate their teenager's anger, and therapists may need to work with parents (without their teenager present) to explore these restraints. For instance, restraints may arise from parents feeling guilty; or from having experienced harsh parents themselves; or from wanting their teenager to like them. One way of uncovering restraints is to ask what parents imagine might happen if they set limits. For example, the therapist could ask, '*If you were to become firmer, what do you think would happen?*' or '*If you were to become firmer, how do you think it would affect your relationship with your teenager?*' Once these restraints have been uncovered, they can be countered by asking parents to envisage the future if they do not take action now. For example, the therapist could ask, '*What do you think will happen if your teenager continues in the way your teenager is behaving?*', '*Is it more likely that your teenager will grow out of it; or is it more likely that you will need to act to get your teenager on the right track?*', or '*If you don't act now, do you think it will be easier or harder to help your teenager change in the future?*'

A significant proportion of young people (25%; Howard, 2008) have witnessed domestic violence against their mother from a father figure. In such cases, disrespect of the mother has been modelled by the father figure, and this makes it difficult for these mothers to assume a position of hierarchy with their teenager. As well as this, trauma from an attachment figure can compromise the capacity of an adolescent to regulate emotion and deal with distress (Kinniburgh, Blaustein, Spinazzola, & van der Kolk, 2005; van der Kolk, 2006). While not all teenagers who witness domestic violence grow up to be aggressive, many of these teenagers will have greater difficulty managing emotions and may need additional help from their parents to regulate their feelings. Their experience of hurt often needs to be addressed before the parent can regain authority. This may involve coaching a non-abusing parent – often the mother – to hear the painful story of how the violence affected the teenager while, at the same time, this parent still needs to set limits on the teenager's aggression. Again, framing this as taking a caring position may help overcome any feelings of guilt that might restrain such a parent.

Sometimes siblings other than the aggressive adolescent are involved in hitting or verbal abuse, and, in these cases, the therapist needs to seek a 'no hitting or abuse' commitment from everyone. To do this, the therapist helps the family to create a vision of how their family would be different if there were to be 'no hitting' in the family. The therapist asks each family member the hypothetical question, *'What would it be like in your family, if I could wave a magic wand and there was no hitting?'* and the therapist unpacks this vision. For example, if children say their mother wouldn't be stressed, the therapist can ask, 'How would your mother be different?' The therapist can also ask how the sibling relationships would be different if there were 'no hitting'. Once this vision has been explored, the therapist asks family members to make a commitment or promise not to hit. If all agree, it can be useful to mark this by getting the family members to shake hands on this commitment. Consequences need to be set for breaking the 'no hitting' commitment, and involving children in having a say about consequences can lessen resistance when they are used. The therapist then needs to review progress with the commitment in subsequent sessions.

In summary, dealing with aggressive adolescent behaviour requires the therapist to discriminate between expressive and instrumental aggression and to be alert to adolescents' needs around both attunement and limits. As parents establish boundaries, it is important to maintain a connection to their teenager so that parents are seen to come from a position of caring rather than being punitive. It can be easy to underestimate the restraints that may operate for parents with addressing this problem; however, once a normal parent–adolescent hierarchy is established, other problem behaviours usually become easier to resolve.

Substance abuse

Treatment of adolescent substance abuse is often individually focused but there is strong evidence to suggest that family-based treatment in conjunction with the mobilisation of wider system supports is the most effective way of addressing this problem (Catalano et al. in Carr, 2000; Liddle, Rowe, Dakof, Henderson, & Greenbaum, 2009). Working individually with adolescents is of limited usefulness unless the adolescent is motivated to address the problem, which typically is not the case. Even when this is the case, the adolescent usually needs help, because substance abuse is a problem that is very difficult for a teenager to handle alone.

Effective treatment of adolescent substance abuse first involves getting a good picture of the extent of the problem and then considering any restraints (and strengths) that might operate in the adolescent's family and the wider system.

Typically, there are four stages along a continuum. The first stage is when an adolescent starts with curious experimentation; then the adolescent may move on to the next stage of using drugs for relaxation and fun; then usage can become daily; and the final stage is where there is uncontrolled, constant drug use (Dimoff & Carper, 1992).

In stage 1, an adolescent experiments with easily available (gateway) drugs such as parents' alcohol or cigarettes, and the initial drug use is unpleasant. The motivation is mostly adventurous curiosity about the 'forbidden fruit'.

The adolescent enters stage 2, when getting high becomes a motive. There is something enjoyable about the use of drugs or alcohol, and the adolescent may get relief from the new, intense feeling states associated with adolescence. Drugs or alcohol are used to feel relaxed, and parties are no longer fun without them. The adolescent develops increased tolerance and may move on from the gateway drugs to other, stronger substances. An adolescent has entered stage 2 when substance abuse becomes a regular habit. There can be noticeable behaviour changes and school performance may drop; truancy may increase; and the adolescent may begin to enter a shadowy world where one of the things that bind peer groups is a common interest in illicit substances.

An adolescent enters stage 3 when life begins to revolve around drugs and there is daily drug use. Such an adolescent is likely to be an older adolescent, and the drugs are likely to be more potent substances, such as ice and cocaine,[16] but it may also be extensive use of other substances such as alcohol or cannabis. Getting money to buy drugs becomes an ongoing issue, and an adolescent may turn to stealing from home or outside or selling drugs to obtain drug money. Behaviour worsens, police incidents may occur, and the adolescent is usually failing at school. The adolescent's general health deteriorates, and suicidal thoughts may start to emerge.[17]

An adolescent has reached stage 4 when drug use is constant and uncontrolled, and tolerance is high. It is important to help young people before they reach this stage because recovery from this point is extremely difficult.

Once the stage of substance abuse is determined, the parents and the therapist can adopt various therapeutic positions to help the adolescent (Table 8.2). Thus, if an adolescent is in stage 1 – and this occurs with most adolescents – it is important for parents to react and set clear limits regarding drug use rather than turning a blind eye and minimising the behaviour. Here, it is helpful for the therapist to inquire actively about the adolescent's drug use and educate the parents about the risks and the importance of taking a stand against any form of drug use rather than normalising the behaviour.

With stage 2, parents need to be more proactive by learning about drugs and the indicators of drug use; by setting clear rules; and by monitoring their adolescent's behaviour. This means checking on where their adolescents are going and with whom they mix, as well as establishing good networks with other parents. If they are not confident about their adolescent's drug use, one way of ensuring their adolescent is not using drugs is to institute random drug tests (inexpensive drug-testing kits and breathalysers are available on the internet).

Random tests need to be discussed with the adolescent before being implemented, with clear consequences established beforehand if the adolescent fails or refuses to be tested. Random room searches can also be undertaken (with the adolescent present), and obtaining a clear drug test result can also be a way an adolescent can recover parents' trust. Here,

Table 8.2 Stages of substance abuse

	Stage 1	Stage 2	Stage 3	Stage 4
Adolescent	Experimenting	Partying	Plotting	Failing
Parents	Reacting versus minimising	Networking versus normalising	Taking charge versus enabling	Rehabilitating versus resigning
Therapist	Inquiring & educating versus reassuring & normalising	Escalating & confronting versus normalising	Empowering versus tolerating	Strengthening versus resigning

the therapist needs to take a position that directly addresses substance abuse as an issue by asking the parents to invest their energy into addressing this problem until they are in charge. The therapist also encourages the parents to strengthen their networks and work with other parts of the wider system, such as relatives, other parents, and school authorities (Henggeler, Schoenwald, Borduin, Rowland, & Cunningham, 2009).

If an adolescent reaches stage 3, the parents usually recognise the substance abuse and the associated behaviours as a problem, but there are likely to be significant restraints operating, which have prevented them from taking charge. The therapist's task here is to assist them with addressing these restraints and developing creative strategies (Sells, 2004).

An adolescent at stage 4 requires supervised in-patient drug rehabilitation, and the therapist's task usually involves addressing the family dynamics that allowed this situation to develop in the first place.

In practice, family therapy where substance abuse is an issue involves assessing how big a problem it is and making a tactical decision about how to tackle it. This involves understanding how the problem might be functioning within the system and what restraints might be operating to stop the parents from being effective. Therapists need to also look at the wider system and assess whether to intervene in other domains of the adolescent's life, such as friends and school. It can also be useful to ask what an adolescent likes about a particular drug to determine the psychoactive effect the adolescent may be seeking, for example, reduced anxiety, increased excitement, or the deadening of feelings. If drug use is a way of coping with distressing feelings, it may be important to address the cause of the distress.

Commonly, parents may not be confident about how to deal with this problem: they may be fearful of driving underground or making things worse if they act. A crucial feature of successful therapy involves establishing a good therapeutic alliance with parents by exploring their fears and building their motivation and confidence. A useful strategy is to dedicate a session to brainstorm how they anticipate their adolescent might react to their getting tougher, explore possible responses they might make, and then predict how they think their adolescent might respond to their responses. In doing this, parents become more united, and they can explore what to expect from each other.

In some cases, it might be necessary to remove adolescents from their environment to disrupt networks and also to detoxify them by taking them away on a 'holiday' for a week or two. As in other situations of taking a firm position, it is important to balance increased toughness with increased efforts at maintaining connection. Parents often feel more comfortable assuming this role if it is framed as their being more caring. They can be coached to frame punitive action as caring by saying, for example, '*I love you so much that I am going to do all I can to stop you becoming dependent on drugs*'. Taking the energy to address substance abuse means parents also must be more 'present' for their adolescents, who will recognise this even if it is hard for them to acknowledge it.

School problems

School problems with adolescents often go unaddressed until they become too big to avoid, because school authorities may view this area as primarily a responsibility of parents, while parents may see it as in the school's realm. A more useful approach is to conceptualise the situation in terms of an all-encompassing system that contains both the family subsystem and the school subsystem. From this perspective, the family and the school are seen as embedded in a larger system where all the typical system dynamics (such as circular patterns, triangles, and so forth) operate. The work then involves actively intervening in this wider system to bring the school subsystem and the family subsystem into an aligned alliance (Henggeler et al., 2009). The key to managing school problems effectively with adolescents is collaboration between school and parents, and collaboration with school authorities enables parents to extend supervision of their children into the realm of school, so that the wider system reinforces and amplifies their 'authoritative' parenting position (Baumrind cited in Henggeler et al., 2009, pp. 56–57).

First, it is important to get an accurate understanding of the problem. Whether it be poor school performance, school misbehaviour, truancy, or school refusal, it is usually useful to get the school's perspective. So, a good first step is to organise a meeting with key school personnel, such as year advisers and any counsellors who may operate in the school system. The therapist's job then is to coach parents about how to gain the school's cooperation by seeking a good understanding of the school's point of view and what each side needs from the other. Ideally, the therapist should attend this meeting to provide moral support for the parents and to help keep the meeting focused. It is unhelpful for the adolescent to witness any disagreements between the school and parents, so it is best if the adolescent remains outside the meeting room until a united plan of action is agreed. This can then be presented to the adolescent.

As part of gaining an accurate picture of the problem, it is important to explore with the teenager whether there might be any learning difficulties or other things, such as being bullied, that are making school hard. Parents should seek the opinion of school staff about this and, if there are gaps in information, request the school's assistance with finding out. This can then be a first step towards asking the school to remedy any problems that are the school's responsibility.

Once the problem has been clearly defined, the two features of an effective plan are communication and accountability. Establishing good communication means creating a system where parents can monitor their adolescent at school. One effective strategy for this is to set up a daily logbook where class attendance, homework, and class behaviour are recorded, and it is the adolescent's responsibility to get signed by teachers after every class. Establishing good accountability means that clearly understood consequences are put in place for the adolescent, consequences that will be enforced by the parents without the need to rely on busy school personnel. In the first meeting with the school, specific and measurable goals should be written up. Scheduling a second meeting to review progress keeps the plan and its goals front of mind for everyone and also ensures that any improvements are noticed.

Parental supervision and consequently the study habits that teenagers learn at home seem to be the main factor in good academic performance (Watkins & Noble, 2008). If a teenager is not doing homework, an effective strategy can be to insist that the teenager sit at a table under the direct supervision of a parent, who may still undertake normal home activities such as preparing the evening meal. Similarly, if a teenager is truanting, an effective strategy is for a parent to escort the teenager to and from school. If the teenager still manages to cut classes, the parent can escalate the intervention by attending classes with the student, which, of course, needs to be undertaken in consultation with the school. Usually this only needs to happen once for teenagers to get the message that their parents are going to invest whatever energy is required to get them back on track with school.

When it is difficult for teenagers to attend school at all, this is a more complex problem and different from truancy. Truancy is usually hidden from parents, but school refusal occurs when an adolescent wants to stay at home and does not hide not wanting to go to school from parents. Sometimes the problem can be the product of an adolescent being non-compliant, and so the situation requires that the parents re-establish firm limits, but, more typically, school refusal is associated with anxiety about things at school or at home or both. It is more likely to happen at times of change, such as, for example, starting high school, or if parents are separating and the teenager's anxiety may be accompanied by depression. It is important to get the adolescent back to school as soon as possible, because the longer this goes on, the harder it is to turn around.

Therapy for teenagers not attending school involves gaining an accurate understanding of what is worrying the adolescent in the first place, systematically addressing these things, and then developing a plan to ease the adolescent back into the school routine. Often a lack of structure may underlie an adolescent's anxiety. For instance, an adolescent may not be well organised around homework and may feel anxious about being behind. As with other phobic situations, care needs to be taken in developing a plan for the adolescent's gradual reintroduction to the difficult situation. It should strike the right balance between gaining mastery and not feeling overwhelmed, and it may be useful to graduate the re-entry by, for instance, organising for the adolescent to attend for a half-day at first or walking in with a friend. Parents need to remain attuned to their adolescent's feelings while being quietly insistent about implementing re-entry to school. In other words, they need to remain connected while taking control.

Depression and self-harm

Adolescent depression occurs in 4–8% of the population, but in specialist mental health settings, this percentage is likely to be much higher. Given that depression is a significant factor in adolescent suicide as well as other forms of self-harm, the stakes are high. Empirical evidence supports the use of cognitive behaviour therapy, interpersonal therapy, and the cautious use of antidepressant medication as standard treatments for adolescent depression. However, what happens in families can be significant in the development and progress of adolescent depression, and there is evidence that the use of family-based interventions can be helpful, either as a separate intervention or integrated with other treatments (Diamond & Josephson, 2005; Larner, 2009).

Adolescent depression can be associated with self-harm, which may take the form of either self-destructive (suicidal) behaviour or self-inflicted injury, such as cutting. However, a distinction needs to be drawn between these two forms of self-harm. A person who considers suicide seeks to end all feelings (Fisher, 2017), whereas a person who does self-inflicted injury seeks to feel better and gain relief from emotional distress by this behaviour (Favazza, 1996). Consequently, the interventions for each are different. Adolescents can present with these problems overtly, or else they may be concealed or unrecognised, so therapists should routinely screen for their presence.

The causes of adolescent depression are varied. Family factors that can be involved include physical and sexual abuse; neglect; attachment failure; psychiatric illness in a parent (particularly maternal depression); family conflict; stress and breakdown; poor parent–adolescent relationships; and ineffective parenting (Larner, 2009). As well as these, external factors such as school bullying can be potent triggers. There are several reasons why a family-based approach is useful. It establishes an arena in which to engage with family-based causes; it creates a space for repairing disjunctions in relationships; and it provides a framework in which to coach parents on how to assist their distressed adolescent around regulating feelings.

One technique a therapist can use for identifying the causes of distress for a teenager is to ask the teenager to draw a circle and then to divide the circle up in proportion to the issues that are affecting her or him – like pieces of a pie. The therapist asks, '*Can you draw a line to indicate how much of what is upsetting you is to do with home and how much is outside?*'. Then the therapist asks the teenager to subdivide the largest segment of the circle, '*Can you help me understand this big slice: what makes it up?*' The teenager then divides up the largest segment and labels each piece so that a clear picture emerges of the things that are troubling.

It is a misconception that asking about self-harm will make things worse, and in the case of self-harm that is self-destructive, it is important to detect suicidal thoughts as early as possible. One way of checking if an adolescent has considered suicide is to ask, '*How bad have things become? Have you ever thought of hurting yourself?*' If the answer is yes, then ask the adolescent what she or he has thought of doing. And depending on the answers to more detailed questions,[18] a picture emerges about the level of risk.

If an adolescent appears to be at risk, a safety plan should be developed that engages key support people, with relevant phone numbers and ideas about how to notice and manage the adolescent when distressed. Therapists should automatically discuss such cases with their supervisor, and it may be important to seek a more formal assessment and treatment plan from an expert in this field, such as a psychiatrist. If an adolescent has even vague thoughts of suicide, it needs to be taken seriously, because it has become part of the adolescent's way of thinking, to which she or he may now be more inclined.

Scaling questions can be particularly useful in this context. They accustom the adolescent to quantifying her or his experience; this allows both therapists and parents a simple way of regularly monitoring the risk, as well as providing a means of getting an indication of the adolescent's emotional state. Thus, parents can be coached to ask their adolescent, '*On a scale of 1 to 10 (with 10 meaning feeling good, and with 1 meaning feeling bad), where would you score yourself today?*' '*On a scale of 1 to 10, how much do you feel like hurting yourself today?*'

Depression and self-harm thrive on isolation and disconnection (Bickerton, Hense, Benstock, Ward, & Wallace, 2007). Establishing a relationship discourse creates a framework within which relationships can be reworked. Here, the central organising principle is the goal of establishing at least one parent as a reliable attachment figure (Diamond & Siqueland, 1998). This means someone who is safe, trustworthy, and dependable, someone who acts as a secure base from where the teenager can explore her or his own competence and autonomy. Establishing a parent as a reliable attachment figure first requires getting an understanding of the current constellation of relationships, and a good way of doing this is by undertaking a 'relationship scan' (see Chapter 2). Therapy then involves establishing a connection.

To do this, the therapist can ask parent(s) what they think stops their teenager coming to them when she or he is feeling low; what they miss about the relationship they used to have with their teenager; and what sort of relationship they would like to have with their teenager. If parents are to become good attachment figures, it is they (not their adolescent) who must take the first step in reaching out to reconnect. This usually means encouraging parents to spend one-to-one time with their teenager. Parents typically find this challenging, and they need to draw confidence from the therapist, who coaches them around anticipating feeling awkward and rejected. In some instances, if an adolescent is holding a past hurt, the therapist may first need to elicit an apology from a parent. The procedure for eliciting an apology is the following: the therapist (a) revisits the incident; (b) explores what both parties were intending and feeling; (c) elicits any regrets about what happened; (d) encourages each person to consider the effect on the other and also their relationship; and (e) asks the person who caused the hurt to apologise.

In the case of self-harm in the form of self-inflicted injury (Favazza, 1996; Klonsky, Oltmanns, & Turkheimer, 2003; MacAniff Zila & Kiselica, 2001; Ross & Heath, 2002) the effects are usually concealed, and it most often manifests as cutting; however, it can occur in other less predictable forms across a wide range of behaviours, from scalding to dangerous skateboard riding. With emotionally distressed adolescents, therapists should routinely check for this by asking adolescents and also their parents about whether they ever hurt themselves if they are upset. Self-injury is an indication of an individual's disconnection not only from others but also from self. It is a habitual way of dealing with distress that comes about when an adolescent becomes disconnected from thoughts, feelings, and physical sensations, and the adolescent is likely to be feeling desperately lonely and also ashamed of the behaviour.

Therapy involves creating a space for adolescents to voice their experience of aloneness, then coaching them to recognise their feelings and express them in ways other than by self-injury. If the focus of therapy moves to coaching parents with how they can assist their adolescent access and start to regulate feelings, adolescents usually need help recognising and expressing their feelings, and here the Imago dialogue can be a useful framework. Parents need to adopt a position of warm empathy and help their adolescent to self-soothe when situations are stressful (Stiefel & Renner, 2004). An adolescent should not be put in a position to help parents express their emotions. Rather, parents should take the lead in this process as a way of taking on the role of attachment figures.

Social media devices

Managing Information Technology (IT) devices presents a dilemma for families because, these days, competence with this technology is essential but this same technology can become a disruptive trap. Knowing how to manage this does not come naturally but, with smart limit setting, this problem can be transformed into an opportunity for adolescents to cultivate self-regulation.

The addictive nature of IT devices is now recognised (Gillespie, 2019; Marshall, 2019; Hari, 2022)[19] and not only young people but also parents can be captured by software that is deliberately designed to mesmerise and maintain involvement. It may not always be apparent that IT devices are a problem for a family because either there may not be an obvious link to a presenting problem or infiltration of IT devices may be so pervasive that it is not obvious that other family members may also have a problem. Vigilance regarding the pervasive nature of IT devices ensures the impact can be assessed. With respect to uncovering a connection to a presenting problem, getting a detailed interactional sequence is often sufficient to expose the role of IT devices. However, if other family members are also in the thrall of IT devices, the need to address this may not be apparent to a family.

The first step then is to assess the way IT devices are used within a family by asking questions about how and when everybody uses technology. If it is evident there is a problem, not just for particular children but also for others in a family, then, before embarking on psychoeducation about managing technology – just as with changing other compulsive behaviours in a relationship context – it is crucial to understand how this behaviour functions. It may be a solution to another problem, for instance, dealing with difficulties around intimacy or conflict; so, inviting parents to reduce the use of technology may expose other problems. Exploration needs to be undertaken with care and undertaken without activating fears about the vulnerability of speaking candidly in the presence of other family members; so, sometimes meeting with just the parent subsystem may be better and, with IT technology, it is especially important parents become aligned around goals. Once again, the principles of connection and limit setting provide a reliable approach for helping adolescents where there are problems.

In terms of connection and attunement, the context of IT offers unique opportunities for joining with a teenager either through sharing an activity or simply talking about online material. In terms of sharing an activity, an adolescent's interest in particular apps or games can be a windfall opportunity for connection. While it may not be an adult's first choice of a relaxing thing to do, it may be a teenager's, so showing interest in this (even participating) can be a rapid path into a young person's world via a shared experience.

In terms of simply talking about online material, this can be an opportunity for a parent to orchestrate authentic connection through 'curious conversation'. The difference between a 'curious conversation' and what can be termed an 'operational conversation' is that the latter is likely to be more pedestrian around topics such as the young person's day, whereas a 'curious conversation' involves more focused attention with active listening. Parents often need coaching around adopting curiosity by setting aside predetermined judgements with the intention of genuinely trying to understand. Opportunities for curious conversations are more likely to be successful if care is taken around the set-up (time-of-day, location,[20] the antidote to suspect online information). For example, a parent might ask, '*What do you think is the difference between something online that is sensual and erotic and something that is pornographic?*'

Conversations where curiosity is a feature normalise having discussions respectfully. They have the effect of positioning adolescents to be more open to influence. However, self-regulation does not happen automatically, and parents need to take charge and set limits that the young person can eventually internalise. Setting limits is going to be easier and more effective if a young person's cooperation is enlisted collaboratively through a negotiated agreement. For this, parents may need to be coached or they may need to practise how to do this with in-session enactments.

The first step in reaching a negotiated agreement with adolescents about the use of devices is to invite them to discriminate between the effects of respective platforms. Invite them to reflect on the effect that different IT platforms have on their state of mind (Einstein, 2019). To do this, adolescents can be asked to score on a scale of '1 to 10' their mood after using a particular platform and then be encouraged to name their emotional state. After using harmful platforms that are addictive, adolescents begin to recognise how they usually feel depleted or irritable; in contrast, if the platform has a healthy impact, they may be able to detect a difference in mood where they feel energised or more settled. Parents need to be cautioned about the timing of these sorts of conversations; on the one hand, interrupting a young person while engaged in an addictive activity is likely to elicit an unexpectedly angry response (much like what happens when someone interrupts a movie at a dramatic moment); on the other hand, the impact of the experience needs to be recent enough to be available for reflection; so these sorts of conversations may need to be titrated episodes and tailored to particular platforms. The goal is to enable adolescents to learn to control their attention, manage their time, and switch off from urges, in other words, to enable them to learn self-regulation.

But, once hazardous platforms are identified, how to set limits? Recommendations about restrictions are usually for an upper limit of 2 hours per day on school days (Einstein, 2019; Marshall, 2019). The important thing is that there is a specific measure for what constitutes 'non-educational' screen time. Negotiation then needs to be undertaken about what IT use will be allowed and which will not fall within the negotiated daily time ration.

What makes the problem of managing IT devices unique is that it comes with its own inbuilt consequences. If access is regarded as a privilege instead of an entitlement, then access can be stopped as a penalty or increased on weekends as a reward. So, while adolescents may initially become reactive, provided parents maintain their motivation, adolescents quickly experience that resistance is futile and the big collateral benefit is that it becomes a vehicle for learning self-regulation which is the goal of parenting adolescents in the context of family therapy.

Conclusion

This chapter has outlined how family-based therapies can be effective interventions for many of the common problems that adolescents experience. Individuation is a central feature of adolescent development, but it is often interpreted as the pursuit of independence through separation from family. This downplays the importance of parental connection, which supports an adolescent developing autonomy. Teenagers may appear to be like adults physically, but their brains are on a path of growth that takes more than 10 years to complete. They need help with processing their experience of the world, and they need to feel that there is someone bigger and stronger than they are who can guide them through the process of growing up. Parents are best placed to do this by maintaining attuned connection to their teenagers and by providing security through the structure of limits. Successful therapy typically involves helping parents enhance these areas. Some family structures are better than others for adolescent development (namely, those in which parents are in a hierarchical position), and family therapy is a unique vehicle for understanding how the web of family relationships operates. Working with families is often the best pathway for change with adolescents.

Acknowledgement

The material in this chapter was developed at RAPS Adolescent Family Therapy and Mediation Service, a program of Relationships Australia (NSW). RAPS was established in 1990 at Parramatta with funding from the Australian Commonwealth Government. A major influence in shaping the program's approach has been the clinical consultant Dr Laurie MacKinnon.

Notes

1 Here the term 'parent' refers to a person who assumes the role of psychological parent, and in some situations, this may be a caregiver other than a biological parent, such as a stepparent, relative, or foster parent.

2 'Sex' usually refers to biological differences (chromosomes, etc.); 'gender' usually refers to the social construct aggregated around all the features usually associated with sex.

3 'Affect is … a sensorimotor, physiological representation that generates a felt sense', which is subsequently categorised or labelled ('signified') as a specific emotion (Hill, 2015, p. 6).

4 Mentalizing is 'an individual's awareness of mental states in himself or herself and in other people, perceiving and interpreting the feelings, thoughts, beliefs and wishes that explain what people do' (Fonagy, 2019, p. 3).

5 'Acting out' means performing an action in contrast to managing difficult feelings, such as happens, for example, with a temper tantrum of a toddler.

6 Neuroscience research suggests that the ability to name a painful feeling actually alleviates the experience of it: 'name it to tame it' (Siegel, in Codrington, 2010).

7 Foucault's concept of a 'discourse' (Foucault, 1977) is here linked with the idea of 'relationships' as a framework (MacKinnon, 1998), which then determines that individuals see themselves as relationship 'subjects' (Althusser, 1971).

8 An enactment is a structural family therapy technique designed to bring the actual process of interactions into the therapy room; in other words, interactions are enacted. As the therapist witnesses this, family members can be coached about better ways of interacting.

9 Teenagers need more sleep than children or adults, and this is associated with brain maturation (Dahl & Lewin, 2002). A typical 14-year-old needs nine hours' sleep (Wolfson & Carakadon, 1998).

10 Symptoms can range from somatic reactions, such as headaches, to more serious behaviours, such as self-harm behaviours such as cutting.

11 If there are couple issues, but the parents have come to therapy because of their adolescent, it can be risky to reframe it as a marital issue. At one level, couples usually recognise that there is a couple problem, but it feels safer to seek therapy around the adolescent's problem behaviour. Moving to a new frame of couple therapy is likely to trigger anxiety, which may lead to dropout. It is usually safest to address the couple issues using the frame of 'building a better parenting team to get their teenager on track' while much of the therapeutic work may, in fact, be couple therapy.

12 Adolescents begin to think differently to children; Piaget (1950) described this change as a shift from concrete operational thinking to formal operations where adolescents are able to move beyond the immediacy of experience and can think in terms of 'form' or process rather than just concrete content. Teenagers are able to reason in abstract terms: to think about what 'could be', not 'what is'. As adolescents attain this form of thinking, their experience of reality is different, and they experience the world anew.

13 Adoptees may wonder whether there was something wrong for the biological parent to give them away and there may be an underlying sense of shame and loss (Verrier, 1993).

14 Scott Sells' book, 'Treating the Tough Adolescent' discusses the idea of 'buttons' in detail. The book is a useful resource that provides a repertoire of strategies for managing difficult adolescent behaviours, and parts of the text are available on the internet.

15 Therapists need to be able to tell parents the age when the justice system deems offenders 'juvenile' or 'adult', and what happens to police records of juveniles, which are usually handled with more discretion than those of adults. The information for particular jurisdictions is usually accessible through the internet.

16 'Ice' is a crystal methamphetamine that is more potent than other forms of amphetamine, such as 'speed'.

17 One of the pernicious effects of many of these substances is that they induce depression, and a vicious cycle can develop where an adolescent uses a substance to obtain relief from feeling depressed, only to feel more depressed afterwards.

18 If the answer is 'yes', then the therapist can gently assess the risk of suicide by exploring how well formed the adolescent's thoughts are about this. First, the therapist can ask if the

adolescent has a clear plan (which indicates greater risk than if the thoughts are vague); then ask whether the adolescent thinks she or he could carry out these plans; and finally, whether the adolescent has already tried to do anything harmful. From this, a picture emerges about the level of risk.

19 Devices are now regarded as addictive, especially for developing teenage brains, because they stimulate dopamine production (Gillespie, 2019: 40).

20 The term 'critical thinking' involves evaluating information and assumptions instead of thinking which can be categorised as 'uncritical' and which relies on nothing but assertions.

References

Althusser, L. (1971). *Lenin and philosophy*. London, England: Monthly Review Press.

Baumrind, D. (1991). The influence of parenting style on adolescent competence and substance use. *Journal of Early Adolescence, 11*, 56–95.

Bickerton, A., Hense, T., Benstock, A., Ward, J., & Wallace, L. (2007). Safety first: A model of care for working systematically with high risk young people and their families in an acute CAMHS service. *Australian and New Zealand Journal of Family Therapy, 28*, 121–129.

Biddulph, S., & Biddulph, S. (2003). *The complete secrets of happy children*. London, England: Penguin.

Blakemore, S. (2018). *Inventing ourselves: The secret life of the teenage brain*. London, England: Doubleday.

Carey, T., & Oxman, L. (2007). Adolescents and mental health treatments: Reviewing the evidence to discern common themes for clinicians and areas for future research. *Clinical Psychologist, 11*, 79–87.

Carr, A. (Ed.) (2000). *What works with children and adolescents? A critical review of psychological interventions with children, adolescents and their families*. London: Routledge.

Carr, A. (2009). The effectiveness of family therapy and systemic interventions for child-focused problems. *Journal of Family Therapy, 31*, 3–45.

Codrington, R. (2010). A family therapist's look into interpersonal neurobiology and the adolescent brain: An interview with Dr Daniel Siegel. *Australian and New Zealand Journal of Family Therapy, 31*, 285–299.

Codrington, R., Iqbal, A., & Segal, J. (2012). Lost in translation? Embracing the challenges of working with families from a refugee background. *Australian and New Zealand Journal of Family Therapy, 32*, 129–143.

Cottrell, D., & Boston, P. (2002). Practitioner review: The effectiveness of systemic family therapy for children and adolescents. *Journal of Child Psychology and Psychiatry, 43*, 573–586.

Dahl, R., & Lewin, D. (2002). Pathways to adolescent health sleep regulation and behaviour. *Journal of Adolescent Health, 31*, 175–184.

David-Ferdon, C., & Kaslow, N. (2008). Evidence-based psychosocial treatment for child and adolescent depression. *Journal of Clinical Child and Adolescent Psychology, 37*, 62–104.

Diamond, G., & Josephson, A. (2005). Family-based treatment research: A 10-year update. *Journal of the American Academy of Child and Adolescent Psychiatry, 44*, 872–887.

Diamond, G., & Siqueland, L. (1998). Emotions, attachment and the relational frame: The first session. *Journal of Systemic Therapies, 17*, 36–50.

Dimoff, T., & Carper, S. (1992). *How to tell if your kids are using drugs*. New York, NY: Facts on File Inc.

Einstein, D. (2019). *The dip: A practical guide to take control of screen addiction and reconnect your family*. Sydney, Australia: Distinct Psychology.

Eliot, L. (2009). *Pink brain blue brain*. London, England: Oneworld publications.

Favazza, A. (1996). *Bodies under siege: Self injury and body modification in culture and psychiatry*. Baltimore, MD: Johns Hopkins University Press.

Fisher, J. (2017). *Healing the fragmented selves of trauma survivors: Overcoming internal self-alienation*. New York, NY: Routledge.

Fonagy, P., Luyten, P., Allison, E., & Campbell, C. (2019). Mentalizing, epistemic trust and the phenomenology of psychotherapy. *Psychopathology, 52*(2), 94–103. https://doi.org/10.1159/000501526

Foucault, M. (1977). *The archaeology of knowledge*. London, England: Tavistock.

Giedd, J. (2015). 'The amazing teen brain', *Scientific American*, June.

Gillespie, D. (2019). *Teen brain*. Sydney, Australia: Pan MacMillan Australia.

Gottman, J. (1999). *The marriage clinic: A scientifically based marital therapy*. New York, NY: W.W. Norton.

Gottman, J., & DeClaire, J. (1997). *Raising an emotionally intelligent child*. New York, NY: Bloomsbury.

Gottman, J., & Silver, N. (1997). *The seven principles for making marriage work*. Guernsey: Guernsey Press.

Hari (2022). *Stolen focus: Why you can't pay attention*. London, England: Bloomsbury.

Hendrix, H. (1988). *Getting the love you want*. New York, NY: Macmillan.

Hendrix, H., & LaKelly Hunt, H. (1997). *Giving the love that heals: A guide for parents*. New York, NY: Atria.

Henggeler, S., & Schaeffer, C. (2010). Treating serious emotional and behavioural problems using multisystemic therapy. *Australian and New Zealand Journal of Family Therapy, 31*, 149–164.

Henggeler, S., Schoenwald, S., Borduin, C., Rowland, M., & Cunningham, P. (2009). *Multisystemic therapy for antisocial behavior in children and adolescents*. New York, NY: Guilford Press.

Hill, D. (2015). *Affect regulation theory*. New York, NY: W.W. Norton.

Hoffman, L. (1982). A co-evolutionary framework for systemic family therapy. *Australian Journal of Family Therapy, 4*, 11–15.

Hogue, A., & Liddle, H. (2009). Family-based treatment for adolescent substance abuse: Controlled trials and new horizons in services research. *Journal of Family Therapy, 31*, 126–54.

Howard, J. (2008). It all starts at home: Male adolescent violence to mothers. *Inner South Community Health Service and Child Abuse Research Australia*. Melboure: Monash University.

Imber-Black, E. (1988). *Families and larger systems*. New York, NY: Guilford Press.

James, K. (2007). Differentiation in couple therapy: Revisiting the Schnarch–Hendrix debate. In E. Shaw, & J. Crawley (Eds.), *Couple therapy in Australia: Issues emerging from practice*. Kew, VIC, Australia: PsychOz Publications.

James, K., & MacKinnon, L. (2010). The tip of the iceberg: A framework for identifying non-physical abuse in couple and family relationships. *Journal of Feminist Family Therapy, 22*, 112–129.

Kindlon, D., & Thompson, M. (2000). *Raising Cain: Protecting the emotional life of boys*. New York, NY: Ballantine.

Kinniburgh, K., Blaustein, M., Spinazzola, J., & van der Kolk, B. (2005). Attachment, self-regulation and competency. *Psychiatric Annals, 35*, 424–430.

Klonsky, E., Oltmanns, T., & Turkheimer, E. (2003). Deliberate self-harm in a non-clinical population: Prevalence and psychological correlates. *American Psychologist, 9*, 353–388.

Larner, G. (2009). Integrating family therapy in adolescent depression. *Journal of Family Therapy, 31*, 213–232.

Lebow, J. L. (2014). *Couple & family therapy an integrative map of the territory*. The American Psychological Association. Washington, DC: Maple Vail Press.

Liddle, H. (2010). Multidimensional family therapy: A science-based treatment system. *Australian and New Zealand Journal of Family Therapy, 31*, 133–148.

Liddle, H., Rowe, C., Dakof, G., Henderson, C. E., & Greenbaum, P. E. (2009). Multidimensional family therapy for young adolescent substance abuse: Twelve-month outcomes of a randomized controlled trial. *Journal of Consulting and Clinical Psychology, 77*, 12–25.

MacAniff Zila, L., & Kiselica, M. (2001). Understanding and counseling self-mutilation in female adolescents and young adults. *Journal of Counseling and Development, 79,* 46–52.

MacKinnon, L. (1998). *Trust and betrayal in the treatment of child abuse.* New York, NY: Guilford Press.

Marshall, B. (2019). *The tech diet for your child & teen.* Sydney, Australia: HarperCollins.

McKay, S. (2018). *The Women's brain book.* Sydney, Australia: Hachette.

Piaget, J. (1950). *The psychology of intelligence.* London, England: Routledge & Kegan Paul.

Rippon, G. (2019). *The gendered brain.* London, United Kingdom: Penguin Random House.

Robinson, E., Power, L., & Allan, D. (2010). What works with adolescents? Family connections and involvement in interventions for adolescent behaviour problems. Australian Family Relationships Clearing House Briefing Paper No 16. Melbourne, Australia: Australian Institute of Family Studies.

Robinson, E., & Pryor, R. (2006). Strong bonds project: Promoting family-aware youth work practice. *Developing Practice, 15,* 28–35.

Ross, S., & Heath, N. (2002). A study of the frequency of self-mutilation in a community sample of adolescents. *Journal of Youth and Adolescence, 31,* 67–77.

Schave, D., & Schave, B. (1989). *Early adolescence and the search for self.* New York, NY: Praeger.

Segal, J. (2010). Therapeutic process as a means to navigate impasse? Reflections on a complex case of cross-cultural adolescent family therapy. *Australian and New Zealand Journal of Family Therapy, 31,* 266–274.

Sells, S. (2004). *Treating the tough adolescent.* New York, NY: Guilford Press.

Siegel, D. (2014). *brainstorm: The power and purpose of the teenage brain.* Brunswick, Australia: Scribe Publications.

Silverstein, O., & Rashbaum, B. (1994). *The courage to raise good men.* New York, NY: Viking.

Sprenkle, D., Davis, S., & Lebow, J. (2009). *Common factors in couple and family therapy.* New York, NY: Guilford Press.

Stern, D. (2019). *The infinity of the unsaid: Unformulated experience, language and the nonverbal.* New York, NY: Routledge.

Stiefel, I., & Renner, P. (2004). Beyond behaviour: The importance of communication in parenting 'defiant' children: Pilot study and program. *Australian and New Zealand Journal of Family Therapy, 25,* 84–93.

van der Kolk, B. (2006). Clinical implications of neuroscience research in PTSD. *Annals of the New York Academy of Sciences, 1071,* 277–293.

Verrier, N. (1993). *The primal wound: Understanding the adopted child.* Lafayette, CA: New South Wales Post Adoption Resource Centre.

Watkins, M., & Noble, G. (2008). *Cultural practices and learning: Discipline and disposition in schooling.* Sydney, Australia: University of Western Sydney.

Wolf, E. (1994). Self object experiences: Development, psychotherapy and treatment. In S. Kramer, & S. Akhtar (Eds.), *Mahler and Kohut: Perspectives on development, psychopathology and technique.* NJ: Jason Aronson.

Wolfson, A., & Carakadon, M. (1998). Sleep schedules and daytime functioning in adolescents. *Child Development, 69,* 875–887.

Chapter 9

The Why and How of Separate Parent Sessions in Family Therapy

Kerrie James and Laurie MacKinnon

Introduction

A distinguishing feature of family therapy is the default position that everyone in the household attends the therapy sessions. Holding to this position avoids the tendency to slide into what is an apparently easy but in the long run problematic practice: conducting sessions with only those family members who can attend at times convenient for the therapist and only those most motivated to come. In many settings this slide means that therapists only see the mother and problem child, leaving out key actors in the family drama – the disengaged father, the older parentified sibling, or the favoured child. While holding to this default position, family therapists may also decide at times that it is important to work with a subsystem, very often the parental subsystem. This chapter focuses on knowing why and how to meet with parents separately and the risks involved in doing so.

Why see parents separately?

How therapists conceptualise family relationships informs their decision as to whether to meet separately with parents. Both Structural Family Therapy and the Milan Systemic approach address the way a child's symptoms and problems are produced and maintained within the system of family relationships. The therapist intervenes in dyadic and triadic sequences to change patterns of closeness/distance, inclusion/exclusion, and dominance/submission that characterise family relationships (Jiménez, Hidalgo, Baena, León, & Lorence, 2019; Minuchin, 1974). Triadic patterns may indicate the negative involvement of a child in the parents' relationship: triangulation, detouring, and cross-generational coalitions.

Triangulation is when both parents seek a coalition with a child, putting the child in a loyalty bind which may lead to the child showing symptoms or behavioural difficulties (Bowen, 1978; Minuchin, 1974). Detouring is when parents over-focus on a child as a way of avoiding conflict between them as a couple, resulting in the child having emotional or behavioural difficulties that are reinforced by their parents' attention (Minuchin and Fishman, 1981). Cross-generational coalitions occur when one parent joins with a child against another parent, resulting in problems for the child and the excluded parent (Haley, 1987; Madanes, 2009).

Cross-generational coalitions result in hierarchical problems, problems in the balance of power in a relationship. A hierarchy is called "incongruent" when one parent forms a coalition with a child against the other parent resulting in the child having an inappropriate amount of power in the family (Haley, 1987).

DOI: 10.4324/9781003490104-10

Dyadic patterns may indicate underlying relationship issues. In a complementary pattern, the behaviour of one person elicits the opposite behaviour of the other. When unchecked, complementary patterns become polarised positions of pursue/withdraw, over-functioning/ under-functioning, dominant/submissive, and hard/soft parenting (Madanes, 2009; Watzlawick, Beavin, & Jackson, 1967). In symmetrical patterns, the behaviour of one person elicits similar behaviour from the other person. When unchecked, negative behaviours such as attack/attack or criticise/defend result in escalating conflict associated with parents in the throes of separation and divorce (James, 1989).

Most often family therapists deal with all of the above relationship patterns during the family session with the child present (Minuchin, 1974). There are, however, several reasons *why* a family therapist would decide to meet with parents without the children present.

"De-triangulating" children from couple conflict

There are times when the couple's relationship is in serious jeopardy and one of the parents is not willing to give up seeking the support of the child against the other parent. The couple may be on the verge of separation, there may be domestic violence, or a parent may be seriously depressed. Parents may then "triangulate" a child into their conflict, each trying to gain support from the child for their position or attempting to turn the child against the other parent. In these instances, therapists may choose to see the parents separately to clarify their capacity and willingness to deal with couple issues freeing the child from their triangulated position.

Identifying and addressing couple issues

A child's problems may be related to their parent's relationship conflict in ways other than their triangulation. The child's problematic behaviour may be connected to a parent's preoccupation and emotional distance; exposure to parental conflict, abuse, and violence; or the absence of one parent or the over-involvement of the other. In family sessions, the therapist explores the dyadic or triadic sequences that involve the parents and the problem child and addresses the attachment relationship between the child and each parent. In separate sessions with parents, the focus is on resolving couple issues (Guerin, Fay, Burden, & Kautto, 1987, 1996).

Identifying and challenging soft/hard splits between parents

Parents often present with differences in parenting styles that lead to conflict between the parents or between parents and children, particularly when one parent is authoritarian and the other is indulgent or permissive (Baumrind, 1978). Commonly referred to as a "soft-hard" split, one parent, the "toughie", has higher expectations and a stricter style of discipline, while the other, the "softie", has lower expectations and lacks consistency in following through with discipline. In this interactional pattern, "softness" in one parent escalates in response to the "hardness" of the other and vice versa. When a parent-child coalition or couple conflict is driving the "softie", then over time the tough parent becomes more distant from the child and the other parent. If this complementary pattern has escalated to the point where the tough parent has given up and withdrawn or become abusive, separate parent sessions might be indicated.

In this situation, the goal is to soften the tough parent while firming up the soft parent. After assessing the extent of "toughness" to rule out abuse or violence, the therapist can use separate parent sessions to help the parents come to an agreement on how to respond to issues. Getting the parents "on the same page" by helping the soft parent implement rules and consequences puts distance between the soft parent and the child, challenging the coalition between them. The therapist encourages the "toughie", now relieved of his or her role, to develop a warmer relationship with the child.

Respecting personal boundaries

There are some issues that parents regard as "out of bounds" and that they will resist talking about in front of their children. These may be problems personal to them such as intimacy issues, illness, mental illness, depression, or substance abuse. They may also be reluctant to reveal unresolved trauma that is triggered by parent-child conflict. When these issues impact the parent's ability to function as a parent, the family therapist must decide the appropriateness of exploring these issues with the children present taking into account the parent's willingness and the possible effect on the children.

Challenging a pattern of "over functioning"/"under functioning"

One parent, perhaps suffering from depression, anxiety, mental illness, or substance abuse problem, may initially present in therapy as incompetent, irresponsible, or not coping. The other parent presents as the polarised opposite, appearing super responsible and competent. This complementary pattern escalates both parents' behaviour: one parent feels burdened while the other becomes more symptomatic; one parent becomes over-involved with children and the other parent becomes disconnected. In this mix, a child, worried and anxious, can become "parentified" looking after the under-functioning parent, or become symptomatic, seeking to distract and mobilise the parent.

Professionals may reinforce a parent's "under-functioning" by diagnosing mental illness, prescribing medication, and inadvertently aligning with the over-functioner. The family therapist can choose to use separate couple sessions to help the over-functioning parent take a back seat and make room for the other parent. Confronting the rigidity of the parents' roles, the therapist elicits the over-functioning parent's experience of stress and vulnerability and challenges the under-functioning parent to take more responsibility, demonstrating his or her latent capacity (Minuchin and Fishman, 1981).

Confronting parents' negative or abusive behaviour

Family therapists may decide to meet with parents separately to confront parents' harsh, abusive, neglectful, or controlling behaviour if the therapist is concerned that the parents would feel shamed or undermined if the children were present. By confronting them privately, the therapist demonstrates respect and is more likely to maintain engagement. This does not mean that therapists are neutral about abuse when children are present, but simply that therapists hold to a principle of not shaming or undermining parents in front of their children.

Strengthening parent-therapist alliance

Although therapists aim to engage all family members equally, therapists do not always feel equally sympathetic to both parents. Perhaps one parent is more committed to therapy and open to the therapist, while the other may be reluctant to engage. Therapists may at times have a strong negative or positive reaction to one parent's personality or opinions. Separate parent sessions or individual sessions with each parent can help the therapist to solidify his or her engagement with the parent with whom they feel less engaged.

Facilitating change when therapy is at an impasse

When therapy fails to make headway, changing the constellation of who attends the session may create a shift in family relationships, unleash new information, or increase the parents' commitment to changing their own behaviour.

Different family constellations

Different family constellations influence a therapist's decision as to the why and how of meeting separately with parents. Single parents, feeling alone and unsupported, turn to therapists as sounding boards in making parenting decisions. A therapist may offer separate sessions to a single parent, temporarily becoming a de facto "other parent". Soft-hard splits are common between parents in stepfamilies with the biological parent typically described as "too soft" and the stepparent as "too hard". As outsiders in the triangle of biological parents and their children, stepparents are vulnerable to feeling rejected and criticised. By meeting with parents separately, the therapist can challenge a stepparent's harsh behaviour while helping him or her to save face in relation to the children. The therapist can then assist the biological parent to exercise more authority, freeing the stepparent to develop a warmer relationship with the children.

Child protection issues

Therapists may use separate sessions to engage parents who are forced to come to therapy by legal or child protection authorities. In setting the stage for therapy, the therapist meets with the parents for an "initial meeting" to hear their experience of professionals and give them a choice about whether to proceed with therapy (MacKinnon, 1998). When parents have used hitting or other forms of abuse to punish a child, the therapist can use separate sessions to challenge the parents and to obtain their commitment to using non-abusive practices. If the parents have used harsh or abusive practices, the parent-child relationship is unlikely to improve until the parents have changed their parenting style, reduced their reactivity, and ceased to use violence or physical discipline. If a parent has hurt or betrayed a child, a new relationship can be forged by helping the parents apologise to the child (James, 2007; MacKinnon, 1998). With the therapist's support, confrontation, and coaching, parents are enabled to lean into the child's experience and to apologise.

How to plan and conduct separate parent sessions

The first step in setting up a parent session is to think through the purpose of the session and to clearly formulate objectives. The session may be a one-off opportunity to see the parents by themselves and to gain the most from it the therapist must be prepared. If one of the objectives is to assess for possible depression or mental illness, the therapist needs to be prepared with appropriate questions and assessment tools to make effective use of the time.[1]

The therapist's next step is to develop a rationale or frame for the separate parent session, one that the parents will find acceptable, and then to present it to them. The separate session might be framed as ordinary, "*What we usually do as our next up is meet with the parents separately*" or "*This is the way I work with families – I meet with everyone together and then in different groups including the parents separately*", or the therapist may say that the session has a specific purpose that will make sense to the parents.

In the actual parent session, the therapist, guided by the objectives, weaves between and manages the overlap of parenting and couple conflicts. Many parenting conflicts are intricately connected to couple relationship issues. Sometimes the parenting conflicts exacerbate existing couple problems or cause problems for the couple in their relationship. Other times pre-existing couple relationship issues prevent the parents from working together. It is the therapist's task to make connections between the child's issue and the parent's couple conflicts in a way that parents find acceptable and can acknowledge. If parents acknowledge the existence of couple conflict, then these issues, to the degree to which they interfere with the parents' ability or willingness to cooperate with each other in setting limits, need to be addressed.

Following the parent session, the therapist maintains an overview of the process of therapy and evaluates the impact of the parent session. Have the parents followed through on agreements made in the session? How did the parents' relationship change? To what extent did resolving a parenting issue positively impact their couple relationship and vice versa?

Case study

A mother with an Italian surname phoned for an appointment, concerned about the behaviour of her 13-year-old daughter, Sophie, who was failing school, truanting, and being charged with stealing from a shop.[2] The mother, in her early 50s, worked full time as a beautician, and her husband, in his 60s, had worked for many years in a struggling small business. Their four children ranged in age from 13 to 26 years old and the two eldest children were no longer living at home. The maternal grandmother, in her 80s, lived nearby (Figure 9.1).

In the first few sessions, the mother had revealed that she was preoccupied with the illness of her own mother and still grieving the death of her father who had died two years earlier. Feeling unsupported by her husband, she had distanced from him. He had turned to Sophie who perceived her father as more amenable and accessible than her mother. This soft/hard split escalated when the father undermined the mother by giving in to Sophie's demands. This led to arguments between the parents and the mother becoming more hostile towards both her husband and Sophie.

In the family sessions, the parents could not come to an agreement about how to manage Sophie. When they talked to each other, Sophie persistently interrupted their conversation and the father turned to Sophie, inviting her opinion, drawing her into the parents' conversation. The therapist decided to offer the parents a separate session for them to work out their "game plan" without interruption.

The therapist developed a frame for the problem that did not blame the parents and gave a rationale for a separate parent interview

At the end of a family session, the therapist said, "*Parents often have things they would like to talk to me about with just the adults present. This is something I offer to parents routinely.*

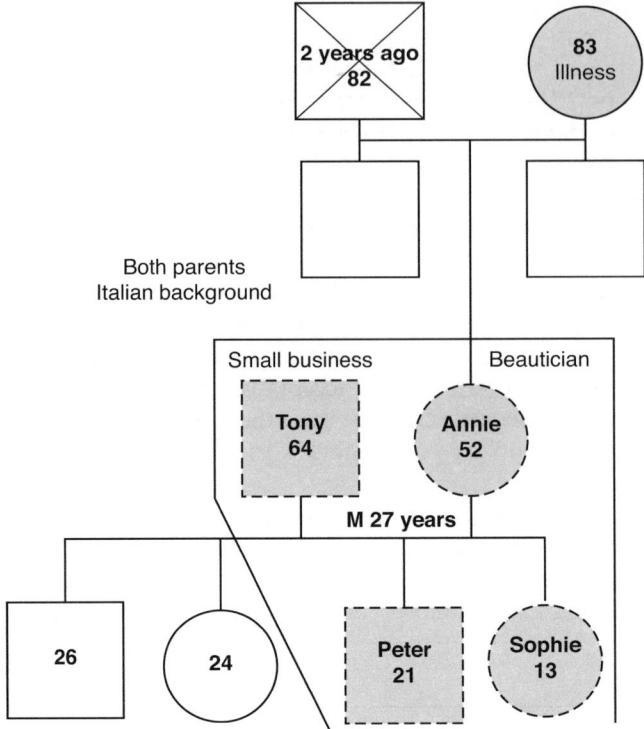

Figure 9.1 Genogram.

In your situation, I think by meeting with just the two of you it will be easier to work out your game plan without Sophie interrupting you".

The parents agreed, both saying yes; they thought this was a very good idea. The therapist also had other reasons for offering this meeting. Because she found herself liking the father more than the mother, she worried about her neutrality. She wondered if the mother's harsh persona masked underlying sadness and depression and hoped that a separate meeting would allow her to develop more empathy for the mother's situation. The therapist was also concerned about the parents using physical force themselves, or, allowing others to use physical force against Sophie and she knew that in a separate session she could explore this issue without the parents losing face.

The therapist developed a clear set of objectives for the separate parent session

In consultation with a colleague, the therapist planned and wrote down the following objectives for the parent session:

- To strengthen her engagement with the mother by listening empathically to her distress concerning the loss of her father, the terminal illness of her mother, and the acting out behaviour of her daughter.
- To assess whether the mother is clinically depressed.

- To secure the parents' commitment to not using or allowing any form of physical discipline or violence.
- To coach the parents so that in a subsequent session they will be able to hear and respond empathically to Sophie's hurt and anger at them for using physical discipline and allowing the brother to hurt her.
- To coach the parents so that in a subsequent session they will be able to make a congruent apology to Sophie and commitment to her to not use or allow physical discipline or violence.[3]

The therapist assessed the parents for individual problems and mental health issues

The therapist began the session by saying that when parents are faced with a teenager's challenging behaviour, it is very wearing and stressful on them individually and on their relationship as parents. She asked if they would be willing to complete a questionnaire that would give her some sense of the degree of stress they were both experiencing in their lives right now. They agreed and when they had done so, she quickly checked the results, noticing that the father's scores were all in the normal range and the mother's scores were indicating moderate depression and extreme stress. She explained the results to the parents and asked them if the results matched their experience.

The therapist joined with the mother by eliciting her experience

The mother replied, "*The last year has been really tough. I guess it's really worn me out running back-and-forth between home and my mother. And it's never enough. When I try to get things done at home, I feel guilty that I'm not over there looking after her. And when I'm with her, I feel stressed about all I'm not getting done at home. I have trouble sleeping. And then these problems with Sophie on top of it all*".

"*It's too much for one person to take on*," said the therapist beginning to genuinely feel more empathy for her.

"*It really is*," said the mother and she began to cry. "*And I don't know how long we'll have Mum for, either. I feel like she's slipping away everyday*".

"*You're afraid you're losing her*", said the therapist. "*And so soon after losing your father*".

"*It just seems like yesterday that he died*", said the mother.

The therapist talked at length with the mother about the losses she was facing. The mother softened, opened up, and the therapist felt a strong connection with her. "*Maybe you're also feeling scared that you are losing Sophie too*", the therapist said.

The mother nodded, tearing again, "*I feel like I've lost the little girl I had*".

"*She's pushing you away*", said the therapist.

"*She was a wonderful little girl before she went to high school*", said the mother and she went on to talk about her memories of Sophie as a little girl.

The therapist obtained the parent's commitment to making an apology and to planning the apology session

By this stage the therapist felt very connected to both parents and felt that it was the right time to broach the subject of the violence.

"I'm thinking about what Sophie said in the last session, that she thinks you condoned her brother beating her up", said the therapist addressing both parents. *"I'm worried that so long as she thinks that, she will keep pushing you away. As long as she thinks you could let someone hurt her again, she will never trust you"*.

"It's over. It's behind us", said the father. *"She has to let go of it and move on"*.

"I think so too", said the therapist. *"But we have to find a way of helping her let go of it. We have to find a way of letting her know she can trust the two of you again"*.

The parents nodded in agreement.

"But how?" asked the mother.

"First" the therapist answered, *"we have to give her the space to say out loud her hurt and anger about her brother hitting her and you not stopping him. We have to just listen and let her say it. Are you prepared to do that? With my support?"*

"Of course", said the father, *"if that's what it takes"*.

"If that's what it takes", said the mother.

The therapist helped the parents commit to non-violence

Happy with the progress made so far in the session, the therapist sensed that it was now time to "seal the deal" by asking the parents to commit to non-violence. *"It will take more"*, said the therapist. *"It will take a commitment from both of you to protect her and a commitment to never using or letting anyone else use physical violence with her. Can you make that commitment? With me now?"*

"But then how do we get through to her?" asked the mother.

"I will help you find other ways. Ways that work but that don't make her want to retaliate against you. But first she needs to know that you'll never go back on the old ways. You'll never let anyone hurt her. Do I have your commitment to that?"

Having obtained a clear "yes" from both parents, the therapist spent the rest of the session coaching the parents on how they would respond to Sophie in the next meeting.

A week later, the therapist helped Sophie tell her parents about her hurt, anger, and sense of betrayal. They listened quietly and then paraphrased back what she had said. When Sophie finally said there was no more to say, the parents apologised to her, making a commitment to protect her and to find non-physical means of resolving their difficulties.

In the next session with Sophie present, the therapist returned to the issue of the parents coming to an agreement about how to handle Sophie's behaviour. This time, the parents reached an agreement.

When they returned the next week, however, they said that the father had broken the agreement and given in to Sophie's demands. Several things were now pointing to relationship difficulties between the husband and wife: their inability to stick to agreed upon rules and consequences; the ease with which the father gave in to the daughter, siding with her against the mother; and the father's criticism of the mother in the session. Although the therapist would have been pleased had the parents been able to stick to their agreements, she also knew that had it been so easy to do so, the problem would not have been so extreme and the parents might never have sought therapy.

The therapist arranged another session with the parents by themselves and formulated the following objectives for the session:

• To understand in more depth why the father could not follow through with what he had agreed to do.

- To uncover relationship issues that fuelled the father's turning away from the mother and towards the daughter.

Beginning the session with an enactment, the therapist asked the parents to talk to each other.

"*What I'd like you to do is to talk to each other about what happened to the plan you made the last time you were here*".

"*I admit it's my fault*", said the father, addressing the therapist. "*But that plan sounded a lot easier last week than it was in real life*".

Looking down at the floor, ignoring his bid for eye contact, the therapist said, "*Talk to each other, not to me*".

The mother said, "*We had an agreement when we walked out of here last time, Tony. **You knew** what **you** were supposed to do, so why at the last minute did you cave-in and let her go out anyway?*"

"*Look, Annie*", said the father, "*I'm just **so sick** of the arguments*".

"*Well **I'm** sick of looking like the bad guy. I'm **sick** of having to do it **all** myself. Sick of being the only one who worries*".

"*You're not the **only** one who worries. And if **you** weren't so hot headed you wouldn't look like the bad guy*".

"*I've had it. I'm exhausted. That's why I'm hot headed. **You** leave **everything** up to me. We both work full time and you leave all of the cooking and cleaning and washing and shopping up to me. You think it's women's work. You come home late, turn on the TV and put your feet up. And now with Mum sick, it's just impossible. Sometimes I just feel like leaving*".

"*Don't talk like that, Annie, why do you **always** blow things right out of proportion?*"

"*It's **not fair**. It's not right that you leave it all up to me*".

When the parents continued to argue for the next few minutes, the therapist intervened. "*Annie, tell Tony what you need from him for you to feel his support*".

"*I need you to take on some of the work in the house. I mean take **responsibility** for it, not do it as a job to help me*".

The therapist asked: "*And what do you need to feel his emotional support?*"

"*I need you to listen to me when I'm upset or worried about Mum. There used to be a time when we could talk*".

The father sighed, "*It's hard to talk when you're so angry all the time*".

The therapist identified the parents' triangulation of Sophie into their relationship conflict

Turning to the father, the therapist said: "*When you think Annie is acting 'hot headed', how much do you think this has to do with Sophie and how much does it have to do with you?*"

"*Annie directs it towards Sophie*", said the father, "*but I feel like, underneath, she's really directing it at me*".

"*And do you ask Annie about that at the time?*"

"*Oh, no. That would make it worse. Throwing petrol on the fire*".

"*So maybe, instead, you support Sophie. Sophie stands up to Annie and fights your battles for you*".

"*Maybe she does*".

For the next 15 minutes, the therapist and parents discussed how Sophie's involvement in their conflicts made the situation between them worse. The mother disclosed that she was often so angry with the father for supporting Sophie against her that she had taken to sleeping in the lounge room. The father acknowledged he was angry at his wife's sexual withdrawal and this fuelled his support of Sophie against her. The mother admitted that although it must have seemed that she was rejecting him, she had lost interest in sex following the death of her own father.

The therapist helped the parents solidify a plan for change

The therapist pulled the session together by saying: "*It would be good to have a plan about what you're going to do differently to support each other during this rough time. If you both feel supported by each other, you'll be able to stick together when you make an agreement about how to handle Sophie. So let me ask you, Annie, what are three things, any one of which if Tony were to do, would make a difference to you in terms of the issues we've talked about today?*"[4]

"*Well, on a practical level*", said the mother, "*it would make a huge difference if Tony would take over the responsibility for some of the work in the house. Like the washing or the grocery shopping. The second thing would be if he was willing to visit my mother on his own some evenings. She adores him and it would make her very happy and it would mean I wouldn't have to go that evening. The third thing would be if Tony sat down with me every evening for twenty minutes so that I had a chance to talk about some of the things that are weighing me down*".

To ensure that the father had understood the mother's three requests, the therapist asked him to paraphrase the mother's requests back to the mother. He did this successfully.

The therapist then asked, "*Could you agree to one of those requests, Tony?*"

"*Sure. In fact I can agree to all three. I'm willing to take on the washing and the grocery shopping. I don't mind at all going and visiting her mother. And I think it would be a good thing for us to talk together every night*".

"*OK. All three?*"

"*Yeah, all three*".

The mother smiled and, looking at the therapist, said, "*I told you he was a marshmallow*".

"*He's sweet all right,*" replied the therapist. "*It's nice to see that softness working in your favour too. But Tony, can you stick to your commitment this time?*"

"*I can*".

Handing the father her pen, the therapist said, "*I think you can, too. Here, Tony, how about you write down what exactly you are committing to do*".

Tony smiled and took the pen.

Then the therapist asks, "*Tony, what three things would you like to ask of Anna?*"

"*I can only think of two. It would mean a lot to me if she would come back to sleeping in our bed. The other thing is that if she would cut back on yelling at Sophie*".

"*Try for a third*".

"*OK. A hug in the morning before I leave for work*".

The therapist asked the mother, "*Can you commit to one of Tony's requests?*"

The mother smiled and reached over, placing her hand over his. "*I'll come back to the bed and a hug is easy. The shouting, I'll have to work on*".

"*You'll get there*", said the therapist and then concluded, "*This is a hard time in your lives. But there is a lot of good will and a deep love between the two of you*".

At the beginning of the following session, the therapist saw the parents alone before bringing in Sophie and her brother, checking in with the parents about the agreements they had made to each other. The mother, looking softer and less stressed, reported that the father had fulfilled his promises, helping around the house, doing the shopping, and visiting her mother. They had talked most evenings. The father said they were closer, more affectionate, and that they were sleeping together again. The mother had raised her voice to Sophie but had refrained from yelling.

In this session, the parents worked out another agreement about how to respond to Sophie's rebellious behaviour. This time Sophie, who seemed calmer and less reactive, did not interrupt the parents nor did the father invite her into the discussion. Over the next few months, both parents kept to their agreements despite Sophie's many challenges. The mother said that she felt supported by the father and the parents reported a closer relationship. Sophie and her mother began spending more time together with Sophie saying was now easier to talk to her mother.

Conclusion

While this chapter has focused on the benefits of separate sessions, it is important to outline the risks involved when therapists see parents separately. The most common risk therapists encounter is that of receiving too much information. Parents may reveal secrets that they want the therapist to keep from their children: the father is not the biological father; the "mother" is in fact the "grandmother"; the "parents" are in fact the "adoptive parents". A parent may be dealing with a terminal illness or the parents might be planning to separate. Therapists face the dilemma of whether or not to encourage the parents to reveal their secrets, taking into consideration the impact on the therapy, engagement with the parents, and the effect on the children.

Another risk is that parents may perceive separate sessions as the therapist implying that the parents are, or that their couple relationship is, the cause of the child's problem and that they are therefore to blame (Brown, 2008). If the therapist does indeed believe that couple relationship issues impede the parents working together as a team, then the therapist must explore the connection between the child's problem and the parents' relationship in a way that demonstrates this connection to the parents as exemplified in the above case study. Otherwise, separate sessions that focus on couple issues *do* imply that the parents are to blame for their child's problem and the therapist does risk losing engagement.

On the other hand, given the opportunity to discuss their couple relationship separately, some parents may open the floodgates and therapists may make the mistake of proceeding with de facto couples' therapy while the child's presenting problem remains unresolved. Within the context of family therapy, couple sessions should be seen as a means towards the end of freeing the child from the parents' relationship. Once this is accomplished and the presenting problem resolved, the parents may be referred or the therapist may recontract for couple therapy.

This chapter has illustrated how strategically timed meetings with parents within the overall context of family sessions can help parents save face, speak openly about individual and couple problems, strengthen the parental alliance, and free the identified patient from a triangulated position. Separate parent sessions need to be carefully integrated into the overall process of family sessions. By developing clarity about the "why" and "how" of separate parent sessions, therapists can progress therapy while ensuring that sessions with the whole family remain the main game.

Notes

1 Therapists should have access to and familiarity with screening instruments for anxiety and depression such as the Beck Depression Inventory or the Depression and Anxiety Scale (DAS).
2 This case is a compilation of several cases. Any similarity to actual families is coincidental.
3 For further elaboration on apology sessions, see MacKinnon (1998) and James (2007).
4 See Luquet (2006) for information on "behaviour change requests" from Imago Couples Therapy.

References

Baumrind, D. (1978). Parental disciplinary patterns and social competence in children. *Youth and Society*, *9*, 238–276.

Bowen, M. (1978). Family therapy in clinical practice. New York, NY: Aronson.

Brown, J. (2008). We don't need your help, but please fix our children. *Australian and New Zealand Journal of Family Therapy*, *29*, 61–69.

Guerin, P., Fay, L, Burden, S., & Kautto, J. (1987). *The evaluation and treatment of marital conflict*. New York, NY: Basic Books.

Guerin, P., Fay, L., Burden, S., & Kautto, J. (1996). *Working with relationship triangles; the one, two, three of psychotherapy*. New York, NY: Guilford Press.

Haley, J. (1987). *Problem-solving therapy* (2nd ed.). San Francisco, CA: Jossey-Bass Pub.

James, K. (1989). When twos are really threes. The triangular dance in couple conflict. *Australian and New Zealand Journal of Family Therapy*, *10*(3), 179–189.

James, K. (2007). The interactional process of forgiveness and responsibility: A critical assessment of the family therapy literature. Ch. 10. In C. Flaskas, I. McCarthy, & J. Sheehan (Eds.), *Hope and despair in narrative and family therapy* (pp. 127–138). UK: Karnac Press.

Jiménez, L., Hidalgo, V., Baena, S., León, A., & Lorence, B. (2019) Effectiveness of structural–strategic family therapy in the treatment of adolescents with mental health problems and their families. *International Journal of Environmental Research and Public Health*, *16*(7), 1255.

Luquet, W. (2006). *Short-term couples therapy: The Imago model in action*. New York, NY: Brunner/Mazel.

MacKinnon, L. (1998). *Trust and betrayal in the treatment of child abuse*. New York, NY: Guilford Press.

Madanes, C. (2009). *Relationship breakthrough*. New York, NY: Rodale Books.

Minuchin, S. (1974). *Families and family therapy*. London, UK: Tavistock Pub.

Minuchin, S., & Fishman H. C.(1981). *Family therapy techniques*. Cambridge, MA: Harvard University Press.

Watzlawick, P., Beavin, H., & Jackson (1967). *The pragmatics of human communication*. New York, NY: W.W. Norton.

Chapter 10

Family of Origin Sessions

Why, When, and How

Hugh Crago

What is the purpose of family of origin sessions?

Family therapy must balance adult clients' concern to 'fix' a young person who is presented as the problem against the strong likelihood that the adults themselves are part of the problem, inadvertently maintaining the young person's behaviour by their behavioural responses to it, or by interpretations of the behaviour that are not helpful. Since the early days of family therapy, we have understood that if we challenge parents' perceptions of the problem too overtly and too early, we risk losing the family. Intervention must acknowledge that the child does present real difficulties for parents and/or stepparents, while not closing the door to the possibility that the adults may in time learn different responses to the young person, and, simultaneously, come to accept more of a share of responsibility for what has gone wrong.

This would suggest that family of origin interventions, directed at adults, would usually be deferred until the later stages of therapy, where some improvement in the presenting problem has already been achieved, and parents are ready to focus on themselves. But what constitutes 'later stages' will of course vary widely from family to family. For some families, months might need to elapse before the focus can begin to shift to the adults.

Sympathetic investigation of parents' families of origin can often be crucial to enhancing their empathy for their 'problematic' young person. It can promote understanding of their own reactions and motivate them in the direction of change. Information about the adults' family of origin experiences can assist in reframing current difficulties and accessing suppressed or denied suffering which has unconsciously shaped their own parenting beliefs and practices. Additionally, a family of origin questioning sometimes uncovers untimely deaths, secrets, or 'shameful' events which may directly bear on the development of symptoms in a young person (Imber-Black, 1994).

What is the theory behind family of origin sessions?

Structured family of origin questioning has been a recognised assessment tool since the early days of family therapy (e.g., Satir, 1967), a systemic equivalent of 'taking a history' in traditional psychiatric practice. Over a 20-year period, Monica McGoldrick and her colleagues have developed a standard framework for questioning, and for recording and interpreting family of origin information (McGoldrick & Gerson, 1985; McGoldrick, Gerson, & Shellenberger, 1999; McGoldrick, Gerson, and Petry, 2008). Software programs exist for constructing genograms and incorporating data into them.

DOI: 10.4324/9781003490104-11

A genogram is not only an assessment tool. Constructing it with the family is itself an intervention. Genogram sessions can also lead to other interventions, including 'family of origin coaching', as described by Murray Bowen (1978) and his school, or investigations of 'imbalances in the family ledger' across generations as described by Boszormenyi-Nagy and Spark (1984) and Boszormenyi-Nagy and Krasner (1986). In Boszormenyi-Nagy's terminology, young people can demonstrate 'invisible loyalty' to an ancestor they may not have met, or who died before they were born (in my view, both genetic and environmental factors probably play a part in such occurrences). A handful of psychoanalytically influenced investigators have posited predictable 'generational repeats', linked to specific marker events in the life of a member of one generation, which then 'reappear' in the form of a crisis (benign or malign) in an individual of the next generation, when that individual reaches the same chronological age at which his same-sex parent experienced the original marker event (Earnshaw, 1998; Schutzenberger, 1998). This phenomenon may be related to the so-called 'anniversary reactions' long noted by psychoanalytic scholars (e.g., Engel, 1975).

But, perhaps because of its association with 'grand theory' and modernist assumptions of objective truth, the genogram seems to have fallen from favour over the past 20 or so years. Some current family therapy approaches, particularly those influenced by social constructivism, avoid it altogether. They argue that drawing a genogram, like writing a letter that offers the therapist's interpretation of clients' situation, can sometimes impart 'authority' or 'realness' to what has hitherto only been spoken about. To my mind, however, asking the adults questions about their own families of origin and drawing up a genogram based on their answers remain key interventions when working with two or more generations.

There is an enormous difference between asking clients family of origin questions in individual therapy and asking clients the same questions in a conjoint interview with partners and/or children. Psychologically sophisticated clients often say they have 'already worked on' their family of origin or 'come to terms with all of that'. What this often means in practice is that they have convinced an individual therapist of the correctness of their stance of blame, hurt, and disappointment, leaving the family of origin status quo unchanged. Many individual therapists do not even suggest the possibility that their clients might engage with parents or siblings to refashion previously problematic relationships. The assumption is that such attempts will inevitably fail or may 'damage' the client. Some therapists believe that there are 'toxic' parents and supporting a client to avoid or work separately is the only feasible approach.

Clients' recollections of their childhood and upbringing are bound to be subjective. The constructivist approach to memory has emphasised that memories are refashioned every time they are recounted and that the social context in which a memory is talked about will invariably influence the details that are recalled (Engel, 1999; Spence, 1982). And we possess empirical data on how differently family members may describe key events and relationships (e.g., Dunn & Plomin, 1990). To my mind, none of this necessarily invalidates the genogram, which is ultimately a representation of one family member's reconstructed 'reality' and does not necessarily claim to be objective truth. Careful questioning by a therapist who is outside the family system can often uncover new perspectives on family members whom the client may have idealised, judged harshly, or dismissed as unimportant. Genogram questioning thus aims for a fuller or 'thicker' description (Geertz, 1973) of the family of origin than the one that has guided clients in the past.

However, even when therapists can see the usefulness of gaining family of origin information, many adults in Western cultures resist the notion that problems in their own relationships of choice, or problems in the lives of their children, may be directly or indirectly related to events, personalities, and behaviour patterns in their families of origin. So thoroughly have we trained ourselves to value being 'independent' of our parents, to see our lives as separate from theirs, that the idea of a connection may seem counter-intuitive, even far-fetched. By contrast, many non-Western cultures see problems in one generation as the direct result of 'the spirit of an ancestor' influencing a young person's behaviour (Andary, Stolk, & Klimidis, 2003; Medland, 1988).

When should I conduct this part of the therapy?

Common impasses within client families that lend themselves to family of origin exploration include the following:

- An adult has become 'stuck' in a dysfunctional pattern of behaviour towards a young person – the same pattern in which she/he was 'stuck' with his/her own parent(s). The adult is now in his/her own parent's position, and 'instinctively' or unquestioningly replicates the parent's behaviour, even though it felt bad when he/she was on the receiving end of it.
- An adult is unable to form a satisfactory attachment bond with a child or connects with the child only under certain conditions (e.g., if the child is 'good' and does not show anger or distress). In these cases, the adult is often replicating the kind of attachment (or lack of it) that she or he had with her/his own caregiver (Karen, 1998).
- Relatives in the older generation (e.g., grandparents) are over-involved in the family of their offspring, advising, blaming, offering financial support, or threatening to withdraw it, and taking over responsibilities which are rightfully those of the younger generation. Alternatively, those in the younger generation are cut off from legitimate sources of support (e.g., with childcare), feel isolated, and are overhung by feelings of anxiety, guilt, or anger towards their families. Thus, the parents' impaired relationship with their own parents (and, often, siblings) forms a context in which it is more difficult for them to offer secure attachment and appropriate parenting to their offspring.

When the therapist senses that one or more of these impasses may be at issue, one or more family of origin sessions may prove extremely productive. However, the more rigidly the adults insist on focussing on the problematic young person, and the more they manifest anxiety, defensiveness, or irritation at any shift away from this focus, the less likely they are to be receptive to family of origin questioning in the early stages of therapy. Hence, it is usually best to work initially with the family unit as the clients themselves have defined it, normally the two-generation 'nuclear' family, but often minus one of the biological parents of the 'problem' young person. Exceptions may be made where grandparents – or other relatives – regularly act as caregivers for children because of the parents' incapacity or unwillingness to take the primary parenting role.

This means that family of origin questions are deferred until you get a sense of how the immediate family are affected by the presenting problem, and how they interact around it. Even if you strongly suspect that family of origin issues may be important, it still makes sense not to ask about them straightway. Clients need to feel that the problem, as they see it, is being taken seriously. It is also common for adult clients to resist early questions about family of origin because they know there are shameful or upsetting things 'back there', which they have never told their children about, and certainly don't wish to air in front of a stranger. The worker must respect this while building a level of trust with clients that will allow exploration of family of origin to take place later.

Other things being equal, I'd usually expect to start thinking about family of origin questioning from around the fourth session onwards. This means that the therapy has survived the 'third session challenge' (Crago, 2006, pp. 50–53; Crago & Gardner, 2019), and hopefully, some foundations have been laid for a therapeutic alliance. You will need to judge for yourself, or in discussion with your supervisor, whether the right time has come by the fourth session, or whether it is still far too early. As always, it is your clients' behaviour – the way they are responding to you and to each other – that will provide your best source of information as to whether they are 'ready' for something or not. No manual can tell you that.

What if the clients themselves mention family of origin in the first session? If something is raised by clients early in therapy, it needs to be acknowledged as important, even if not dealt with immediately. If a child, rather than an adult, raises the question of the involvement of an extended family member, this can sometimes be dealt with by a 'checking in' with the caregiver, as in the following examples.

Therapist:	So you guys are with Mum and James (step-Dad) most of the time, and you see Dad at weekends every now and then. Is that right?
Tim (aged nine):	Grandma says Mum shouldn't be with James cos she thinks he's a creep.
Therapist:	OK, I see. I just want to check with Mum here. [*Turns to Mum*] Janine, what do you reckon? Is this something we should be talking about right now, or is it more important to talk about the stuff with the school, and how Jodie's getting into strife with the teachers?
Janine:	Look, Tim's just a smart-arse, don't take any notice of him, he's just attention seeking.

The therapist registers Tim's comment as probably accurate, and worth coming back to in later sessions, but gets the message loud and clear that now is not the time to explore it.

Alternatively,

Janine:	It's true what he says, Mum's always getting between me and James. I hate it and it's not fair – she wants to split us up, and it's none of her business.
Therapist:	OK, so Tim's put us onto something quite important, hasn't he? Let's come back to Grandma a bit later on, but for now, I'd like to spend a bit more time on Jodie and the things you're worried about with her.

The therapist registers that Janine has confirmed Tim's perception and 'owned' it as an issue. However, she does not rush to explore it. Instead, she returns to the family's original presentation of Jodie's behaviour.

In this, as in many other ways, it is very difficult to be too prescriptive about how, and when, to use family of origin questioning. For example, it is perfectly feasible to incorporate the drawing-up of a genogram into the first or second session as part of the assessment phase of therapy, but to defer more searching questioning around family of origin until a later stage, where trust in the therapy process has been established, and once the adults have given some indication of the significance of wider family relationships. Alternatively, family of origin questioning may be introduced for the first time much later, where it has become clear that the family is 'stuck', and a widening of the context may be necessary to provide new momentum.

Systematic family of origin questioning is an option, not a necessity. Some families are better served by interventions directed at behaviour change in the present than by potentially threatening enquiries into family of origin.

Where there have been hints about abusive or traumatic experiences in one or both adults' families, you may have a sense that your clients are avoiding anything that might come near those experiences. Clearly, setting aside adults-only sessions will help in this regard (see below) but though it may lessen client concerns, it will not take them away. If I pick up the unspoken message, 'This is just too hard—I can't face it', then the therapist might pose a strategic dilemma:

Therapist: Mmm., I need to tell you about a problem I have here. Janine, I'm very aware that you've hinted at some pretty bad things that happened in the family you grew up in. I'm aware that to talk about these things might be extremely painful for you, and I certainly don't want you to feel that you have to revisit these things. On the other hand, what we know is that sometimes, understanding bad things that happened to us in childhood can really help us to be better parents. It's sort of like a key that unlocks the door – when the door's been locked until now. I'd like to be able to talk with you about your childhood, and what happened, and the part that other people in your family played in all of that. But I don't want to cause you pain. What do you think I should do?

Janine: I'm shit scared to talk about that stuff. But I know I need to. I'm just scared I'll cry for a week. But if it could make it easier between Jodie and me – I'd do anything to make that happen.

Implementation: How do I do it?

Family of origin work may involve a variety of approaches – constructing a genogram, conducting dedicated 'family of origin sessions', discussing specific homework based on information obtained in the sessions, and, more rarely, inviting adult clients' relatives to special 'consultation' sessions. It is impossible to reduce this diversity to a single set of principles or 'strategies', so I have organised this section around the kinds of questions that trainees typically ask:

You seem to be assuming that I should set aside whole sessions for these questions, but what about just weaving them in session by session as they seem relevant?

Manualised approaches and step-by-step models can sometimes conflict with the kind of flexibility that working with a family (indeed, with any client) ideally demands. Clearly, both 'dedicated' sessions and 'questions as you go' have advantages and disadvantages.

'Questions as you go' might be more suited to the 'level one' family I have described in my *Couple, Family and Group Work* (Crago, 2006, pp. 151–156). Such families come into therapy with more flexibility, more openness, and more motivation than the majority. Adults in these families will be able to handle some 'to and fro' between past and present and can tolerate the possibility that their behaviour with their children might be influenced by their own past experiences. Adult couples are more likely to be interested and support-ive of each other when sensitive material from the past is disclosed. Their level of conflict is manageable.

By contrast, sessions dedicated to family of origin exploration can be useful when there is a high level of conflict between adult partners, and they maintain rigid, polarised posi-tions regarding the young person. The therapist can frame the sessions as set apart from the 'main issues' and can introduce them as, 'a chance for me to find out more about where you're both coming from, and maybe work out some of the experiences that are influencing how you relate to one another'. Specific ground rules can be set for these ses-sions, for example,

Therapist: In this session, I'll be speaking just to you, Janine, for the first half hour. After that, I'll be speaking just with you, James. I've set aside time for each of you to tell me about the families that you grew up in, and that means no interrup-tions from the other one. You'll be listening, and later, I'll be glad to hear any comments you might have.

Having special sessions 'just' for drawing a genogram and asking the family of origin questions can sometimes feel, for clients, like a relief from the hard work, tensions, and conflicts of family therapy (Hoang, 2005). On the other hand, for some clients, it may loom as more threatening, and more shameful, than exploring their current nuclear fam-ily issues (see above section 'When should I conduct this part of the therapy?'). Again, in deciding which way to go, you need to pay attention to how your clients respond to the direction you are embarking upon.

Is there anything that the kids might benefit from hearing about?

Often there is, but I have generally found it best to ask the sensitive questions in an adults-only session, and then consult the adults as to how, and when, they would prefer to share some of their discoveries or disclosures with the young people. Developmental consid-erations obviously apply. Younger children may not be able to understand certain things, whereas many teenagers can take the same things in their stride. If the information to be disclosed relates directly to the child's behaviour and feelings, then its potential impact on the young person needs to be considered.

Parents in overly close families (Salvador Minchin used the term 'enmeshed'; see Mi-nuchin, 1974, pp. 54–56) tend to overprotect their children (and other family members), assuming that their kids may be traumatised by information (e.g., about who their 'real' parent is, or about the existence of half-siblings they have never met). Parents in distant or 'disengaged' families (Minuchin, 1974, pp. 54–56), which sometimes correspond with the 'neglectful' families encountered in child protection work, may do the opposite, lacking sufficient empathy to sense that a child may be overwhelmed by a sudden disclosure that overturns its previous unquestioned assumptions about the family.

It is up to you, as a therapist, to monitor these variables, and to step in with words of caution or encouragement if appropriate. Your judgement and sensitivity in such matters will be much more reliable if you have yourself engaged in family of origin work as part of your therapy, your training, or both (see the following section 'Equipping yourself to ask family of origin questions').

Should I put a genogram up on a whiteboard, or just draw it on my own notepad?

The genogram should normally be prominently displayed so that all the clients can see it. Whiteboards are good in that additions can be rapidly made and incorrect information erased. I sometimes draw up a mini genogram on a notepad if clients start volunteering family of origin information before I had planned to deal with it. Later, this can form the basis for the 'public' genogram. If I've constructed a partial genogram in one session, I often put this up so it can easily be seen and then invite clients to help me fill in the gaps and answer questions I, or they, might have.

Are there creative alternatives to 'whiteboard and marker' versions of the genogram?

There are all sorts of alternatives. Clients can be encouraged to use ready-made magnetic genogram symbols and to construct their own genograms on the board. Or they can cut out figures and shapes from magazines and paste them into a collage. The most recent edition of McGoldrick's text (McGoldrick, Gerson, & Petry, 2008) includes colour plates illustrating the use of small figurines. Clients will often talk away while selecting and positioning these figures, much as young children do in sand tray work or play therapy, and their talk will be less 'consciously controlled' and 'censored' than if they were simply responding to your questions.

What questions do I start with?

The great thing about genograms is that you have plenty of starting points. I start with something 'safe' and for the opening phases, I concentrate on just getting the facts and dates. The principle here is: always proceed from the 'easy' to the 'hard', from the factual to the emotional. Avoid starting straight in with hard-hitting questions about painful areas. Work around them and proceed gradually. Of course, once you know your clients well, and sense that they feel safe with you, you can afford to be a bit less careful – but that will not usually happen until you and they have been meeting for some time.

Later, I can ask the more 'unsafe' (that is, more personal, more emotionally loaded) questions, for example:

OK, so your parents got married in 1974, and your sister came along quite soon after that, and then you were born a few years later. How did your parents get on, when you were growing up? How would you describe their relationship at that time?

You said that your parents split when you were thirteen. What do you remember from around that time? What was that like for you? How did you manage your feelings about it?

You left home when you were fifteen. What made you leave at that time? Do you think it was more your decision, or more their decision?

I am not above prompting, if clients are reticent, but if my questions result in 'stonewall tactics', then I usually prefer to back off:

Therapist: So you said that your brother was the one your Dad really treated as special. Where did that leave you?
Client: Wouldn't know. You don't think about that sort of thing when you're a kid. You just get on with life.
Therapist: I guess I was just wondering if maybe you sometimes felt left out or wished your Dad would spend a bit more time with you?
Client: Nup. Never occurred to me.
Therapist: Well, that's pretty normal. Let's talk about your Mum.

As always in therapy, simply asking the question can be an important intervention, regardless of whether the client chooses to answer it. By asking a question about some key area, we acknowledge its existence. Sometimes, clients will voluntarily return to such areas much later if we don't push them too hard to answer our questions the first time. An excellent demonstration of a calm, persistent approach to genogram-construction and questioning (informed by a Bowenian perspective) can be found in a 1989 Menninger Clinic videotape, *Family Systems Theory with an Individual: Conducting the First Two Sessions.*

How do I know what the 'important' information is? What do I leave out?

Your understanding of family dynamics (and your experience of having thoroughly explored your own family of origin) will help you to sense what is more central, and what is peripheral. Sometimes adults will go into detail about the nature of their parents' employment, or sporting involvement, or some other aspect of life. As they talk about these apparently peripheral topics, I listen for signs of emotional or relational significance. I notice what they leave out, as well as what they put in. Then I may ask:

What was the satisfaction for your Mum in getting involved in fostering those kids? What do you think it meant for her? Why did she keep doing it, even after she didn't need the extra income any more?[1]

So your uncle and your Dad worked the farm together, right? What do you know about that partnership? Did they get on well? Or did they run into a bit of difficulty working together? You know, just because you're family doesn't mean you always see eye to eye, does it? It is important to have a repertoire of 'normalising statements' to help clients feel that it's OK to say something that may feel 'critical' or 'disloyal' to the family they grew up in. 'Close' families generate intense 'loyalty', which manifests as a shared belief that, while individual family members may be criticised within the family, it is improper and shameful to voice such criticism to outsiders. In this way, families in Western cultures may continue to act in ways anthropologists associate with 'shame-oriented' or 'face-governed' cultures.

If the other partner butts in and contradicts the partner I'm questioning, what should I do?

It is important to preserve the ground rules of the session: each partner should have the space to talk about his/her family without interruption. I would normally turn to the interrupting partner and say,

Sounds like you see it very differently. I'll be interested to hear about that later. But right now, she's the one who has the floor, because it's her family. When it's your turn, I'm not going to let her interrupt you, OK? When you read these words, they may sound quite abrupt and controlling, but remember that they will be spoken quietly and calmly, and not in a hectoring or chiding manner.

Of course, partners' interruptions are not necessarily 'power plays'. In families where there is a higher level of mutual understanding and supportiveness, the partner's contribution will often be accepted by the speaker. I would briefly acknowledge these contributions, but then turn back to the client whose family is the topic and invite them to continue.

What happens in a blended family? Do I involve the non-biological parent, or not?

You do. The partner will be influenced in his/her parenting attitudes, values, and practices by what he/she grew up with, just like the biological parent. Moreover, clinical evidence indicates we are attracted again and again to the same kind of person, so even though a new partner may appear very different from the children's biological father or mother, there are likely to be some similarities in personality, and some replication of key dynamics. Thus, in listening to the experiences and perceptions of the new partner, we may even gain some insight into the children's biological parent, and we can safely assume that the new partner, like previous ones, will represent a personality type that 'fits' with the family of origin of the children's biological parent.

What if one of the adults doesn't know anything?

It is common for people to know a lot more about one side of their family of origin than the other. Typically, it is the mother's family that is known about, while the father's is 'in the shadows', because women are typically more invested in maintaining relationships and try to keep up some contact, even when family members are separated by distance or the temporary fracturing of emotional bonds. Men, by comparison, typically display a lack of interest in relatives they have rarely seen and will not initiate renewals of contact as readily as women. As my own father once memorably grumbled, 'You don't know them, and you've got nothing in common with them. Why would you bother?' I was wise enough by then to refrain from saying, 'Well, if you knew them, maybe you'd find you did have things in common with them, and then you would bother!'

If one of the adults in the session has 'gaps' of this nature on one side of their genogram, this fact is often worth asking about:

What ideas do you have about why you know so little about your Dad's family? How would a situation like that come about? Who do you think might have decided that you should grow up without knowing anything about your Dad's parents?

Of course, these questions need to be asked calmly and in a spirit of genuine enquiry, rather than coming across as accusatory. I often add a 'normalising' comment to remove any sense that the adult is being criticised or pathologised for knowing little about one side of the family:

> Well, what you're describing isn't all that uncommon, you know. I think often we grow up knowing more about one side than the other. And when you're a kid, you just accept it – you know, that's the way it is. Often we don't even question it until much later.

Again, it is the impact on the client of the 'missing pieces' which should be the focus of the therapist's attention: *Have you ever wondered why you know so little about your Dad's side? What impact do you think it might have had on you, that you know quite a few family members on your Mum's side, but nobody at all on your Dad's? If your Dad had known how this would affect you, how do you think he might have felt?*

These questions open areas which may previously have been unknown. Some clients will rise to the challenge of exploring them further, others will not, but either way, as I explained above, it is still useful to ask them. For a minority of us, questions demand answers, and 'missing pieces' must be found (Crago, 1992); for the majority, it seems better to 'let sleeping dogs lie'.

What about a parent who was adopted?

Usually, adopted clients will tell you which family they consider important. Those who have extensive knowledge of their biological family (probably a minority) may want both on the genogram; many will not (as an adopted cousin of mine once observed, 'I've already got a family—why would I want another one?'). It is important to be guided by clients as to what they consider the formative influences on their development. Some adoptees will insist that their biological heritage counts for very little; others will be aware of genetic traits they share with their biological parent(s) and may want these considered. Adoptees who were told from very early about their adopted status may have a very different perspective from those who did not learn of it until they were almost grown up (this was once quite common, although rare today). Those whose biological parent (usually their mother) seeks them out and wants to resume a relationship with them will have very different experiences from those who, as adults, themselves initiate contact with their biological parent. Mike Leigh's movie *Secrets and Lies* (1996) is a particularly poignant portrayal of the realities of adult recontact (as opposed to the fantasies that many adoptees, and biological parents, entertain before such recontact is accomplished). Goodwach (2003) provides a useful introduction to this whole area.

How much should I join with an adult client against an abusive family member, or a family member that they hate?

When your questions elicit a torrent of loathing towards a parent or sibling, you will experience a powerful 'pull' to join the client in her/his stance, especially if violence and sexual abuse have been involved. However, simply 'siding with the client' can be problematic, especially as the whole story does not necessarily emerge the first time the topic is raised, and it may later turn out that your strong alliance with the client has not been wholly justified. It is useful to master phrasing like, 'Well, it sounds like you experienced your relationship with him as pretty awful. As you remember it, he never understood you, or had time for you'. Here the careful choice of words conveys a measure of 'wait and see', while at the same time giving your client the impression that you are hearing her and taking her feelings seriously.

It can also be useful to say, 'So that's how it felt when you were growing up. Have you noticed any changes in your relationship with him since you've had kids of your own, or has it stayed much like as it was back then?'

What does it mean if adults insist that they had a 'wonderful childhood', when that seems improbable?

There is no point in struggling with clients over how 'wonderful' their childhood really was. However, I have found that narcissistic clients who idealise their families will nevertheless admit to wounding or humiliating experiences *at school* (e.g., teasing, bullying, ostracism) and this can provide an important 'way in' to empathising with their childhood pain and (often) loneliness.

Other clients may idealise their childhood and family relationships because of dissociative defences formed early on against trauma. It is generally easy enough to tell when idealisation is occurring, because the portrayal of both individuals and relationships is global and unspecific, with little or no mention of their personal feelings:

Client:	Dad was a great person. He really cared about us. Everyone loved him.
Therapist:	How did he show you that he cared about you? What sort of things did he do? [*Therapist pushes for an account of actual behaviour rather than value judgements*]
Client:	Oh, I don't know. He just cared. Everyone remembers him as a caring person. Hundreds of people came to his funeral, you know. [*Client refuses the invitation to be more specific and shifts the ground to a less personal arena.*]
Therapist:	Sounds like people really respected him and admired him. I wonder, did he ever disappoint you, or make you mad? You know, maybe when you were a teenager? [*Therapist directly suggests the possibility of conflict or negativity.*]
Client:	Never. He was always just there. That's what people appreciated. [*Return to the global and the impersonal.*]

In this case, the client may be protecting not only themselves (from distressing memories) but also the family member in question ('Never speak ill of the dead') or the whole family's reputation. It seems highly unlikely that any parent would be as 'perfect' as this father is portrayed to be. Even intelligent, high-achieving individuals may display quite primitive, irrational behaviour in relation to their family of origin, behaviour which they would never manifest in their work lives.

If clients can't remember anything about their childhood, does that always mean they were abused?

Not necessarily, but you need to entertain that as a possibility. Remember, it is quite common for people to have relatively sparse memories of their early childhood years (prior to age five), and most of us have none of the pre-verbal period. Also, clients may sometimes 'blank out' details due to anxiety; the fact that they can remember little when asked the first time need not necessarily mean that have no memories at all. Important questions are worth asking a second and a third time. Later in a therapy, clients may feel safe enough to answer them more fully.

What do I do with the genogram once I've got it? Does it lead on to anything?

It is only novice therapists, or therapists who are lacking in empathy and curiosity, who could fail to see the possibilities inherent in almost any genogram. Again, you will be far more aware of these possibilities if you have done your own family of origin work. Here are some of the possible ways to 'follow up' the genogram (all of which, of course, depend upon indications from the client that she/he is interested and motivated to move in such a direction):

- A client may contact another family member (typically a sibling, sometimes a cousin, uncle, or aunt) to compare their perceptions of the family environment with his/her own. This sometimes occurs when clients realise for the first time that perhaps someone else, apart from themselves, may have been subjected to sexual abuse in childhood.
- A client may initiate contact with another family member (typically a parent) where there has been a problematic or conflicted relationship in the past, but where there now seems more possibility of reaching a mutual understanding.
- A client may open lines of communication with previously 'cut off' relatives (Bowen, 1978), realising that such cut-offs often arise out of misunderstandings and rigid judgements, and tend to 'roll' unquestioned from one generation to the next.
- A client may enter into a dialogue with his/her child, revealing for the first time significant events in his/her own childhood.
- A therapist may suggest that an adult client invite parents, siblings, or other significant relatives to one or two sessions of 'consultation'. See the separate subsection below.

Simply answering family of origin questions can be 'work'. However, I agree with Bowen and his school that family of origin work in the true sense involves real-life dialogues between clients and their relatives. When a client can enter into 'adult to adult', non-blaming conversation with parents, siblings, or other relatives, she can achieve a higher level of 'differentiation of self' (see Brown, 2017; Kerr & Bowen, 1988; McGoldrick, 1995; Titelman, 1987). Under ideal conditions, clients will initiate such moves unprompted by the therapist, or with only minimal encouragement. In other cases, it is sometimes necessary to offer a good deal of support and advice to assist clients to 'go home again' (McGoldrick, 1995). This is what Bowen famously described as family of origin 'coaching', to distinguish it from 'therapy' (Bowen, 1978, pp. 540–541).

If I ask a client to approach a family of origin member for information, or to resolve something, what do I need to be careful about?

When a therapist invites a client to approach a relative with whom there has been a conflicted or cut-off relationship, clients typically assume that the goal of this intervention is to 'change the other person'; I always explain that the real goal is to change yourself by doing something different from what you've always done. The other person may change as a result (that's a bonus) but you must not enter the task with the expectation that this will happen. Of course, some clients will then refuse to undertake the task, equating it with 'accepting the blame'. If the other person isn't likely to change, they reason, then why should they themselves do anything different?

Emotionally labile clients or those prone to disintegration under extreme stress are not good candidates for direct approaches to family members with whom things have been difficult in the past. Attachment theory provides an invaluable interface with family therapy in this regard, and you should be aware of the three main attachment strategies (Karen, 1998), particularly the Type C strategy, in which the child (and, often, the adult he/ she becomes) alternates between angry blaming and helpless dependency. Adult clients whose infant attachment was of this type often find it difficult to approach family of origin encounters without becoming hijacked by intense anger or distress and readily become 'hooked in' if their initial moves are met with defensiveness or blaming from the other party. I suggest letters as a first step for clients who have difficulty staying non-anxious. If the letter can be relatively short, and tactful, then it stands a chance of 'opening a door', and a meeting may then follow. I generally offer to read their letter before they send it. Otherwise, clients may produce long, rambling letters which slather the recipient with feelings, and try to cover so many 'loaded' topics that their chance of achieving a respectful reception is minimal.

Many clients' parents who have mild or severe personality disorders become even more rigid as they grow older, whereas less disturbed parents are more likely to 'soften' as they approach the end of their lives. Hargrave and Anderson (1992) provide a clearly written and highly practical guide to interactions between adult clients and ageing parents, making an important distinction between 'reparation' and 'forgiveness'. As mentioned earlier in this chapter, we should never jump too quickly to the assumption that a client's parent is 'beyond hope' simply because the client presents them this way. Black-or-white judgments must always be regarded with caution: they represent a primitive kind of thinking, normal for preschool children, but immature and potentially destructive in adults.

So, is it ever a good idea to invite family of origin members to a joint session?

As anticipated above, suggesting that adult clients invite one or more family of origin members to an actual session (or sequence of sessions) is an option, although a very underutilised one, in family therapy. Freeman (1992) has offered clear, persuasive examples of what can happen when adult clients are prepared to invite their siblings, parents, or other relatives into a session. In my experience, one or two consultations with extended family members can sometimes dramatically 'unstick' a long-standing impasse within the nuclear family. Of course, your client must be on side, and even then, it may be tough for them to persuade their relatives to attend a session that 'has nothing to do with them'.

Diplomatic phrasing (*'My therapist says that he would like to hear from you directly, instead of just asking me what you think'* or *'My therapist is happy to phone you in person if you have any questions about how this might work'*) is essential, and of course, if relatives refuse to cooperate, this must be respected. But surprisingly often, at least some family of origin members will take the risk and accept the invitation. They must be treated with respect and courtesy in the ensuing consultation session so that there is no suggestion that they have been hauled in to 'take their punishment' for what they've done to your client! Just asking for information, and being interested in it when offered, is often sufficient. Sometimes you will be able to facilitate a productive dialogue between your client and a sibling, or an ageing parent, and this can be extremely rewarding for all concerned.

Are there times when doing a genogram might make things worse?

Occasionally, yes. I have already mentioned that it does not pay to focus on family of origin work if clients are still rigidly focussed on the 'problem' young person. But over and above this guideline, I have learned that families who have a deterministic and pessimistic outlook on life generally tend to interpret genogram data in the same way. For them, the therapist's identification of a 'repeating pattern' across generations, or a therapeutic reframing of problematic behaviour as 'loyalty' to a relative in the past, can be risky. Some parents simply assimilate such interventions into their existing schema ('there is bad blood in this family') and end up even more deeply entrenched in pessimism. If families seem to be reacting in this way, it is important to shift emphasis onto family strengths and positives and tread lightly around dysfunctional patterns from the past.

Evidence provided in recent years by epigenetic research (Yehuda et al., 2014) strengthens the likelihood that traumatic experiences in one generation may indeed be transmitted to the next (the genes themselves remain unchanged, as evolutionary theory has always believed, but 'tags' attached to the genes can modify their expression). Personally fascinated by such phenomena, I have had to realise that, for most people, any exploration of cross-generational repetition of personality and behaviour remains very sensitive and sometimes threatening and can be vehemently rejected.

How it looks in practice: Excerpt from a hypothetical session

Janine, in her mid-thirties, has sought counselling because of problems with her daughter Jodie, now 14. Jodie has been in trouble for defiant behaviour with her teachers and has a conflicted relationship with Janine's current partner, James, as well as with Janine herself. Whenever the children visit their Nanna (Janine's mother), Jodie and her younger brother Tim (nine) return seeming angry and upset, and according to Janine, Jodie 'comes back and picks a fight with James'. Janine cannot understand this, because, she says, 'James has always respected Jodie, and he actually likes her, only Jodie can't see it'. In an individual session, Janine discloses that she 'finds it hard to like Jodie—I mean, I love her, and that— I'd do anything for her, but when she gives me grief, I just can't seem to give her any rope. I just shut down and yell at her. I feel like she's trying to split me and James, and James is the best thing that ever happened to me'.

The therapist suggests a session with Janine and James, with the aim of having a look at their respective families of origin. Janine is reluctant (see above) but agrees that it might be worthwhile 'if it could help Jodie and me understand each other better'.

In the following extract, draft genograms of Janine's and James' families of origin have already been drawn up, and the therapist has started the session by approaching the 'loaded' topic of Janine's relationship with her parents by first asking similar questions of James, who has presented as less anxious around family of origin issues than Jodie. We enter the session at a point where James has been talking about how he must have been a difficult teenager, and how he now has a better relationship with his dad than he did then:

James: Dead right, I did put a wall up, I shut him out. I can see I did that, now. I guess I've tried to sort of show him that I trust him more now than I did. It took a while, I suppose it took a few years of trying to get through to him, but now I think we get on pretty well. Most of the time, anyway [*laughs*].

Therapist: Janine, what are you thinking, as you're listening to James talk about this?

Janine: [*Bitterly*] Some people have it lucky!

Therapist: It all sounds a bit too good to be true, right? You had a pretty difficult experience, didn't you, with your dad?

Janine: Yeah, with my dad but more so with my mum, really. I mean, dad was a hard man, and he drank and stuff, but we were all used to that. The worst thing was that mum didn't understand me, she'd never take my side, and if he exploded, she'd say it was my fault. That felt—

Therapist: Must've been bloody awful. You really needed her to support you, stick up for you, and she just didn't seem to be able to do that. [*Therapist is careful to use language to leave open the possibility that this is Janine's perception and that there may be a good reason why Janine's mother acted as she did.*]

Janine: Too right she wasn't. It just wasn't in her to give me what I needed. I don't think she really cared about me, or saw me, and I was just invisible as far as she was concerned. Her whole fuckin' world revolved around that bastard…

Therapist: [*recognising that Janine has reverted to black-and-white, condemnatory language and realising that a deeper level of empathy is called for*] You really needed her to care about you, to see you, and she couldn't. She only seemed to see him. Do you know why she did that? Revolved her life around him?

Janine: I never thought about it then. Now, I reckon she was scared of him. Scared to cross him, set him off, you know.

Therapist: Why do you think she was so scared of him? Did he knock her around? Threaten her?

Janine: No, that's the funny thing, he didn't. He'd yell, you know, and bang things around, but he didn't raise a hand to her [*pause*] I think she was scared he'd walk out, that she'd lose him. He was very jealous of us kids, you know, and didn't want her to be talking about us or showing too much interest.

Therapist: Looking back on it now, you can see that she was scared of losing him. Sounds like maybe he was important to her. I know that's hard, 'cos, you know, she wasn't giving you what you needed, not at all, so it was pretty natural for you to just hate her, back then. But as the age you are now, what do you reckon about the way she had to be so careful around him? Do you know why he was so important to her? Why she made him the centre of the universe?

Janine: Probably because he … I dunno. She did say once, it was after I got married to my ex, she did say then that he was very good to her when they first met, you know, she had a child and she wasn't married, and he took that on board and didn't judge her for it. She said 'He accepted me for who I was. He's a good man, it's just that sometimes he does bad things'.

Therapist: Is that so? Really? When you think back to that, to what she said, it sounds like nobody had ever supported her before, or something …

[*Therapist picks up on a glimpse into the painful past experiences of Jodie's mother, experiences which might help to explain why she felt so unable to relate lovingly to Jodie.*]

Janine: Well Nanna and Pop –I mean, my Nanna and Pop, not the kids' Nanna and Pop—they were pretty strict. I 'spose they wouldn't have given her much praise or anything…I mean back in the olden days, it was 'kids should be seen and not heard', wasn't it?

Therapist: So you're telling me that your Mum wouldn't have got much support from her parents. And she probably felt pretty much on her own. And then she got pregnant and had a baby, and I guess they didn't approve of that; she might've felt pretty terrible about herself. [*Therapist supplies some 'scaffolding' to assist Jodie to see more of what her Mum may have felt.*]

Janine: Yeah [*pause*] I hadn't ever thought about it that way. She probably – she probably felt [*starts to cry*] like Jodie does now [*weeping*].

Therapist: [*quietly*] You really feel for Jodie, don't you? Even though she gets up your nose. You know just what she feels like. Do you think she knows that?

Janine: I don't know. I think she does. But we never talk about it. We just yell at each other [*cries*]. I wonder sometimes if she hates me.

James: She doesn't hate you, Janine! She loves you. She's just got a funny way of showing it. [*A supportive partner, who has genuine goodwill, can often supply the 'reality check' that a client needs.*]

Janine: [*cries quietly*]

Therapist: Well, it sounds as though we've got three women here who felt left out and misunderstood – your mum, and you, and now Jodie. And it's nobody's fault, really, these things just happen in families and nobody realises what's happening until it's all happening and it's hard to stop it. [*Normalising statement*] What's it been like, talking about this stuff in here? [*Very important to ask this, not simply because emotion has been shown, but also because Jodie was initially hesitant about embarking on this discussion. Jodie must be given the kind of compassionate listening and consideration that her mother failed to give her.*]

Janine: Hard. I dreaded coming here today, 'cos I knew I'd said I needed to talk about it.

Therapist: It's been really, really hard. But you know, people have to be pretty brave to do what you've just done.

James: Janine's the bravest person I know. She'd take on any challenge. If it's to help her kids, or me, she'd do anything, she'd take anyone on. [*Again, James supplies strong support, which means that the therapist does not need to supply it.*]

Therapist: Janine, when you think about what we've talked about today, your Mum, and her family, and the family you grew up in, how your Mum behaved to you, and how she behaved around your dad, what do you reckon now? [*Open question, allowing a wide field for possible responses, but taking Janine out of emotion, into 'reflective thinking'.*]

Janine: I just thought mum hated me. I suppose she didn't hate me, really. I can't forgive her for what she did to me. But I can see why she would've wanted to hang onto dad. I never thought about that. She was scared to lose him, 'cos he was the best thing that ever happened to her. Poor thing. [*Janine achieves some measure of compassion for her mother, a real breakthrough. This may lead to her softening towards Jodie, with or without an actual conversation with Jodie about the subjects raised in the session.*]

Equipping yourself to ask family of origin questions

You should not embark on family of origin focussed interventions with clients without having experienced them yourself. Questions which seem innocuous to you might be deeply threatening to some clients. By contrast, some questions which you might hesitate to ask, because of sensibilities stemming from your own family background, may not distress or disturb your clients nearly as much. You need to know how it feels to hear words come out of your own mouth which you have never said before, and which suddenly reveal to you a feeling or attitude that you had not realised you held. This is how your clients are sometimes going to feel when you start asking them family of origin questions.

You need to have experienced your own 'resistance' to questioning, and your own automatic 'family loyalties', which make it difficult for you to see a loved parent objectively, or to see that a loathed parent might have some redeeming features. McGoldrick's general audience book *The Genogram Journey: Reconnecting with your family, (2011) is* probably the best introduction to doing your own family of origin work even though it was published some time ago. Titelman (1987) also collects several first-hand accounts of such work and *Growing Yourself Up* (Brown, 2017) is a more recent Australian guide for both clients and trainee therapists.

A full exploration of your own family of origin, under the guidance of a trained Bowenian practitioner, is the systemic equivalent of the 'training analysis' students of psychoanalytic psychotherapy are required to undertake. It will take at least a year and probably more. It will make you a far 'safer' person for families to sit with, when talking about painful conflicts of loyalty within their own kinship networks, or when trying to reconcile their childhood perceptions of parents with the more objective appraisals now available to them.

Note

1 Any of these questions, asked on its own, might elicit the kind of information a therapist needs. Generally, it's best to avoid 'double-barrelled' questions; they are included here only to save space.

References

Andary, L., Stolk, Y., & Klimidis, S. (2003). *Assessing mental health across cultures.* Bowen Hills, Australia: Australian Academic Press.

Boszormenyi-Nagy, I., & Krasner, B. (1986). *Between give and take: A clinical guide to contextual therapy.* New York, NY: Brunner-Mazel.

Boszormenyi-Nagy, I., & Spark, G. (1984). *Invisible loyalties: Reciprocity in intergenerational family therapy.* New York, NY: Harper & Row.

Bowen, M. (1978). *Family therapy in clinical practice.* New York, NY: Jason Aronson.

Brown, J. (2017). *Growing yourself up: How to bring your Best to all of life's relationships* (2nd ed.). East Gosford, NSW, Australia: Exisle Pub.

Crago, H. (1992). Becoming the family Archivist. *Australian and New Zealand Journal of Family Therapy*, *13*, 191–210.

Crago, H. (2006). *Couple, family and group work: First steps in interpersonal intervention*. Maidenhead: Open University Press.

Crago, H., & Gardner, P. (2019). *A safe place for change: Skills and capacities for counselling and therapy* (rev. 2nd ed.). Brisbane, Australia: Interactive Publications.

Dunn, J., & Plomin, R. (1990). *Separate lives: Why siblings are so different*. New York, NY: Basic Books.

Earnshaw, A. (1998). *Time bombs in families, and how to survive them*. Sydney: Spencer Publications.

Engel, G. L. (1975). Death of a twin. *International Journal of Psychoanalysis*, *56*, 23–40.

Engel, S. (1999). *Context is everything: The nature of memory*. New York, NY: Freeman.

Family systems therapy with an individual: conducting the first two sessions VHS 297: BF637. C6 F25 (1989) Counselling and therapy in video. https://alexanderstreet.com/products/counseling-therapy-video-library

Freeman, D. (1992). *Multigenerational family therapy*. New York, NY: Haworth.

Geertz, C. (1973). Thick description: Towards an interpretive theory of Culture. In *The interpretation of cultures: Selected essays*. New York, NY: Basic Books, a division of Harper Collins

Goodwach, R. (2003). Adoption and family therapy. *ANZJFT*, *24*, 61–70.

Hargrave, T., & Anderson, W. (1992). *Finishing well: Aging and reparation in the intergenerational family*. New York, NY: Brunner-Mazel.

Hoang, L. (2005). I thought we came for therapy! Autobiography sessions in couple work. *ANZJFT*, *26*(2), 65–72.

Imber-Black, E. (1994). *Family secrets: Implications for theory and therapy* [videotape] New York, NY: Guilford.

Imber-Black, E., Lerner, S., Cullen, G, Wyatt, R., & Seid, E. (2006) Family secrets : implications for theory and therapy. Video Works, Inc, Guilford Publications, Inc,Psychotherapy.net, LLC, San Francisco, CA, ©2006

Karen, R. (1998). *Becoming attached: First relationships and how they shape our capacity to love*. New York, NY: Oxford University Press.

Kerr, M., & Bowen, M. (1988). *Family evaluation: An approach based on Bowen theory*. New York, NY: W.W. Norton.

Leigh, M. [director] (1996). Secrets and lies [movie], distributed by Network Entertainment.

McGoldrick, M., (2011) *The Genogram journey: Reconnecting with your family*. New York, NY: W.W. Norton.

McGoldrick, M., & Gerson, R. (1985). *Genograms in family assessment*. New York, NY: W.W. Norton.

McGoldrick, M., Gerson, R., & Petry, S. (2008). *Genograms: Assessment and intervention* (3rd ed.). New York, NY: W.W. Norton.

McGoldrick, M., Gerson, R., & Shellenberger, S. (1999). *Genograms: Assessment and intervention* (2nd ed.) New York, NY: W.W. Norton.

Medland, J. (1988). Working with the Wahmer Aboriginal and Torres Strait Islander people. *Australian and New Zealand Journal of Family Therapy*, *9*, 33–35.

Minuchin, S. (1974). *Families and family therapy*. Cambridge, MA: Harvard University Press.

Satir, V. (1967). *Conjoint family therapy: A guide to theory and technique* (2nd revised ed.). Palo Alto, CA: Science and Behavior Books. [First edition 1964.]

Schutzenberger, A. (1998). *The ancestor syndrome: Transgenerational psychotherapy and the hidden links in the family tree*. Trans. Anne Trager. London, England: Routledge. [First published in French, 1993.]

Spence, D. (1982). *Narrative truth and historical truth*. New York, NY: W.W. Norton.

Titelman, P. (1987). *The therapist's own family: Toward the differentiation of self*. Northvale, NJ: Aronson.

Yehuda, R., Daskalakis, S. P., Lehrner, A., Desarnaud, F., Bader, H. N., Makotkine, I., Florey, J. D., Bierer, L. M., & Meaney, M. J. (2014). Influences of maternal and paternal PTSD on epigenetic regulation of the glucocortical receptor gene in holocaust survivor Offspring. *American Journal of Psychiatry*, *171*(8), 872–880.

Chapter 11

Embracing Differences

Transforming Family Therapy Through Diversity and Inclusion

Kerrie James and Jane Mowll

Introduction

Family therapy emerged in the 1950s and 1960s as a revolutionary force in mental health. It brought a new perspective, arguing that symptoms in an individual were not an isolated phenomenon but the result of, and maintained by, intricate dynamics within family relationships. This was a bold departure from the then-prevailing psychoanalytic approach, which attributed mental illness to internal psychic conflicts and insisted on prolonged individual therapy as the cure. Steadfast in its foundational defiance, family therapy has consistently distanced itself from the conventional biopsychosocial paradigm of diagnosis and medical treatment that reigns supreme in psychiatry.

With deep-seated connections to social work, systemic practice, and a cybernetic approach to communication, family therapy embraced the systems metaphor. The primary focus of family therapy was the examination of family member interactions and communication, role clarity, and overall relationship functioning. This systemic approach brought about interventions that shifted the pathology from the individual – often labelled the "identified patient" – to the collective familial unit, seeking resolution through the transformation of family relationships, leveraging the collective participation and strengths of family members. The evolution of family therapy in the 1980s saw the development of diverse models such as structural, strategic, Milan, Bowenian, solution-focused, and narrative approaches. These models were initially sculpted by a homogeneous group – predominantly white, male, and middle-class Western men, many of them psychiatrists.

In the first section "Family therapy and social movements", we explore how this original family therapy literature and discourse evolved over the years to be more inclusive of diversity, social justice, and social context. We look at how family therapy has been influenced by major social movements resulting in changing social landscapes in the USA and Australia. In the second section "Practice skills for incorporating diversity into family therapy", we address the question of how family therapists translate an understanding of diversity, social justice, and social context into their therapy with families.

Family therapy and social movements

The 1950s and 1960s in the USA were marked by the Civil Rights Movement, striving to end racial discrimination against African Americans. Concurrently, the Indigenous Rights Movement in Australia focused on the rights of Aboriginal and Torres Strait Islander peoples. These movements underscored the need for family therapy to address racial

DOI: 10.4324/9781003490104-12

equality and develop cultural sensitivity. The 1970s saw a surge in movements addressing diversity issues. In Australia, discussions on immigration and multiculturalism intensified post the White Australia policy, highlighting challenges in housing affordability, economic inequality, and refugee treatment. Simultaneously, the Disability Rights Movement in both countries advocated for the deinstitutionalisation and societal participation of people with disabilities, later broadening to include accessibility and employment discrimination. These movements brought to the forefront the importance of inclusivity and accessibility in therapeutic practices.

From the 1960s onwards, the Feminist Movement, followed by the #MeToo movement in the 2010s, campaigned for equal pay, reproductive rights, gender equality, and combating sexual harassment and assault. Their impact on family therapy highlighted the necessity of integrating gender-sensitive approaches in treatment. The Black Lives Matter movement in the USA beginning in 2013 challenged racism and police brutality towards people of colour and this movement continues to be supported in family therapy circles. (See the Ackerman Institute's media release, https://www.ackerman.org/blog/statement-on-black-lives-matter/2020.) The LGBTQ+ rights movement, starting in the 1970s, achieved significant milestones, including the legalisation of same-sex marriage in 2015 in the USA and in 2017 in Australia. This era emphasised the importance of addressing LGBTQ+ issues within family therapy, respecting diverse family structures and relationships. Finally, the late 20th century to the present has seen a growing awareness and advocacy for disabilities including neurodiversity in both countries, focusing on identity, acceptance, and support.

These social movements, focussing on issues ranging from racial and gender equality to neurodiversity and immigration, reflect the ongoing efforts within both the United States and Australia to confront a wide array of complex social challenges. Their profound impact on family therapy underscores the importance of understanding and integrating these evolving societal contexts into therapeutic practices. By analysing family therapy's intersection with these social issues, we aim to understand its role in reflecting and addressing the complexities of contemporary societal challenges. This exploration seeks to unravel whether family therapy has kept pace with the rapidly changing social landscape or if it has lagged in embracing the diversity and multiplicity of human experiences. In the following sections, we examine family therapy in relation to sexism and power, cultural diversity and racism, social class and inequality, First Nations people, sexuality and gender, and disability and discrimination.

Sexism and power

During the early years of the approach, family therapists largely failed to consider the broader societal, structural, and cultural dimensions impacting family life. This oversight was particularly evident in the field's handling of gender inequalities and power abuses within family structures. At a time when disciplines spurred by the feminist movement, like sociology and women's studies, were actively exploring women's subjugation within patriarchal systems, family therapy's literature seemed largely indifferent to these issues. It often neglected to confront gender-based violence or to consider how societal inequities influenced familial bonds and individual resilience. A few lone feminist voices published articles in the family therapy literature pointing out this failure (Goldner, 1985; Hare-Mustin, 1978; James, 1984; James & McIntyre, 1983, 1989).

The 1970s and 1980s were marked by a significant societal transformation in Western countries. Women were challenging male dominance and questioning traditional gender roles. Influential works like Simone de Beauvoir's "The Second Sex" and Sylvia Plath's "The Bell Jar" were emblematic of this era, highlighting how patriarchal structures contributed to widespread depression and substance abuse among housewives. Despite this growing awareness, family therapy literature from this era was largely silent on issues like domestic violence, sexual abuse, and child abuse, often failing to integrate the intersectionality of gender and other identity factors within family dynamics (for critiques, see Asiimwe, Lesch, Karume, & Blow, 2021; James, 2007; James & MacKinnon, 1990). Even though family therapy models acknowledged systemic and historical and intergenerational influences, the literature from this era often overlooked broader societal contexts. Such contexts include crucial issues such as gender disparity and power dynamics within families, a significant omission considering the concurrent feminist movements highlighting the oppression of women in patriarchal family structures.

The narrative began to shift with the increased involvement of women in the family therapy field. Scholars like Rachel Hare-Mustin, pivotal in this change, began publishing works that addressed the social context and societal injustices within families. Hare-Mustin's seminal 1978 paper "A Feminist Approach to Family Therapy" marked the field's initial engagement with gender issues. Following this, feminist family therapists critiqued the prevailing literature for perpetuating traditional gender roles and ignoring the realities of violence and power imbalances in families (Goldner, 1985; James & McIntyre, 1989; MacKinnon & Miller, 1987). The *Journal of Feminist Family Therapy*, established in 1990, emerged as a pivotal platform that significantly broadened the discourse in family therapy. It provided an essential space for both women and men to deeply examine family dynamics through the critical lenses of gender, power, and, subsequently, culture and race, thus enriching the field with diverse perspectives.

Also in 1990, Virginia Goldner and colleagues published "Love and Violence: Gender Paradoxes in Volatile Attachments", which advocated for the integration of feminist perspectives with systemic, social constructionist, and narrative frameworks in understanding couple dynamics, especially in abusive relationships. This approach enabled therapists to directly acknowledge and address violence and power abuses, while still considering the interactional patterns within which abuse occurred (Goldner, Penn, Sheinberg, & Walker, 1990). The evolution of family therapy into a more inclusive and socially aware practice represented a profound change. It was a shift towards acknowledging and challenging power dynamics integral to understanding and improving family relationships. It allowed for a richer, more nuanced approach to family therapy, incorporating both systemic and feminist perspectives.

Cultural diversity and racism

The integration of race and ethnicity into family therapy literature reflects broader cultural shifts and the recognition of diversity as a pivotal element in therapeutic practice. This evolution was significantly influenced by critical voices from women of colour, including bell hooks, who in her book "Ain't I a Woman: Black Women and Feminism" (bell hooks, 1981) criticised mainstream feminism for its failure to fully address racial oppression. Such critiques underscored the necessity of incorporating issues of ethnicity and race into family therapy (Falicov, 2007). Monica McGoldrick and colleagues' groundbreaking book, *Ethnicity and Family Therapy* (McGoldrick, Giordano, & Garcia-Preto, 2005) first published in the 1980s, marked a watershed moment in this regard. It was instrumental in emphasising the importance of cultural competence in family therapy, highlighting how ethnic and cultural backgrounds profoundly influence family dynamics, beliefs, and behaviours. In their paper "Uncommon Strategies for a Common Problem: Addressing Racism in Family Therapy", Laszloffy and Hardy (2000) further advanced this discourse by exploring the impact of racial trauma on individuals and families, which was pivotal in encouraging therapists to acknowledge and address the psychological wounds inflicted by racial trauma. McGoldrick's work, along with her colleague, Kenneth Hardy (see McGoldrick & Hardy, 2019) challenged the field's Eurocentric biases, bringing a greater understanding of the diverse family structures, values, and interaction patterns across different cultures. They urged therapists to integrate factors such as race, ethnicity, and cultural heritage into the therapeutic process, fostering a more comprehensive and empathic approach to a family's unique challenges and strengths. These authors' advocacy for a greater understanding of clients' cultural contexts has been essential in shaping a more inclusive and socially aware approach to therapy, ensuring that racial dynamics are acknowledged and addressed as a fundamental part of the therapeutic process.

As family therapy grew into a global phenomenon, with significant developments in countries such as China, India, Peru, and African nations (Asiimwe, Lesch, Karume, & Blow, 2021; Roberts et al., 2014), the importance of engaging effectively with diversity and cultural differences became increasingly recognised in the counselling and psychology fields (for a review, see Hook, Hodge, Sandage, Davis, & Van Tongeren, 2023). In the Australian context, with the claim for diversity as a multicultural society, there was a call for therapists to engage with multicultural understandings and responsiveness (Sisko, 2021). Importantly, however, as Dadras and Daneshpour (2018) argue, discourse on multiculturalism in family therapy and mental health has been limited, and there is a danger of superficiality in failing to address deep-seated inequities and structural racism.

In a sense, each therapeutic session is inherently cross-cultural, with therapists and family members bringing their own culturally shaped experiences and values. Tsang (2017) emphasises the importance of therapists enabling clients to share their stories without therapists reducing them to preconceived stereotypes. In understanding the uniqueness of each family, however, it is important that we don't minimise the social and structural oppressions, including racism that can perpetuate inequities (Cottrell-Boyce, 2022). Therefore, we should work to understand the social and structural conditions that shape people's lives and the problems that bring them to therapy. It's important for us to interact with and grasp the dominance of our own and others' commonly accepted ideas, values, and assumptions. Comprehending white privilege, particularly for therapists from dominant white cultures (Combs, 2019), is crucial for being sensitive to clients' experiences with discrimination and racism and recognising societal and structural oppressions, including ethnocentrism and racism, that contribute to inequality. This is especially crucial when considering past interactions these families may have had with white professionals. It is vital, therefore, for white therapists especially to be conscious of how their clients perceive their whiteness and inherent privilege, and how these factors influence their therapeutic relationship.

Research suggests that a therapist's "cultural humility" can positively impact therapy outcomes (Zhang et al., 2022). Cultural humility includes attributes like openness, self-awareness, ego-lessness, and a commitment to understanding cultural identities (Foronda,

Baptiste, Reinholdt, & Ousman, 2016). Therapists must maintain reflexive awareness of their biases and strive to understand clients' perspectives (Nguyen, Naleppa, & Lopez, 2021), cultivating curiosity and a collaborative spirit in tuning into both their own mental processes and those of family members (Hernandez-Wolfe, Acevedo, Victoria Eugenia, & Volkmann, 2015). The integration of cultural awareness and humility into family therapy represented a significant shift towards a more inclusive and comprehensive approach, acknowledging the crucial role that race and ethnicity play in shaping family dynamics and therapeutic outcomes.

Social and structural inequality

Family therapy, as a discipline, has evolved over the decades to recognise the importance of social class in both theory and practice. The initial focus was on family dynamics and communication, with little attention to the wider social and economic contexts. Families are deeply embedded within socio-political and economic contexts, which significantly intersect with the issues brought to therapy (MacKinnon, 1993) McDowell, Knudson-Martin, & Bermudez, (2019). Social class and economic status crucially impact mental and physical health, influencing daily life, autonomy, decision-making, and overall safety and security (Dadras & Daneshpour, 2018). Social and structural factors such as financial hardships, lack of social capital, limited access to resources such as housing and food security, affordable childcare, and transport compound and intensify the problems that lead families to seek therapy. Lack of affordable, available, and accessible services see many families locked out of access to the supports that they may need particularly in regional, rural, and remote areas.

Ignoring the role of social and structural inequities in therapy can perpetuate systemic injustices. A focus solely on individual or family responsibility for change may reinforce "internalised oppression", where individuals struggling with poverty and hardship mistakenly attribute their difficulties solely to personal failings, due to a lack of awareness of the broader class-based societal structures that influence their situation (Dadras & Daneshpour, 2018). Despite historical acknowledgment within family therapy of the need to consider socio-structural contexts and adopt equity-focused, anti-oppressive practices (McDowell, Knudson-Martin, & Bermudez, 2019), many therapists work within frameworks that prioritise psychological explanations for problems, thereby overlooking the role of social and environmental factors in causing or exacerbating illness and emotional distress.

Contemporary family therapy approaches are now more likely to incorporate social and structural contexts as a critical element in understanding family dynamics and challenges. Such approaches also focus on multicultural and intersectional aspects, recognising how social class, for example, intersects with other identity factors like race, ethnicity, and gender (McDowell, Knudson-Martin, & Bermudez, 2022). Systemic and ecological models highlight the impact of broader social and economic systems on families, acknowledging factors like poverty, unemployment, and social inequality. Research and scholarship have expanded to explore the intersections of social class, poverty, and family life, informing both practice and policy (Dadras & Daneshpour, 2018). However, challenges remain, including calls for the field to address systemic inequalities more robustly and to integrate social and structural considerations more thoroughly into all aspects of family therapy practice. Training and education for family therapists now often include components on culturally responsive practice and social justice, encompassing an understanding of social and structural issues. In summary, the evolution of family therapy reflects a growing understanding of the profound impact of socio-economic and structural resource factors on family life, highlighting the importance of addressing these issues to provide effective, relevant, and equitable therapy to families across the social spectrum.

First Nations peoples

Family therapy's involvement with First Nations peoples marked a critical and evolving juncture in the discipline, highlighting an increasing emphasis on culturally attuned and knowledgeable mental health interventions. Recognising the distinct challenges of First Nations communities is central to developing therapy approaches that are both relevant and effective (Bennett, 2019). These communities grapple with deep-rooted impacts from historical colonial violence including socio-economic impacts, limited healthcare access, educational disparities, and poverty, which significantly impact mental health and family dynamics.

In response to the prevalent trauma within these communities, many family therapists incorporate trauma-informed care, which aims to be sensitive to how violence impacts individuals and families, tailoring therapy to address these profound effects. At the same time, central to working alongside First Nations families is that therapists understand historical violence and oppression and its intergenerational repercussions, stemming from colonisation, forced assimilation, and displacement, which continue to affect mental health, family dynamics, and community well-being (Bennett, 2019). Family therapy literature is often deficient in recognising how mainstream family therapy might inadvertently continue to marginalise First Nations people. The enduring influence of settler colonialism, particularly in countries like Australia, the USA, and Canada, is evident in the perpetuation of colonial narratives that often overshadow Indigenous identities, languages, and cultures (Bennett, 2019; Green, Bennett, & Betteridge, 2016; McDowell & Hernández, 2010). This Western-centric perspective in family therapy can lead to misinterpretations and the imposition of cultural norms that do not align with the experiences of First Nations individuals and families.

The importance of understanding and integrating cultural identities and values in therapy is increasingly recognised. Therapists, accustomed to individual frameworks may find it challenging to fully appreciate perspectives that place the "self" in a communal context (Tsang, 2017). Addressing these colonial biases in family therapy is vital to prevent the further marginalisation of First Nations peoples and to foster a therapeutic approach that respects and incorporates the richness of Indigenous cultures. Bennett (2019) highlighted the significance of historical consciousness in therapy, particularly in Australian contexts, where acknowledging the impacts of colonialism is crucial for developing responsive and effective practices. Such an approach requires ethical and reflective practice, including training and supervision that encompasses an understanding of the histories and narratives of the people and land where therapy occurs.

Green (2019) advocates for a model of cultural support beginning with acknowledgement of power dynamics and self-reflection, particularly when working with Australian First Nations clients. Echoing this, Sisko (2021), alongside Bennett (2019), urges the adoption of decolonising perspectives that recognise the ongoing effects of colonialism, as well as associated power and privilege. Such perspectives challenge therapists to extend their focus beyond interactions between family members, understanding how inequalities are embedded in systems that disproportionately benefit a minority at the expense of many. A decolonising lens is essential for therapists, prompting them to confront and address systemic injustices in their practice.

Sexuality and gender

Family therapy, like many fields in mental health, has evolved over the years in its approach to reflect broader societal changes and an increased understanding of the unique challenges faced by LGBTQI+ individuals and families. Homosexuality was considered a mental illness by the American Psychiatric Association until 1973. The declassification of homosexuality as a mental disorder marked the beginning of a significant shift in the therapy world. In the earlier stages of family therapy, LGBTQI+ identities were pathologised or not recognised. Gradually, there was a growing acceptance in the family therapy community that LGBTQI+ identities were not pathological but part of human diversity. This shift aligned with broader changes in social attitudes and the growing advocacy of LGBTQI+ rights. Many contemporary family therapists adopt LGBTQI+ affirmative approaches. These approaches recognise the validity of identities and the importance of understanding the specific challenges faced by LGBTQI+ individuals and families, such as coming out, discrimination, and the process of forming non-traditional families. Contemporary family therapy emphasises the need to consider systemic and structural issues that affect LGBTQI+ individuals. This includes examining societal prejudices, legal and policy barriers, and the impact of these factors on family dynamics and mental health.

Despite progress, there are still challenges and critiques regarding how family therapy addresses LGBTQI issues. Transgender people may face significant discrimination and abuse, often without the legal protections afforded to cisgender people, as highlighted by Morgan (Petty-John, Tseng, & Blow, 2021). This stark reality challenges some family therapy practices. Traditional tools, like the genogram, used to map family structures and relationships may unwittingly embed heteronormative or cis-normative biases, failing to recognise or accurately represent clients' self-identified gender and sexuality (Blumer, Gavriel Ansara, & Watson, 2013).

Practitioners may still hold biases or lack sufficient training in LGBTQI+ affirmative therapy. Moreover, there's a call for more inclusive research that represents the full spectrum of LGBTQI+ experiences, including those of transgender and non-binary people.

In conclusion, family therapy's approach to LGBTQI+ issues has evolved from a pathologising stance to a more affirming and inclusive one. However, the field continues to develop, with ongoing efforts to improve cultural competence, broaden research, and ensure that therapy practices effectively address the diverse and complex needs of LGBTQI+ individuals and families.

Disability and discrimination

In its early stages, family therapy was influenced heavily by the medical model of disability, which viewed disability primarily as a medical problem residing within the individual. Families with disabled members were often approached from a perspective of managing or "fixing" the disability, rather than understanding the broader psychosocial dynamics.

The early professional literature pathologised families with members who lived with a disability. A disability was viewed as a source of stress or dysfunction within the family system, with little attention being paid to the strengths or adaptive capacities of these families.

Family therapy then shifted towards a more systemic understanding of disability within the context of the family. This approach considered how disability affects and is affected by family dynamics, communication patterns, roles, and relationships, moving beyond the individualistic view of disability. The disability rights movement, which gained significant momentum in the 1970s and 1980s, had as a central tenet the social model of disability, which distinguishes between the limitations caused by a person's impairment and the social limitations caused by societal barriers and attitudes. The focus on family dynamics, MacKinnon and Marlett (1984) argued, still failed to view the family within the larger social context in which people with intellectual and developmental disabilities have faced historical patterns of oppression, marginalisation, and neglect that are at the source of the problems that families may experience. Perhaps particularly people with intellectual and developmental disabilities are recognised to have experienced histories of oppression, marginalisation, and neglect and in both systemic and individual ways that have only been relatively recently acknowledged in the family therapy sphere (Rhodes, 2002).

Many family therapists now approach disability from an empowerment perspective, focusing on inclusion, accessibility, and advocating for the rights and needs of individuals with disabilities and their families. This shift aligns with broader societal movements towards greater inclusion and accessibility for people with disabilities. Understanding the social model of disability is useful for family therapists as it delineates between the impairments with which people live and the attitudes, prejudices, and social, structural, and communication barriers which negatively impact their disability or their lives generally. While contested as a theory that can potentially neglect the nuanced realities of people's lived experience, Barnes (2019, p. 24) and others argue for the pragmatism of the empowerment perspective, noting importantly that how people deal with impairments is determined in many ways by their access to social and material resources. This need not limit the need for understanding the unique needs of the individual and family. Contemporary family therapy emphasises collaborative and strength-based approaches when working with families with disabled members. These approaches recognise the unique strengths, resources, and resilience of these families, rather than focusing solely on challenges or deficits.

Given that people with disabilities often encounter marginalising and devaluing narratives, it's critical for family therapists to amplify the voices and narratives of those living with disabilities (Baum & Lynggaard, 2018). In systemic family therapy, the therapist's role is to facilitate an exploration of different family perspectives while ensuring that the voice of the person with a disability is not overshadowed by others in the therapy room (Baum, 2007). It is essential to create a space to hear their experiences and viewpoints and that they are valued equally, preventing their marginalisation within their own support systems. Despite progress, there are still challenges in how family therapy addresses disability issues. These include the need for ongoing training and education for therapists, addressing implicit biases, and ensuring that therapy practices are inclusive and sensitive to the unique experiences of disabled individuals and their families. In summary, the history of family therapy in relation to disability issues has evolved from a medical and often pathologising perspective to a more holistic, systemic, and empowering approach. This evolution reflects broader changes in societal attitudes towards disability and an increased emphasis on inclusion, rights, and the strengths of individuals with disabilities and their families.

This section has highlighted the evolving influence of social contexts, encompassing class, gender, race, culture, and disability, on individuals and families. These dynamic factors have significantly steered family therapy towards a heightened awareness and incorporation of cultural, social, and diverse perspectives, enriching its understanding and practices.

Practice skills for incorporating diversity into family therapy

As family therapists, it's crucial to incorporate diversity principles into our therapeutic approaches to effectively engage and support families. To aid in applying these principles, we propose a framework of practice skills. These skills are designed to guide therapists and educators in family therapy, helping them contextualise the issues presented by families in therapy.[1] They also emphasise the importance of the therapist's self-reflection in effectively engaging with disadvantaged and marginalised groups. This framework comprises six key areas of competency, each encompassing several sub-competencies or skills to address a process issue related to conducting family therapy sessions. The six areas are power and empowerment; self-reflection; collaboration, dialogue, and reflexivity; using an intersectional lens; considering the role of neutrality; and using a questioning methodology. We first discuss the area and then present summarised skills for each area.

Power and empowerment

The central thread running through the evolution of family therapy is the concept of power. The inherent power held by therapists, due to their professional role, establishes a hierarchy in which clients, particularly vulnerable ones, have less influence over the direction and outcomes of therapy. This power dynamic is intensified when therapists represent cultural dominance, especially when serving clients from disadvantaged backgrounds. The position of power held by the therapist comes with the responsibility to facilitate a space where the family feels empowered to guide the conversation and the course of therapy. This is achieved by attentively exploring each family member's viewpoints, their proposed solutions, and the changes they hope to enact. The therapist's approach should be one of guidance rather than imposition, managing the session to ensure everyone is heard equitably.

Employing a critical social or critical social work perspective (Allan, 2016) can serve as a valuable framework for therapists. This approach emphasises the pursuit of social justice and equality, particularly for marginalised individuals and groups. It involves a keen awareness of power dynamics that contribute to marginalisation and a dedication to challenging and questioning established norms and dominant discourses. Therapists are encouraged to adopt a critical stance towards their practice, analysing problems through the lens of social structures rather than individual pathology. The goal is to foster egalitarian therapeutic relationships and to engage in broader social change efforts (Allan, 2016). Speaking from a First Nations Australian viewpoint, Green (2019, p. 182) stresses the need for therapists to critically engage with power within the therapeutic relationship and to be willing to deconstruct traditional methods in favour of culturally aware, sensitive, and responsive practices. The fundamental ethical mandate for therapists is to help without causing harm, but this can only be achieved by first recognising the power imbalance. This recognition steers therapists to be attuned to client vulnerability and the potential for harm that could stem from entrenched societal discourses that marginalise experiences related to culture, gender, or disability. Therapists must be mindful of the power dynamics present within the therapeutic space and work to mitigate them. This is especially pertinent when therapy includes children and adolescents. Therapists should adopt strategies that make sessions accessible and engaging for young clients, ensuring their perspectives are heard and valued. This might involve using age-appropriate language, creative interventions, and ensuring a safe environment where they feel empowered to share their experiences.

Minimising the power that therapists inherently hold in therapeutic relationships is vital to create a balanced, respectful, and effective therapy environment. Research has highlighted therapist behaviours that contribute to negative therapy outcomes and reduced client engagement. Falicov, Nakash, and Alegria (2021) identified three specific behaviours that can inhibit conversation: excessive talking by the therapist, imposing interventions rather than co-creating them with the client, and failing to invite clients to set the agenda for sessions. From our standpoint, we recognise additional behaviours that can undermine therapy, such as the therapist dominating the conversation, not listening, interrupting, using pathologising language, making judgements, or steering clients towards therapist-set goals. These actions reflect a misuse of power and can significantly detract from the therapy's effectiveness, as reported by clients who have had negative experiences. It's imperative for therapists to remain vigilant against these tendencies to ensure that their power is exercised with the utmost respect and care for the client's autonomy and well-being.

It is crucial for therapists, despite their inherent authority, to facilitate an environment where the family takes the lead in guiding the therapy's progression. This is achieved by delving into each member's viewpoints, their proposed solutions, and the outcomes they desire. The therapist's role is not to dictate the therapy's path but to manage the session's flow, ensuring everyone is heard. By synthesising these diverse perspectives, the therapist can then offer insights and knowledge that may prove beneficial. This collaborative approach respects the family's expertise in their lived experiences while leveraging the therapist's professional capabilities to enhance the therapeutic journey.

Skills include:

Consider power dynamics and empowerment in therapy:

- Acknowledge and address the inherent power imbalance in therapist-client relationships.
- Employ critical perspectives focusing on social justice and equality.

Empower families within the therapeutic process:

- Create a therapeutic environment where families feel empowered to guide the conversation and therapy goals.
- Actively listen to and explore each family member's perspectives, solutions, and hopes.

Employ cultural sensitivity and historical awareness:

- Develop culturally sensitive practices, particularly when working with First Nations people and other marginalised groups.

- Be aware of the historical and ongoing impacts of societal discourses on marginalised experiences, including those related to culture, gender, disability, and race.

Facilitate client-centred therapy and respectful communication:

- Create accessible and engaging sessions for all clients, especially children and adolescents, ensuring their perspectives are heard (see Chapter 6 of this volume).
- Avoid therapist behaviours that hinder conversation, such as dominating discussions or imposing goals.
- Foster a collaborative therapeutic environment where clients' views and solutions are prioritised.

Recognise social contexts and systemic injustices:

- Recognise the influence of social injustices, discrimination, and systemic challenges on mental health.
- Integrate discussions on social and structural conditions affecting clients into therapy sessions.
- Advocate for clients within systems and organisations and ensure access to services and resources.

Foster critical reflexivity and sociocultural attunement:

- Maintain awareness of personal biases and the impact of societal contexts on clients.
- Develop "sociocultural attunement" to understand and address the broader societal factors in therapy (Allan, 2016).

Engage in self-reflection

The importance of therapists engaging in self-reflection is well-established, with a growing body of literature advocating for therapists to critically engage with their racial, cultural, and social identities (Dadras & Daneshpour, 2018; Fernando & Bennett, 2019; Green, Bennett, & Betteridge, 2016; Hutton & Sisko, 2021; McGoldrick & Hardy, 2019). Cheon and Murphy (2007). These authors highlight a crucial, often-neglected aspect of therapy: self-knowledge. Therapists may be steeped in theoretical knowledge yet lack awareness of their own cultural positioning and biases.

Self-awareness is pivotal for addressing and dismantling the social and cultural forces that contribute to oppression. Sisko (2021) connects therapist self-awareness with cultural humility, stressing the need for a consistent self-assessment of biases, particularly when working with marginalised groups. Without such reflective practice, therapists risk echoing dominant societal discourses within therapy sessions. Deep reflection involves a critical awareness of one's privileges, cultural history, and potential complicity in systems of colonisation and oppression. It requires confronting uncomfortable truths about ingrained prejudice, especially the ethnocentric beliefs, and racism that white therapists may hold. Engaging in this reflective process is iterative and benefits greatly from dialogue with peers or within supervisory contexts. Solo reflection can inadvertently reinforce existing biases. Reflection, including using a critical reflection framework encompassing a range of reflective methods (see Bennett & Bodkin-Andrews 2021), is required and may include verbal discussions (Totsuka, 2014) and written exercises (Green, Bennett, & Betteridge, 2016).

Ultimately, the goal of such reflective practice is to inform and improve therapeutic approaches, ensuring they are culturally attuned and socially just.

Therapy inherently brings together the cultural backgrounds of the therapist and the client or family, creating an intersection where understanding and respect must be mutual. A fundamental task for the therapist is to delve into the family's cultural framework, especially how they perceive and interpret their challenges. While this may seem like a basic aspect of therapy, it is a critical step for the therapist to understand the family's world and the social issues that impact them. By weaving together the various strands of the family's narrative and then complementing them with their own professional insights, the therapist can provide informed support that respects the family's autonomy and cultural context. This approach embodies the principle of "leading by following", where the therapist leads the therapeutic process by following the family's direction.

Skills include:

Engage in continuous self-reflection:

- Therapists should critically examine their racial, cultural, and social identities.
- Continually assess personal biases and understand how these may impact therapeutic practice.

Develop and maintain cultural humility:

- Cultivate cultural humility by regularly reflecting on and acknowledging personal biases.
- Ensure therapeutic approaches are culturally sensitive and avoid perpetuating societal stereotypes.

Acknowledge and address privilege and bias:

- Recognise and confront personal privileges and biases, especially in the context of systemic oppression.
- Be aware of ethnocentric beliefs and potential racism, particularly relevant for white therapists.

Engage in collaborative reflection with peers:

- Participate in ongoing dialogues with peers and supervisors to challenge and refine perspectives.
- Use diverse methods of reflection, including discussion (Bennett & Bodkin-Andrews, 2021) to deepen understanding.

Understand and respect clients' cultural backgrounds:

- Work to understand the family's or client's cultural framework and how it shapes their experiences and challenges.
- Respect the cultural context and lived experiences of clients in all aspects of therapy.

Integrate family narratives with professional insights:

- Weave together the family's narrative with professional knowledge to provide informed, respectful support.
- Lead the therapeutic process by valuing and following the family's direction, ensuring their autonomy and cultural context are honoured.

Collaboration, dialogue, and reflexivity

In the realm of family therapy, Rober and Seltzer's (2010) use of the term "colonizing" captures the problematic dynamic when a therapist is overly directive or controlling in a session, thereby muting the family's voices and perspectives. Colonising in this context is about the harmful impact of the therapist imposing their understanding or directives on clients, overshadowing the family members' views. Rober and Seltzer (2010) advocate for a collaborative approach, which is considered a cornerstone of systemic practice. This approach involves the therapist engaging in an ongoing reflexive process, constantly attuning to their own experiences while interacting with family members. Such reflexivity might lead a therapist to choose silence over speaking, to actively listen, or to ask open questions, especially to those less vocal in the session. It's about embracing continuous hypothesising – remaining curious, cautious, and attentive to each person, every emerging theme, and concern, all the while incorporating an awareness of social and cultural intersectionality to avoid the narrowness of one's worldview.

Hypothesising serves as a tool for therapists not only to ponder possible dynamics within the family but also to examine their own preconceptions, biases, and potential judgements. It includes scrutinising referral notes for biases of other professionals and considering the quality of prior interactions between practitioners and family members. Often, negative dynamics emerge from families feeling coerced into therapy due to the behaviour or symptoms of a particular member. To establish a better therapeutic relationship, therapists must meet families "where they are at", exploring their journey to the therapy session and their past experiences with professionals and services. This exploration includes hypothesising about each family member's expectations and willingness to engage with the therapeutic process. Therapists must also confront their own biases by reflecting on their experiences with similar cases or personal connections that may influence their perceptions of family dynamics.

As Rober and Seltzer (2010) emphasise, hypothesising is not a static activity but one that evolves throughout the session. It involves the therapist's continual awareness and examination of their visceral and emotional reactions, thoughts, and interpretations of the family's interactions. Through this process, therapists practice reflexivity, adapting to the family's responses while keeping the therapy focused on the family's concerns and needs. This reflective practice ensures that therapists remain culturally humble and responsive, making space for families to feel understood and safe.

Skills include:

Avoid imposing personal views:

- Be mindful not to overpower the family's voices and perspectives with personal interpretations or directives.
- Practice restraint in guiding the session, allowing space for the family's experiences and views to surface.

Foster a collaborative therapeutic approach:

- Embrace a collaborative stance, prioritising the family's input and perspectives in the therapy process.
- Engage in a reflexive process, continually attuning to personal experiences and biases during interactions with the family.

Practice reflexive silence and active listening:

- Consider allowing silences to occur, giving everyone space for reflection and encouraging family members to express themselves (see Seikkula & Trimble, 2005).
- Actively listen and ask open-ended questions, especially to engage less vocal family members.

Employ continuous hypothesising:

- Remain curious and cautious, continuously hypothesising about the family dynamics and themes that emerge during sessions.
- Use hypothesising to challenge personal preconceptions and biases, and to remain open to diverse perspectives.

Scrutinise preconceptions and external biases:

- Examine any existing referral notes or histories for biases from other professionals.
- Reflect on any preconceived notions or judgements that might influence the therapeutic interaction.

Meet families where they are:

- Understand the family's journey to therapy, including their past interactions with professionals and systems.
- Explore each family member's expectations, reservations, and readiness to engage in therapy.

Continuously reflect on the therapist's reactions:

- Maintain an ongoing awareness of personal emotional reactions, thoughts, and interpretations during sessions.
- Adjust therapeutic approaches based on the family's responses, keeping focus on their concerns and needs.

Prioritise cultural sensitivity and responsiveness:

- Ensure that therapy practices are culturally sensitive and responsive to the family's unique context.
- Adapt reflexive practices to create a safe, inclusive space where all family members feel understood and respected.

Use an intersectional lens

In family therapy, understanding intersectionality involves recognising the multifaceted nature of individual identities and how various forms of oppression intersect. Understanding intersectionality is crucial in recognising the complex, overlapping social and cultural dimensions that constitute individual identities. Originating from black feminist scholarship, intersectionality was coined by scholars like Crenshaw (1989) and Collins (2019) to describe how different forms of oppression, such as racism and sexism, can intersect and compound the experiences of individuals. This concept underlines that identities are multifaceted, involving race, ethnicity, spirituality, class, gender, age, sexuality, ability, and more. These elements are not isolated but mutually constitutive, influencing one another to shape an individual's position within society (Butler, 2015; Collins, 2019). An intersectional lens allows for an understanding that eschews either/or binary thinking, instead embracing a both/and perspectivein which various aspects of identity intermingle to form unique personal experiences.

Family therapy practitioners from diverse fields, including social work and psychology, have begun to integrate intersectionality into their understanding of both clients and therapists (Addison & Coolhart, 2015; Petty-John, Tseng, & Blow, 2021). In the therapeutic context, the intersectional identities of both the therapist and the family may be openly acknowledged or remain unspoken (Burnham, 2012). Therapists may show the social signifiers that we embody (such as skin tone) or may choose to disclose aspects of our identities in different therapy contexts (O'Leary, Tsui, & Ruch, 2013). Interpretations of cultural and social commonalities or differences can be laden with assumptions based on these signifiers or initial impressions. Narrative therapy warns against the risks of dominant or single stories that pigeonhole identities through a narrow lens (Peterson, 2021). Khan (2002) cautions against overlooking the diversity within what may appear to be a homogeneous culture, advocating for an appreciation of both intercultural and intracultural differences and commonalities.

The idea of "Social Graces" (Burnham, 2012) has been used in family therapy literature to consider and reflect on power, oppression, and social location for therapists and clients. This checklist, which includes a wide range of identity factors, helps therapists consider the complexity of their clients' and their own social positioning (Burnham, 2012; Butler, 2015). While valuable, if not approached with a nuanced understanding of intersectionality, the "graces" could be seen as oversimplifying the intricate interplay of social differences and similarities (Birdsey & Kustner, 2021; Butler, 2015). An intersectional approach can lead to more insightful questioning, orienting therapists towards the variety of social justice issues a person may face, such as different forms of discrimination. It also highlights the strengths and adaptability that come from navigating such social and cultural challenges. Engaging with intersectionality encourages in-depth reflection, particularly effective when facilitated within peer or group supervision, fostering a richer, more informed therapeutic practice. By incorporating the actions and skills, outlined below, family therapists can more effectively address the unique and overlapping aspects of their clients' identities, leading to more comprehensive and empathetic therapeutic support.

Skills include:

Acknowledge multiple identity factors:

- Understand that identities are composed of various elements like race, ethnicity, class, gender, sexuality, and ability.
- Recognise that these elements are interconnected and shape an individual's societal position.
- Appreciate how different identity factors, such as race and sexual orientation, can interact and influence a client's life experiences and mental health.

Integrate intersectionality in practice:

- Apply an intersectional lens in therapy to understand the complex experiences of clients.
- Be aware of both the intersectional identities of the therapist and the family.

Avoid oversimplification:

- Challenge dominant or single stories that simplify complex identities.
- Appreciate the diversity within cultures and avoid treating any culture as homogeneous.

Utilise social graces thoughtfully:

- Employ the social graces checklist or other reflective tools to reflect on power, oppression, and social location.
- Approach this tool with a nuanced understanding to avoid oversimplification.

Foster insightful questioning:

- Orient questioning towards a variety of social justice issues, recognising different forms of discrimination.
- Highlight the strengths and resilience stemming from navigating social and cultural challenges.

Engage in reflective practice:

- Reflect deeply, especially within peer or group supervision, to enhance understanding and practice.
- Navigate the complexities of each client's identity and experiences with sensitivity.

Observe neutrality

The concept of neutrality in family therapy has been a subject of ongoing discourse, especially in cases involving harm or wrongdoing within the family unit. Traditionally, neutrality is considered a central component of Milan family therapy, where the therapist maintains an equidistant stance from all family members, striving to understand each person's perspective without taking sides (Selvini, Boscolo, Cecchin, & Prata, 1980). This approach is intended to create a safe and balanced space for all voices to be heard, like how a group leader promotes fairness. However, the role of the therapist is not static and can involve adopting various approaches depending on the context of the session. For example, when addressing issues such as intimate partner violence (IPV), therapists may need to move away from neutrality to actively confront and challenge harmful behaviours. In these situations, the therapist might explicitly label behaviours such as aggression as abusive, aligning with a social justice framework to ensure that harmful actions are not overlooked or minimised.

Therefore, maintaining neutrality does not mean condoning destructive behaviours. Therapists have a duty to articulate their professional stance on the impacts of abuse and to advocate for the safety of all involved. In instances where cultural norms or familial patterns are used to justify violence, such as the use of physical discipline as a form of control, therapists must carefully navigate these discussions. While respecting cultural backgrounds, it is crucial to engage in conversations that question and challenge harmful practices, as suggested by James (2010). This may involve educating family members on the negative impacts of such behaviours and exploring alternative, non-harmful ways of interaction. Ultimately, the therapist's role is to facilitate healing and change while ensuring the safety and well-being of all family members, which at times requires an assertive stance against abuse and harm. In family therapy, employing a questioning methodology is essential for exploring family dynamics and individual experiences. By implementing the following actions and skills, therapists can create a more engaging, respectful, and effective therapeutic environment that prioritises the family's needs and perspectives:

Maintaining neutrality

- Balance perspectives by attending to each family member's viewpoint.
- Explore each person's experience, maintaining impartiality, especially in emotionally charged family discussions.

Creating a safe space

- Foster an environment of trust where all family members feel comfortable sharing.
- Mediate interactions to ensure respectful and fair communication among all parties.

Adaptability in approach

- Adjust methods promptly in response to the evolving dynamics of the therapy session.
- Shift strategies when confronting sensitive or potentially harmful situations.

Confronting and challenging harmful behaviours

- Identify and clearly articulate behaviours that are abusive or destructive.
- Intervene decisively to prevent the perpetuation of harmful family patterns.

Advocacy for safety and well-being

- Advocate firmly for the protection and safety of all family members.
- Express a clear professional stance on issues like abuse and its consequences.

Navigating cultural sensitivity

- Respect cultural differences while addressing and challenging harmful practices.
- Incorporate cultural awareness into discussions to enrich family understanding.

Educating and offering alternatives

- Educate family members about the negative effects of certain behaviours.
- Propose constructive alternatives for communication and problem-solving.

Facilitating healing and change

- Encourage open dialogue and mutual understanding among family members.

The importance of questioning and listening skills

In family therapy, the practice of asking questions demonstrates the therapist's curiosity and interest in the lived experiences of family members. People often appreciate being asked questions, as it indicates the therapist's interest in their viewpoints. The use of open-ended questions gives individuals the latitude to respond as they wish, providing either brief or extensive answers. Conversely, closed questions, while limiting in scope, can be beneficial in aiding communication for those who may find open-ended responses challenging.

Adopting a questioning methodology is fundamental to a therapist's ability to explore the unique cultural identities within a family, encompassing race, class, culture, and experiences of disability or mental health conditions. This approach also encourages family members to speak directly to the therapist, which can be advantageous; it allows them to listen to each other's perspectives without the immediate pressure to respond, potentially leading to greater understanding among family members.

While the act of questioning is important, the responses it elicits are of greater significance. It is crucial for therapists to engage in active listening, giving family members sufficient time to articulate their thoughts. This ensures that therapists do not inadvertently steer the session or impose their own focus. By reflecting on the answers before responding, therapists can avoid dominating the conversation and instead take on a "one-down" position, respecting the family's expertise in their own lives. This stance enables family members to take the lead in expressing their views, thereby facilitating a more client driven therapeutic process. At the same time, the therapist maintains control of the session ensuring that the focus of the session is on track and that family members each have opportunities to participate. This approach ensures that the therapist does not engage in specific behaviours that may hinder the therapeutic process. These behaviours include dominating the conversation, failing to listen, interrupting, utilising pathologising labels, making judgements, or coercing the client towards goals set by the therapist rather than collaboratively established ones (Falicov, Nakash, & Alegria, 2021). Such behaviours can contribute to negative experiences for clients in therapy. Here is a list of skills to guide the therapist:

Demonstrate curiosity and interest:

- Use questions to show investment in the family members' perspectives.
- Ensure questions indicate a genuine desire to understand their lived experiences.

Utilise open-ended questions:

- Employ open-ended questions to allow family members the freedom to express themselves fully.
- Ensure these questions provide space for detailed, personalised responses.

Incorporate closed questions when necessary:

- Use closed questions judiciously, especially for those who may struggle with open-ended responses.
- This can help facilitate communication for individuals who find broader questions challenging.

Explore cultural identities:

- Ask questions that delve into the family's unique cultural identities, including race, class, culture, and experiences of disability or mental health.

Foster direct communication:

- Encourage family members to speak directly to the therapist, promoting listening to each other's perspectives.
- Assist family members to ask questions and use active listening when engaging in problem-solving.

Engage in active listening:

- Listen attentively to responses, giving family members time to articulate their thoughts.
- Avoid steering the conversation and respect the family's expertise in their lives.

Reflect before responding:

- Consider the family's answers before responding to avoid dominating the conversation.
- Adopt a "one-down" position, allowing the family to lead the therapeutic process.

Avoid counterproductive behaviours:

- Be mindful not to dominate the conversation, interrupt, use pathologising language, make judgements, or impose therapist-set goals.

Monitor and adjust therapist behaviours:

- Assess talk time to ensure balanced participation.
- Reflect on whether interventions are collaboratively developed.
- Allow the client to set the session agenda, empowering them and tailoring therapy to their needs.

These points serve as a reminder of the fundamental principles that guide effective therapeutic engagement and underscore the importance of the therapist's role in facilitating a client-centred approach. Addressing these areas is crucial for creating a therapeutic environment where clients feel heard, respected, and actively involved in their therapy journey.

Conclusion

In conclusion, this chapter has delved into the evolving landscape of family therapy, underscoring the critical need for therapists to incorporate an understanding of diverse social and cultural contexts into their practice. The profound impact of discrimination, marginalisation, and socio-economic challenges on mental health and family dynamics cannot be overstated. Therapists are tasked with the delicate yet crucial responsibility of engaging families with respect, cultural humility, and an inquisitive mindset that acknowledges and explores the unique cultural narratives of each family. Identifying and addressing abuses of power within family structures is paramount. Furthermore, the practice of self-reflection is indispensable for therapists, as it involves a continuous journey of understanding their own cultural identities, biases, and the "use of self" in therapy. This reflective practice not only enriches the therapeutic process but also fosters a deeper comprehension of the historical, social, and cultural tapestries that shape both the therapists' and the families' lives, thereby enhancing the efficacy and relevance of family therapy.

Note

1 See also Knudson-Martin et al. (2015) who identified competencies for addressing gender and power in couple therapy.

References

Ackerman Institute (2020). Statement on Black Lives Matter News Blog, Statements/May 29. https://www.ackerman.org/blog/statement-on-black-lives-matter/

Addison, S., & Coolhart, D. (2015). Expanding the therapy paradigm with queer couples: A relational intersectional lens. *Family Process, 54,* 435–453.

Allan, J. (2016). Critical social work in action. In D. L. Harris & T. C. Bordere (Eds.). *Handbook of social justice in loss and grief.* New York, NY: Routledge.

Asiimwe, R., Lesch, E., Karume, M., & Blow, A. J. (2021). Expanding our international reach: Trends in the development of systemic family therapy training and implementation in Africa. *Journal of Marital and Family Therapy, 47*, 815–830.

Barnes, C. (2019). Understanding the social model of disability: Past, present and future. In N. Watson, A. Roulstone, & C. Thomas (Eds.). *Routledge handbook of disability studies* (pp. 14–31). New York, NY: Routledge.

Baum, S. (2007). The use of family therapy for people with learning disabilities. *Advances in Mental Health and Learning Disabilities, 1*(2), 8–13.

Baum, S., & Lynggaard, H. (Eds.). (2018). *Intellectual disabilities: A systemic approach.* New York, NY: Routledge.

Bennett, B. (2019). The importance of aboriginal history for practitioners. In B. Bennett & S. Green (Eds.). *Our voices: Aboriginal social work.* London, England: Bloomsbury Publishing.

Bennett, B., & Bodkin-Andrews, G. (2021). Continuous improvement cultural responsiveness measurement tools. Indigenous and Transcultural Research Centre. https://www.usc.edu.au/research/indigenous-and-transcultural-research-centre/building-knowledge-systems

Birdsey, N., & Kustner, C. (2021). Reviewing the social GRACES: What do they add and limit in systemic thinking and practice? *The American Journal of Family Therapy, 49*, 429–442.

Blumer, M. L., Gavriel Ansara, Y., & Watson, C. M. (2013). Cisgenderism in family therapy: How everyday clinical practices can delegitimize people's gender self-designations. *Journal of Family Psychotherapy, 24*, 267–285.

Burnham, J. (2012). Developments in social GRRRAAACCEEESSS: Visible-invisible and voiced-unvoiced. In I. B. Krause (Ed.), *Culture and reflexivity in systemic psychotherapy: Mutual perspectives* (pp. 139–160). London, England: Karnac Books

Butler, C. (2015). Intersectionality in family therapy training: Inviting students to embrace the complexities of lived experience. *Journal of Family Therapy, 37*, 583–589.

Cheon, H. S., & Murphy, M. J. (2007). The self-of-the-therapist awakened: Postmodern approaches to the use of self in marriage and family therapy. *Journal of Feminist Family Therapy, 19*, 1–16.

Collins, P. H. (2019). *Intersectionality as critical social theory.* Durham, NC: Duke University Press.

Combs, G. (2019). White privilege: What's a family therapist to do? *Journal of Marital and Family Therapy, 45*, 61–75.

Cottrell-Boyce, J. (2022). Addressing white privilege in family therapy: A discourse analysis. *Journal of Family Therapy, 44*, 142–156.

Crenshaw, K. W. (1989). Demarginalizing the Intersection of Race and Sex: A Black Feminist Critique of Antidiscrimination Doctrine, Feminist Theory and Antiracist Politics. *University of Chicago Legal Forum*, 139–167.

Dadras, I., & Daneshpour, M. (2018). Social justice implications for MFT: The need for cross-cultural responsiveness. In S. Singh Poulsen & R. Allan (Eds.), *Cross-cultural responsiveness & systemic therapy. Focused issues in family therapy.* Cham, Switzerland: Springer. https://doi.org/10.1007/978-3-319-71395-3_1

Falicov, C. (2007). Working with transnational immigrants: Expanding meaning of family, community and culture. *Family Process, 34*, 373–388.

Falicov, C., Nakash, O., & Alegria, M. (2021). Centering the voice of the client: On becoming a collaborative practitioner with low-income individuals and families. *Family Process, 60*, 670–687.

Fernando, T., & Bennett, B. (2019). Creating a culturally safe space when teaching aboriginal content in social work: A scoping review. *Australian Social Work, 72*, 47–61.

Foronda, C., Baptiste, D. L., Reinholdt, M. M., & Ousman, K. (2016). Cultural humility: A concept analysis. *Journal of Transcultural Nursing, 27*, 210–217.

Goldner, V. (1985). Feminism and family therapy. *Family Process, 24*, 31–47.

Goldner, V., Penn, P., Sheinberg, M., & Walker, G. (1990). Love and violence: Gender paradoxes in volatile attachments. *Family Process, 29*, 343–364.

Green, S. (2019). Social work and cultural support. In B. Bennett & S. Green (Eds.), *Our voices: Aboriginal social work*. London, England: Bloomsbury Publishing.

Green, S., Bennett, B., & Betteridge, S. (2016). Cultural responsiveness and social work – A discussion. *Social Alternatives, 35*, 66–72.

Hare-Mustin, R. (1978). A feminist approach to family therapy. *Family Process, 17*, 181–194.

Hernandez-Wolfe, P., Acevedo, V., Victoria Eugenia, V., & Volkmann, T. (2015). Transnational family therapy training: A collaborative learning experience in cultural equity and humility. *Journal of Feminist Family Therapy, 27*, 134–155.

Hook, J. N., Hodge, A. S., Sandage, S. J., Davis, D. E., & Van Tongeren, D. R. (2023). Differentiation of self and cultural competence. *Practice Innovations, 8*, 50–61.

hooks, bell (1981). *Ain't I a woman: Black women and feminism*. Boston, MA: South End Press.

Hutton, V., & Sisko, S. (Eds.). (2021). *Multicultural responsiveness in counselling and psychology*. New York, NY: Springer Nature Pub.

James, K. (1984). Breaking the chains of gender: Family Therapy's position? *Australian Journal of Family Therapy, 5*, 247–248.

James, K. (2007). The interactional process of forgiveness and responsibility: A critical assessment of the family therapy literature. In C. Flaskas, I. McCarthy, & J. Sheean (Eds.), *Hope and despair in narrative and family therapy* (pp. 128–136). UK: Routledge.

James, K. (2010). Domestic violence within refugee families: Intersecting patriarchal culture and the refugee experience. *Australian and New Zealand Journal of Family Therapy, 31*(3), 275–284.

James, K., & MacKinnon, L. (1990). The "incestuous family" revisited: A critical analysis of family therapy myths. *Journal of Marital and Family Therapy, 16*, 71–88. https://doi.org/10.1111/j.1752-0606.1990.tb00047.x

James, K., & McIntyre, D. (1983). The reproduction of families: The social role of family therapy? *Journal of Marital and Family Therapy, 9*, 119–129. https://doi-org.wwwproxy1.library.unsw.edu.au/10.1111/j.1752-0606.1983.tb01494.x

James, K., & McIntyre, D. (1989). "A momentary gleam of enlightenment" towards a model of feminist family therapy. *Journal of Feminist Family Therapy, 1*, 3–24. doi: 10.1300/J086v01n03_02

Khan, S. (2002). Visible differences: Individual and collective risk-taking in working cross-culturally. In B. Mason & A. Sawyer (2002), *Exploring the unsaid: Creativity, risks and dilemmas in working cross-culturally*. London, England: Routledge.

Knudson-Martin, C., Huenergardt, D., Lafontant, K., Bishop, L., Schaepper, J., & Wells, M. (2015). Competencies for addressing gender and power in couple therapy: A socio emotional approach. *Journal of Marital and Family Therapy, 41*(2), 205–220.

Laszloffy, T. A., & Hardy, K. V. (2000). Uncommon strategies for a common problem: Addressing racism in family therapy. *Family Process, 39*, 35–50. https://doi.org/10.1111/j.1545-5300.2000.39106.x

MacKinnon (1992)

MacKinnon, L. (1998). *Trust and betrayal in the treatment of child abuse*. New York, NY: Guilford Publications.

MacKinnon, L. (1993) Systems in Settings: The Therapist as Power Broker, *Australian and New Zealand Journal of Family Therapy, 14*(3)

MacKinnon, L., & Marlett, N. (1984). A social action perspective: The disabled and their families in context. In E. Coppersmith (Ed.), *Family therapy collections: Families with handicapped members*. Rockville, MD: Aspen Publications.

MacKinnon, L. K., & Miller, D. (1987). The new epistemology and socio-political considerations. *Journal of Marital and Family Therapy, 13*, 139–155.

McDowell, T., & Hernández, P. (2010). Decolonizing academia: Intersectionality, participation, and accountability in family therapy and counseling. *Journal of Feminist Family Therapy, 22*, 93–111.

McDowell, T., Knudson-Martin, C., & Bermudez, J. M. (2022). *Socioculturally attuned family therapy: Guidelines for equitable theory and practice.* New York, NY: Taylor & Francis.

McDowell, T., Knudson-Martin, C., & Bermudez, J. M. (2019). Third order thinking in family therapy: Addressing social justice across family therapy practice. *Family Process, 58,* 9–22.

McGoldrick, M., Giordano, J., & Garcia-Preto, N. (2005). *Ethnicity and family therapy* (3rd ed.). New York, NY: Guilford Publications.

McGoldrick, M., & Hardy, K. (2019). *Re-visioning family therapy: Addressing diversity in clinical practice* (3rd ed.). New York, NY: Guilford Publications.

Nguyen, P. V., Naleppa, M., & Lopez, Y. (2021). Cultural competence and cultural humility: A complete practice. *Journal of Ethnic & Cultural Diversity in Social Work, 30*(3), 273–281.

Nolte, 2007

O'Leary, P., Tsui, M. S., & Ruch, G. (2013). The boundaries of the social work relationship revisited: Towards a connected, inclusive and dynamic conceptualisation. *British Journal of Social Work, 43,* 135–153.

Peterson, J. (2021). Moving beyond the single story: Using a double-storied assessment tool in narrative practice. *International Journal of Narrative Therapy & Community Work, 1,* 70–81.

Petty-John, M., Tseng, C., & Blow, A. (2021). Therapeutic utility of discussing therapist/client intersectionality in treatment: When and how? *Family Process, 59,* 313–327.

Rhodes, P. (2002). Mainstreaming intellectual disability into the history of family therapy. *Australian and New Zealand Journal of Family Therapy, 23,* 211–214.

Rober, P., & Seltzer, M. (2010). Avoiding colonizer positions in the therapy room: Some ideas about the challenges of dealing with the dialectic of misery and resources in families. *Family Process, 49,* 123–137.

Roberts, J., Abu-Baker, K., Diez Fernández, C., Chong Garcia, N., Fredman, G., Kamya, H., & Zevallos Vega, R. (2014). Up close: Family therapy challenges and innovations around the world. *Family Process, 53,* 544–576.

Seikkula, J., & Trimble, D. (2005). Healing elements of therapeutic conversation: Dialogue as an embodiment of love. *Family Process, 44,* 463–475.

Selvini, M. P., Boscolo, L., Cecchin, G., & Prata, G. (1980). Hypothesizing- circularity and neutrality: Three guidelines for the conductor of the session. *Family Process, 19,* 3–12.

Sisko, S. (2021). Cultural responsiveness in counselling and psychology: An introduction. In V. Hutton & S. Sisko (Eds.). *Multicultural responsiveness in counselling and psychology.* Cham: Palgrave Macmillan. https://doi.org/10.1007/978-3-030-55427-9_1

Totsuka, Y. (2014). Which aspects of social GGRRAAACCESSS grab you the most? The social GGRRAAACCEESSS exercise for a supervision group to promote therapists' self reflexivity. *Journal of Family Therapy, 36*(S1), 86–106.

Tsang, N. M. (2017). Otherness and empathy—Implications of lévinas ethics for social work education. *Social Work Education, 36,* 312–322.

Zhang, H., Watkins, C. E. Jr, Hook, J. N., Hodge, A. S., Davis, C. W., Norton, J., …, & Owen, J. (2022). Cultural humility in psychotherapy and clinical supervision: A research review. *Counselling and Psychotherapy Research, 22,* 548–557.

Chapter 12

Working Systemically with Australian First Nation Families

Banu Moloney, Robyne Latham, and Lawrence Moloney

Introduction

A wide range of social and therapeutic interventions into the lives of First Nations individuals and families have been based on a presumption that the intervenors come to the table with superior knowledge and superior skills. This stance of superiority reflects a colonisation narrative, which has dominated much of mainstream Australia's views of its own progress and advancement. The disastrous consequences of these presumptions have been well documented – perhaps the most notorious being attempts to destroy Indigenous languages, culture, and family structure via the systematic removal of First Nations children from their families of origin (Australian Human Rights Commission, 2010).

Within what could be broadly termed the 'helping professions', apologies for these consequences have been made by multiple peak bodies (e.g., Australian Association of Social Workers (AASW), 2004; Australian and New Zealand College of Psychiatrists (ANZCP), 1999; Australian Psychological Association (APS), 2016).

Such apologies typically include statements of intention to adhere to better practices in the future. The most recent from the above professions, for example (Australian Psychological Society, 2017), notes that:

> To demonstrate our genuine commitment to this apology, we intend to pursue a different way of working with Aboriginal and Torres Strait Islander people that will be characterised by diligently:

- Listening more and talking less
- Following more and steering less
- Advocating more and complying less
- Including more and ignoring less and
- Collaborating more and commanding less

This worthy statement of intention speaks to relational skills, which largely reflect elements previously found to be common to all successful therapeutic interventions (Moloney, 2016). That is, multiple studies have found that regardless of the therapeutic model being employed, engagement principles along the lines noted by the APS are at the core of successful outcomes (see, e.g., Duncan, Miller, Wampold, & Hubble, 2016; Wampold & Imel, 2015).

DOI: 10.4324/9781003490104-13

From this perspective, the APS apology signals an intention to work therapeutically with First Nations people in ways that have been shown to be successful with non-First Nations clients. In the light of what is known about the impact of colonisation, however, a question raised in this chapter is whether this 'level playing field' approach is a sufficient response to meaningful and effective engagement with First Nations individuals and families. We suggest in this chapter that a more proactive and more culturally informed response is required. Presumptions of relational equality and equality of resources, we suggest, are not enough. The context of colonisation in which we make this suggestion is briefly addressed in the next section.

The colonial legacy: A brief overview

An overarching impact of colonisation has been that 'Societies, close knit and well-ordered for tens of thousands of years, became fragmented' (McCulloch & McCulloch, 2017, p. 10). The fragmentation led to the marginalisation of Australia's First Nations people and, in many cases, to their subjugation and enslavement. It was fuelled by a virulent form of racism, the origins of which lie in colonisers' presumptions about their own superiority.

As the report noted above points out, the intention behind the systematic removal of First Nations children over a period of 100 years was that they would be absorbed into white society and that their 'Aboriginality' would eventually disappear. This behaviour, along with multiple documented massacres (Centre for Twenty First Century Humanities, n.d.) and the widespread dispossession of the land to which the spiritual lives of First Nations people were intimately connected, has been widely recognised as a form of attempted genocide.

The situation today is that First Nations people have nonetheless survived these multiple attempts to obliterate their culture. Indeed, while they have been reduced to a small percentage of the mainstream Australian population, First Nations numbers are estimated to have increased from 2.8% in 2016 to 3.2% in 2023 (Australian Bureau of Statistics, 2023). There is a growing sense of pride and self-assertion amongst First Nations people, accompanied by a gradually increasing (though yet to be firmly established) recognition by other Australians that First Nations ways of knowing have much to contribute.

At the same time, the costs associated with the survival of First Nations people continue to be considerable. For example,

- In 2018, the First Nations child mortality rate was 141 per 100,000 – twice the rate for non-First Nations children (67 per 100,000; Closing the Gap Report 2018).
- Life expectancy of First Nations men and First Nations women are currently 8.6 years and 7.8 years less than their non-First Nations counterparts (Closing the Gap Report, 2022).
- Incarceration rates are a staggeringly large 2223 per 100,000 (Closing the Gap Report, 2022). This compares with 201 per 100,000 for Australians as a whole (Australian Bureau of Statistics, 2023).
- About 1 in 17 First Nations children are in out of home care. This represents about 24% of all Australian children (Australian Institute of Health and Welfare, 2022).
- In 2018, the First Nations employment rate was around 49% compared to around 75% for non-Indigenous Australians.

Social indicators such as these are of course interlinked. It is well documented, for example, that employment status has associations with outcomes for health, social and emotional well-being, and living standards (Marmot, 2009).

Therapeutic engagement with First Nations people: Thinking beyond mainstream common factors

The common factors associated with effective therapeutic engagement and outcomes, noted above, were first hypothesised by Rosenzweig (1936). Though rigorous research has continued to refine the nature of these factors and how they interact with each other, they can for the purpose of this chapter be summarised as the development of a real relationship, the facilitation of positive expectations, and the incorporation of specific ingredients. The best-studied common factors include paying attention to a therapeutic alliance through the use of empathy, positive regard, and genuineness and demonstrating a close awareness of context. One definition, which speaks to common factors and contextual approach to therapy, has been suggested by the American Psychological Association to be:

> A collaborative enterprise in which patients and clinicians [sic] negotiate ways of working together that are mutually agreeable and likely to lead to positive outcomes. Thus, patient values and preferences (e.g., goals, beliefs, preferred modes of treatment) are central component of [evidenced based practice].
>
> (American Psychological Association Presidential Task Force on Evidence-Based Practice, 2006, p. 280)

Though the American Psychological Association (APA) language retains a medicalised view of therapy (patients and clinicians), the approach nonetheless speaks to an appropriate foundation for therapeutic work with people from both First Nations and non-First Nations cultures. But because of multiple negative experiences associated with colonisation, we suggest that First Nations people would be especially alert and appropriately sensitive to any missteps that may occur in the initial engagement process and in ongoing interactions with the therapist. We suggest that non-First Nations therapists need to begin by recognising that without sustained engagement, they can know little about the lived reality of First Nations people. Non-First Nations therapists must be prepared to begin with a not knowing position (Carlson, 2020); to listen with sensitivity, wait to be asked about what they think or feel, be gently tentative with respect to responses and suggestions they might wish to make, and respond openly to questions about their own experience.

The practical implications of this are both simple and profound. For example, if non-First Nations therapists ask First Nations family members a question about themselves and their circumstances, they must be prepared to answer honestly if they are asked the same question. This flies in the face of a tendency for Western trained therapists to avoid placing themselves in such a vulnerable position. Put simply, Western trained therapists are more likely to hide behind a mask of 'professionalism', reflecting the patient-clinician language used by the APA above. We suggest that a stance of shared vulnerability is especially important from a cultural safety perspective and especially meaningful for individuals who have been marginalised and are attempting to heal from the ravages of colonisation.

In summary, non-First Nations therapists need, in the first instance, to be real, authentic, and themselves – avoiding the sort of pretensions that can be an occupational hazard for professional therapists who may have spent years learning their trade. This means, in turn, being respectfully curious about what First Nations people might and might not want from 'helpers' or from the Service the helpers represent. Generally speaking, First Nations peoples are less impressed with formal qualifications and more reassured by knowing who you are and what grounds you as a person. Are you a mother? Are you a brother? Who are your mob? And what connects you to the place you work in and the land you live on? Shaun Coade, who was a First Nations mentor and cultural consultant to the first author (see Moloney, 2014), put it this way: *You get it right by my people and you will get it right by all people.*

The fit between *Systemic* therapy and First Nations people's ways of knowing

Individually based therapies continue to dominate Western psychotherapeutic practice. The principal focus of these approaches to healing is on the agentic self – that is, the part of ourselves we assume to be acting with autonomy and independence. The focus of *Systemic* therapies, on the other hand, is on our interconnectedness with others and with those things and those interactions that take us beyond ourselves and give meaning to our lives.

Like many human truths, there is a paradox in the distinction between these two approaches to healing. We are, on the one hand, individuals with individual desires and needs. But our individuality has no substantial existence and no solid meaning outside of the group or society that sustains us and which we help to sustain. Both practically and emotionally, the 'autonomous' self relies on supporting and being supported by others.

McLeod's (2013) classic and wide-ranging description of the scope of counselling and psychotherapy reflects a continued concentration on models that focus on individual growth and individual cognitive and emotional distress. Over 464 pages, only one chapter speaks to Systemic models of intervention. Despite this, however, McLeod makes the following significant observation:

> Systemic therapy has taken up the challenge of implementing a relational philosophy based on an understanding that in the end, individualism is not an adequate basis for living a good life.
>
> (McLeod, 2013, p. 284)

Most First Nations people would strongly agree with McLeod's observation. Broadly speaking, individually focused interventions aimed at enhancing personal growth or alleviating feelings of personal distress do not fit naturally into First Nations cultural assumptions. Broadly speaking, the primary frame of reference of Australia's First Nations people is relational. That is, personal strengths and personal problems are seen in terms of how well or how poorly relationships are being supported – with family, with Mob, and with others, but also with animals, plants, and the land by which all are nourished and sustained.

This being the case, there is much to be said for a therapeutic modality with First Nations people that places its focus on patterns of interactions, on the reciprocity of relationships, and on the broader ecological context. These core elements of Systemic practice speak more directly to the collectivist culture, which has sustained First Nations people over many millennia.

Excessive drinking: A First Nations cross-cultural case study

In the case study that follows, a young father of two children is struggling with addiction to alcohol. His own father, who also experienced alcohol addiction as a young man, believes that his son should do what he did, which was to work with a psychiatrist or psychologist to help him control his drinking. But what might be the issues underpinning the son's addiction and is a culturally aware Systemic approach to the problem more likely to be effective?

Case summary

Rebecca is a 32-year-old Wiradjuri-Yorta Yorta woman. She is in a married-up relationship with David, also 32 years old. David was adopted at birth by Tony and Tony's late wife Sarah, who died about three years ago. They knew nothing of David's background at the time but it now appears that he came from a First Nations family.

Rebecca and David have two sons Jarrah aged 4 and Koen aged 2. Until Sarah's passing, Tony and Sarah had been hands-on grandparents. Tony continues to be supportive of Rebecca and David and continues to play an important role as a grandfather.

David has a problem with alcohol misuse. When Rebecca rang the Centre for help with this, she was offered the option of working with Alison Elliott, a First Nations family therapist, and given the further option of bringing whomever she thought might be useful to include in the session. Tony, although somewhat uncertain, agreed to attend. David was also invited but did not turn up for the appointment. Rebecca is not surprised but thinks it might be good to go ahead with the session even without David.

Tony acknowledges he had a drinking problem as a younger man and was helped by individual therapy with a psychologist. Tony believes that all young men drink a bit and that the solution is for David to see a good psychologist or psychiatrist. Rebecca for her part is convinced that David is an Aboriginal man but, like his adoptive parents, was unaware of this until recently.

Rebecca is equally convinced that David's confusion about his identity is a key reason he has begun drinking to excess. She believes David needs to reconnect with his Mob and that this will be a healing experience for him. In her words, 'he doesn't know who he is and doesn't know where he belongs'. Though willing to be part of a family therapy session, Tony is anxious and sceptical that this is the way to go. In essence, it emerges in the therapy session that Tony is worried that he will lose his son if he connects with his Mob.

Selected therapist's input from the session[1]

Opening remarks from Alison, a First Nations Family Therapist.

> I'll just introduce what the session might look like. We can explore if we continue from there – whatever you guys decide. Sometimes family members don't show up, but we can still have a yarn.

> I want to acknowledge that the Centre is on Bunnerong Country. I'm in the First Nations team here at the Centre. I'm actually from Wiradjuri Country.

> I'd also like to pay my respects to you Sis and to your ancestors and to you too Tony and your ancestors.

> I'd like to check about this space we are using. We do have a Healing Garden here outside; but it's a bit wet today to use it.

Comment

Alison emphasises that how and if the session proceeds are up to Rebecca and Tony. She suggests that the fact that David has not come should not necessarily prevent them from having a yarn. As a First Nations therapist, Alison explains who she is and where she comes from and acknowledges where the session is taking place. She also acknowledges the ancestors of both Rebecca and David. Alison addresses the question of the therapy space itself. Does it feel OK? She notes there is a Healing Garden where yarning or therapy can also take place although, on this particular day, the weather would make this option unsuitable.

Alison

Would it be helpful if I find out who is who in the family and if I do a map of who is who?

Comment

Mapping is of course a common practice in family therapy sessions. Getting a clear sense of who is who and the connections between them is especially important in First Nations families. For many reasons, the map, commonly known as a genogram, can be more complex amongst First Nations families. Parenting and other care obligations, for example, can cover a wider group of relationships than might be the case in non-First Nations families. The conventional symbols used in the construction of mainstream family therapy genograms might also be of limited assistance. Much like Aboriginal Artworks which tell the stories of people, places, and events, First Nations genograms are replete with stories of ancestral wisdom handed down to future generations and symbols of connection to land, totems, and waterways (see Figure 12.1).

Alison

If Sarah was here today, would she find that it was useful for us to have a chat, even without David being here?

Comment

Absent family members, including those who are deceased, can have a significant ongoing impact on family relationships and on views about how to proceed. In First Nations families, ancestors have a particular importance. It is both strategic and respectful to remember Sarah in this way. In asking this question, Alison is being true to transgenerational family therapy notions and Systemic family therapy skills of circular questioning. Her comments demonstrate how Systemic family therapy and First Nations ways of being and knowing can be interwoven and coexist.

Alison

Does it feel like it's blaming? What does it feel like?

Comment

Naming a difficult feeling that may be unspoken takes courage. Alison here raises it as a question rather than present it as a statement which is more likely to enhance therapeutic outcomes. In this case, it's important to openly address issues of possible blame. When children are troubled, parents can easily feel blamed. Alison demonstrates how blame can be named and worked with sensitively rather than avoided or minimised.

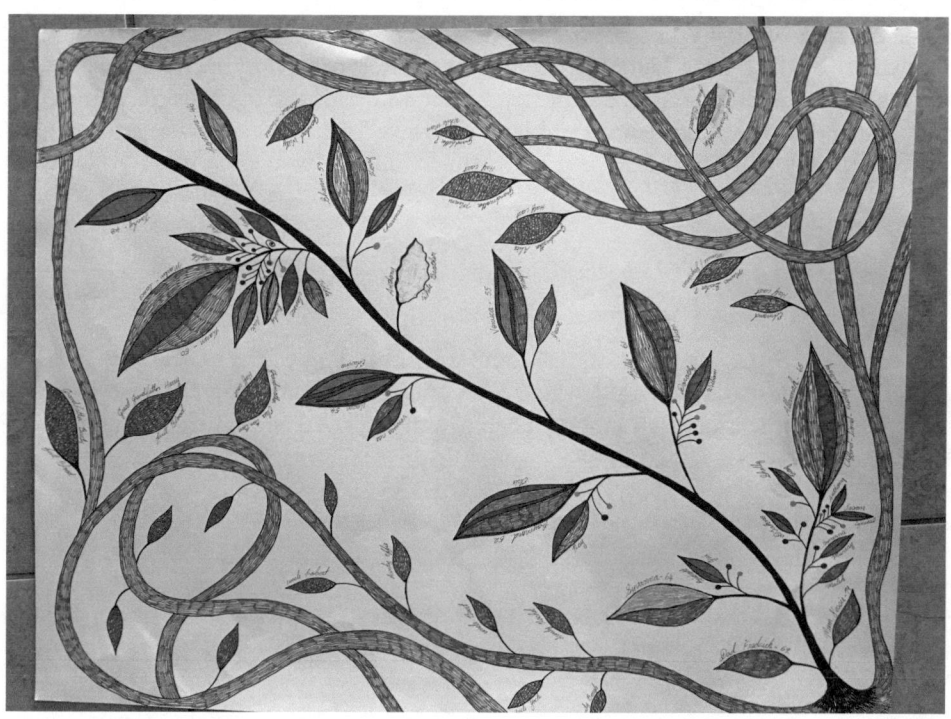

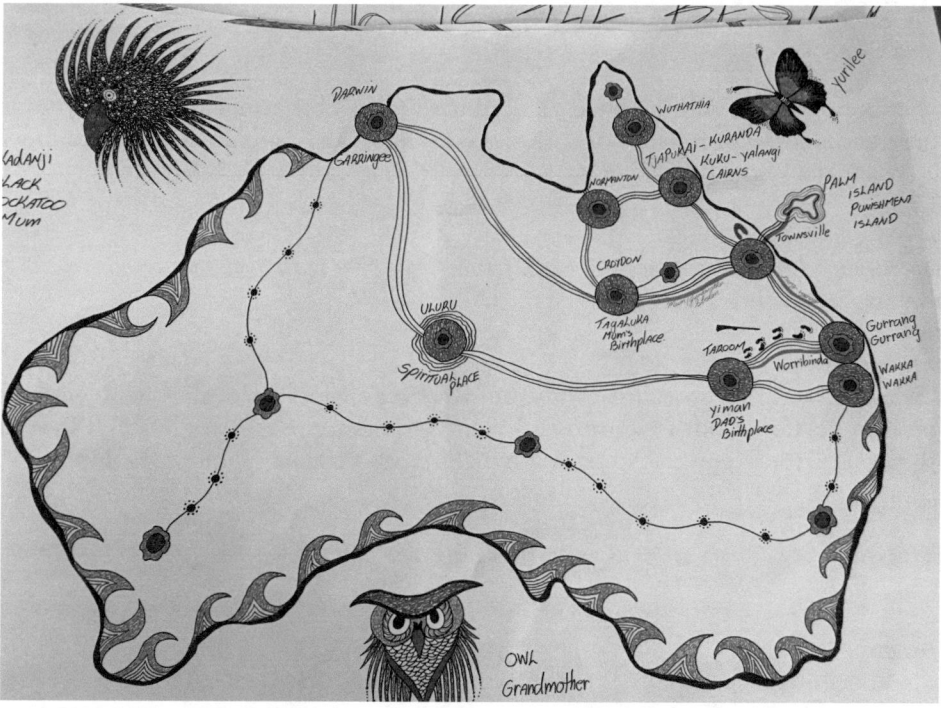

Figure 12.1 Genograms (used by permission of Karen Doolan).

In the context of First Nations families, non-First Nations therapists may not be aware of the extent to which First Nations parents are attuned to having been blamed by society and by a wide range of professionals for their perceived 'failures' to conform to mainstream norms. Not speaking about feelings of blame, however, reinforces this false dominant narrative. Not speaking about it does not make this common lived experience go away.

Alison

Sounds like Sarah was open to supports for all of you.

Comment

In the session, Rebecca was contrasting Sarah's understanding of the situation with what she perceived as Tony's struggle to understand First Nations people's different ways of knowing. Alison brings to the session the support of Sarah, a much loved and respected family member.

Alison

So from your angle, Rebecca, you feel that if he really gets to know his mob …

Comment

In acknowledging differences of opinions and focusing on their shared hopes for David, Alison is normalising differences.

Alison

I'm really curious Tony. When you hear a strong viewpoint from Rebecca about what she's feeling, what would be most helpful from your angle?

Comment

Another comment by Alison aimed at normalising possible conflict by directly addressing differences through the lens of curiosity. This is Milan Systemic therapy idea in which open, evenly delivered curiosity invites a response that legitimises difference.

Alison

Sometimes [different approaches to addiction] can be a really good fit. So, there's no right or wrong with any of these options.

Comment

This is a 'Both and' approach to Tony and Rebecca's views on dealing with addictions. Alison is respectful of both Western and First Nations approaches to healing, thus highlighting a 'Both and' approach first written about by Virginia Goldner (Goldner, 1992).

Alison

David is…. Really wanting to get to know his mob but not wanting to lose his connection with you.

Comment

This is a dilemma if seen as an either-or option. In the context of earlier normalising differences and 'Both-and' statements, Alison is hoping that Tony might begin to see that David could identify with his Mob without losing his relationship with him – his father.

Alison

The fact that you are still here is showing that your connection [with David] is strong.

Comment

Here Alison follows up her previous comment by validating and affirming the strong relationship between father and son. The importance of relationship is valued in both Systemic theories and First Nations ethics and lore.

Alison

Would it be helpful for you to say that to him ... that fear you are going to lose him if he connects with his other family?

Comment

Tony has expressed fear that he might 'lose' David if David identifies with his Mob. This is a turning point in the session. A key question (rather than a statement) is asked in the context of Alison's creation of an accepting and supportive environment. Tony's expression of his fear and the support he receives after acknowledging the fear opens up possibilities that David can explore his First Nations connections with Tony's blessing. Rebecca believes this will impact positively on David's current dependency on alcohol. Alison addresses the issue as a question rather than a statement of fact, a key Strategic idea from family therapy literature (Madanes, 1981).

Alison

It sounds like you (Tony) are a very important person in the life of the little boys. If they were here, what would they be wanting?

Comment

This brings the two boys, Jarrah (4) and Koen (2), into the room. Regardless of the answer, the question affirms the importance of the grandchild-grandparent relationship and affirms Tony's connection to his extended family. It is respectful of First Nations' notions of family in which grandparents typically play an important role in the raising of their grandchildren.[2] More broadly, it further addresses transgenerational issues and ideas of love and loyalty articulated by family therapy theorists such as Boszormenyi-Nagy (1984).

Alison

If Sarah was here, would she be open to this? Would she try to drag you down to meet the Mob Tony?

Comment

Alison is combining both Circular questions from Milan Systemic therapy with acknowledging the significance and importance of an absent family member – in this instance, David's mother and Tony's wife. From a Strategic therapy perspective, this is a question that embeds an idea without formally suggesting to Tony what he might do.

Alison

I'm just wondering Tony how this is going for you ... if you feel that ...?

Comment

A lot is happening for Tony. It's important to acknowledge the work he is doing, seek feedback, and check that things are not going too fast. Tony's continued engagement will be very important if David is to successfully explore his First Nations origins (see generally Duncan, Miller, Wampold, & Hubble, 2016).

Alison

If there is one thing you could take away from today …?

Comment

Alison signals the beginning of the end of the session. Signalling this way allows Rebecca and Tony to tell Alison and to tell each other what was important. Putting this as a question rather than a statement is more likely to be meaningful for Rebecca and Tony than hearing a summary from the therapist. The responses allow Alison to shape the format of the next session and consider how David might participate in the future.

Working with First Nations families: A role for non-First nations therapists?

The case study above provides examples of Alison applying family Systems theory in a situation in which key family members are First Nations people. Alison is one of 180 family therapy graduates from La Trobe University/Bouverie Centre's Graduate Certificate in Family Therapy: First Nations, over the past 15 years.[3]

While this means that more First Nations families have access to First Nations family therapists, it is inevitable that these therapists will not always be available. What then can family therapists trained in mainstream family therapy learn from case studies such as the above if they are to work successfully with First Nations families?

Alison begins with a series of relational and contextual acknowledgments. Who is she? Where is she from? Who are the individuals participating in the session? What important people are not there? The constraints of not having significant family members in the room are managed by using Milan Systemic circular questions. By this means Alison marries family therapy ideas with cultural expectations that she would identify herself and where she fits in.

In addition, Alison speaks of the place in which they are meeting – both the Country and the specific location. She also speaks of options *within* the location, noting the availability of a Healing Garden, weather permitting, and checking that the indoor option on this particular occasion is acceptable.

Finally, in her introductory statements, Alison also acknowledges those who have gone before. Respect for ancestors and the knowledge they have passed on forms an important platform for discussions (yarning) amongst First Nations families. Formally or informally, their voices are likely to carry weight in the session. Of course, presumptions and beliefs handed down from earlier generations (or sometimes reactions against these presumptions and beliefs) are also relevant in non-First Nations families. In non-First Nations families, however, the fact that knowledge of earlier generations may not be so much to the fore can lead non-First Nations therapists to 'forget' the importance of intergenerational wisdoms, assumptions, and tensions.

The introductory statements and interactions are followed by Alison's request to 'map the family'. For First Nations families, this mapping exercise is likely to go considerably beyond the conventional genogram developed over the years by mainstream family therapists (see Figure 12.1). In addition to symbols that acknowledge the connection to land, totems, and waterways, family mapping is more likely to include a broader range of interpersonal relationships for First Nations people. This more extensive form of genogram requires skills and ways of thinking that may not come naturally to some non-First Nations therapists.

Mainstream genograms typically include absent or deceased members, the latter being conventionally marked with an 'X'. The most important deceased family member in the case study is Sarah, David's adoptive mother. Through the use of Milan Systemic therapy circular questioning skills, Alison skilfully acknowledges Sarah's continuing presence in the family. While this is a response learned in her 'Black and White' Bouverie training (Moloney, 2014), Alison would be aware of the potential power such an acknowledgment is likely to have amongst First Nations families. In this family, and especially for Rebecca, Sarah is a significant point of both intergenerational and intercultural connection.

Alison also addresses the question of blame through an open-ended question. Blaming and feelings of being blamed are present in many families seeking therapeutic assistance. As a potential 'elephant in the room', these feelings are better addressed than ignored. While addressing blame must always be carried out with sensitivity, such issues need particularly sensitive responses in the presence of First Nations families, who frequently carry with them a history of being falsely blamed by professionals for their perceived economic and social 'failures', especially failing as parents.

Alison's 'Both and' approach to the intercultural issues, which are at the heart of the differences between Rebecca and Tony, is also an extremely important aspect of the work in this session. Differences may not be able to be fully reconciled. But respect for those differences and acknowledgment that they can coexist and even enrich family life are necessary platforms on the way towards understanding and reconciliation.

As previously noted, the emotional turning point in the session is Tony's willingness to give voice to his fear that he might lose his connection with David if David embraces his Aboriginality. Tony is unlikely to have expressed this vulnerability if he had not connected sufficiently with Alison and was not able to appreciate her 'Both and' approach.

A non-First Nations therapist in a similar situation could of course make use of the same Systemic insight. The efficacy of this insight, however, needs to be linked to a genuinely held appreciation of the likely importance of First Nations Culture in David's life.

The session reveals that Rebecca is convinced that embracing his First Nations culture is David's way forward, both in his life generally and with respect to his problem with alcohol. Tony, however, is more drawn to a mainstream therapeutic approach, which, of course, keeps David more culturally connected to Tony's own experiences.

Perhaps paradoxically, having had the courage to express his fear of losing David, and possibly losing his connection with his grandchildren, a 'Both-and' option has space to emerge. But this option might not have so clearly emerged in a session with a non-First Nations therapist unless the therapist had taken time to learn of and embrace the wisdom of First Nations culture.

Cultural awareness: The key to successful engagement with non-First Nations family therapists

Becoming culturally aware

David was adopted by two loving parents who were ignorant of his cultural heritage. Through David's attraction to a First Nations woman, Rebecca, he came to recognise his own First Nations origins. This awareness has generated risks and opportunities for all family members. The risk is that David will find himself in a cultural vacuum, uneasy in living in the ways of his adoptive parents, yet anxious about embracing the norms and values he recognises in his partner and which he feels are part of his own DNA.

This is a time of crisis, a time of 'dangerous opportunity' for David and for his immediate and wider family. Its expression has come in the form of excessive drinking. But resolution of the crisis begins with awareness of the cultural differences and commonalities at play. These differences and commonalities have the capacity to enrich or destroy.

We suggest that many of us live within our culture in the way a fish lives in water. That is, unless we consciously question or purposefully reflect on the wider world in which we live, we simply regard our assumptions about our laws, language, environment, and personal relationships as 'natural'. We feel a degree of comfort and familiarity with our culture's accepted norms. In short, we feel a sense of belonging without necessarily reflecting on the constraints that our belonging might be imposing.

Becoming culturally aware and acting in ways that are culturally safe requires an unambiguous desire from therapists to learn and to understand ways of thinking and ways of being that take them beyond their comfort zone. The desire must be intrinsically motivated; it cannot be achieved merely through professional rules that speak to mandated or external expectations.

Nor can there be a defined end point to achieving cultural awareness or to acting with cultural safety. This is because as First Nations people embark on the painful process of recovery, there is always more for all to learn. In the meantime, growth towards acting with cultural awareness and cultural safety begins with recognising the reality of past genocide and the fact that this reality continues to be widely denied (Mays, 2020).

Clearly, cultures differ, one from the other, but we suggest that all cultures have fundamental markers such as language, technology, art forms, rites of passage (spiritual beliefs and celebrations), and institutions such as law, health, and education.

Australian First Nation's languages are diverse and are contextually sophisticated in their structure. Technologies include farming practices and aqua engineering, while art forms, which are central to day-to-day living, include song, dance, painting, and craft. Key rites of passage include initiation ceremonies into adulthood for girls and boys. And institutions include lore passed on by Elders with respect to areas such as health, traditional medicine, birthing practices, and education.

An understanding of these key cultural markers can be developed in many ways including online research, viewing documentaries and films, reading literature, and attending cultural events, theatre, and performances created by First Nation's people. However, a deep understanding of another's culture must include more than an intellectual understanding. It is a visceral experience, which can only truly be achieved by engaging with the culture first-hand.

For non-First Nations Australians, this involves working alongside First Nations people while embracing a rigorous interrogation of one's own cultural privileges, values, and biases. Such interrogation enables appreciation of the similarities and differences between cultures. It supports an understanding that a 'normal way of living life' in one's own culture may be puzzling or even incomprehensible to members of another culture, or, if comprehensible, it may be considered inappropriate or unacceptable.

An example in the present context could be the difference between the position of older people in many Western cultures and their position in the Australian First Nations culture. Simplistically put, in many Western cultures, older people can easily be rendered invisible – the subtext being, 'They've had a good life and now have little if anything to contribute'. In the Australian First Nations culture, older people carry the status of Elder and the title of Uncle or Aunty, regardless of familial ties. Elders are highly respected and revered for their life experience, knowledge, and wisdom and are expected to contribute to their community.

In summary, to become culturally aware is a complex and multi layered undertaking and necessitates the development of a Systemic understanding of culture, from the past to the present. Open-minded respect, which entails deep listening (Ungunmerr, 1993) curiosity and empathy which remains devoid of judgement, is integral to understanding the culture of another. When one can stand in this place and develop a visceral as well as a cognitive understanding, one is well on their way to developing cultural awareness.

Making family therapy culturally safe

Cultural safety begins with a physically and psychologically safe environment. This sense of being safe extends to the spiritual, social, and emotional safety of all. An environment containing signifiers of another's culture, such as artworks, provides environmental comfort and reassurance.

As facilitators, family therapists set the tone of the conversations that take place between family members. In the case described above, Alison took time to introduce herself. Though not recorded in the transcript, she asked Rebecca and Tony if they had been offered a drink at reception and asked if there was anything else they needed. She enquired about the suitability of the location, acknowledged ancestors, and acknowledged absent family members.

The default position of family therapy is to be inclusive of all – to nurture and value everyone's opinions and be devoid of judgement or blame. With First Nations people, facilitators must be especially alert to expressions of shame or feelings of guilt associated with not having succeeded in meeting Western expectations. Cultural safety is enhanced through the exercise of shared respect, shared meaning, shared knowledge, and the experience of learning together.

This, in turn, requires the facilitator to recognise the privileges, stereotypes, or biases they themselves carry as part of their own cultural background. Notwithstanding good intentions, unacknowledged privileges and unconscious biases can rapidly lead to misunderstandings. Misunderstandings are likely to be felt before they are articulated. Silence or low levels of responsiveness, for example, might indicate that a boundary has been unintentionally crossed.

Should this happen, it is important to address the issue promptly using words and gestures that signal humility and respectful curiosity. Cross-cultural misunderstandings are to be expected. With goodwill and humility, however, they can be harnessed as a learning opportunity. They can nurture a deepened understanding among the participants and re-establish culturally safety.

Building a cultural bridge

Between all cultures, there is space for shared understanding – a cultural bridge. As with fostering a culturally safe environment, building a cultural bridge can only occur when the environment in which the session takes place is physically and psychologically safe. Like developing cultural awareness, establishing a cultural bridge is primarily a visceral experience. Its foundation stones are empathy, respect, curiosity, open-mindedness, and (again) a deep awareness of one's own cultural biases and privileges. It requires dispensing with judgement and blame as well as alertness to expressions of shame and guilt.

Cultural bridging is predicated upon enthusiasm for learning about another's culture, history, customs, traditions, and values. It looks to cultural similarities while respecting cultural differences. In so doing, it enables learning from each other while preserving the core of one's own beliefs and values.

Somewhat unusually in the case study, the dominant ethos reflects First Nations ways of knowing. The therapist is a First Nations woman. The immediate family consists of a First Nations wife and mother, two First Nations children, and a father who appears to be on the point of embracing his Aboriginal heritage. Tony has connections with First Nations culture via his daughter-in-law and his grandchildren. But he was clearly some distance from embracing the culture and indeed anxious about his son David moving in that direction. Although Sarah had died before getting to know her daughter-in-law well and would have known only one of her grandchildren, Rebecca had a sense that her mother-in-law would have had less difficulty in bridging the two cultures than was the case with Tony.

As a First Nations therapist, it was Alison's responsibility to assist Tony to begin a journey across the cultural bridge. She assisted in this process by, for example, acknowledging the importance of Tony's own ancestors and checking on whether he was comfortable in the environment in which the session was to take place. She also checked on whether proceeding in David's absence was acceptable and later slowed the process down to enquire about how Tony was managing. Alison showed respect for Tony's solution to his son's addiction by acknowledging that mainstream therapies can also be useful.

Whilst checking on absences and checking in on how a client is managing would be expected of all good family therapists, the context of these enquiries, in this case, was clearly one of the significant cultural differences. The fact that Tony was able to acknowledge his fear of losing connection with David in the presence of two First Nations women suggests that Alison was providing at least the beginnings of a cultural bridge. Tony was a long way from embracing the idea of relating to First Nations ways of engaging with the world. But Alison had sown a seed that had the potential for a meeting of cultures and a way forward for David that preserved the best of what was available on both sides.

As a First Nations therapist, Alison has had to deal with dominant Western cultural norms. The challenges in her training included how to adapt those aspects of mainstream family Systems theory to First Nations wisdom.

In such a situation, the challenge for non-First Nations family therapists would be the same in its aims but inevitably very different in its execution. While by no means insurmountable, the challenge for a non-First Nations therapist working Systemically with the problem of David's addiction to alcohol would have been more complex. The therapist would need to be willing in the first instance to experience both the excitement and the discomfort of embracing First Nations wisdoms and, from that place of cultural awareness, to find ways of helping to build bridges that are meaningful and safe.

What can mainstream family therapy learn from First Nations ways of knowing?

A focal point of Bouverie Centre's teaching of family therapy has been, 'The six 'C's' that encapsulate much systemic work – *context, curiosity, connectedness, culture, circularity, and constraints*. We have found that First Nations ways of knowing both reinforce and add to the ways these core Systemic ideas can be appreciated and made use of with families. In this penultimate section, space does not permit exploration of the conceptual richness of each of these constructs. Rather, our intention is simply to provide brief examples of reminders and additions that First Nations cultural norms bring to each.

With respect to *context*, we saw in the case study an example of how Alison took time to set the scene for the work. First Nations people's engagement with their environment and with each other is highly contextual. Each person, place, animal, plant, and 'thing' are in a recognised relationship with each other. Knowledge changes as these multiple variables interact with each other. In the name of efficiency, Western knowledge tends to adopt a more low-context approach in which knowledge tends to span place and time. This more fixed approach to knowledge can mean that less attention is paid when and where a family meets and the circumstances in which family and family therapist meet are afforded less attention.

A First Nations approach also serves as a reminder that *curiosity* is a two-way process. Mainstream approaches rightly place emphasis on remaining open to hearing a range of clients' feelings, narratives, and explanations. The risk, however, is that if the person of the therapist remains largely hidden and or is resistant to the curiosity aroused within family members, his or her capacity to facilitate may be diminished. First Nations ways of knowing serve as a reminder that appropriate personal transparency on the part of the therapist is an important ingredient in Systemic work with family members.

A key idea in mainstream Systems therapy is that of *connectedness* between family members. Milan Systemic theory reminds us that in a family therapy environment, the concept of connectedness includes connectedness with the therapist(s). In Systemic terminology, the presence of the therapist changes the system. Our experience suggests that while Western trained family therapists sometimes need to remind themselves of the importance of this dynamic, this broader notion of interconnectedness fits naturally with First Nations ways of knowing.

In the mind of many Westerners, *culture* is something that others have or is at best regarded as an add-on. In the mind of First Nations people, culture is a living breathing reality that is constantly revisited and reinforced through stories and relationships. From a Systemic perspective, all interactions have a cultural component. A key question that First Nations people bring to mainstream family therapists is whether and in what ways our cultural assumptions are recognised and utilised in the service of healing.

Western ways of knowing can also too easily and too quickly default to presumptions of cause and effect. Systemic theory is closer to First Nations' appreciation of reciprocity in relationships and reciprocal relationships in the broader environment. While the concept of *circularity* in the form of circular questioning has captured this idea in family therapy, it is one that many mainstream students struggle to put into practice. The relative ease with which First Nations therapists grasp the concept is another reminder of the gains that can come from exploring and appreciating these ways of knowing.

Finally, while not exclusive to First Nations individuals and families, an unacceptably high number confront a variety of practical *constraints* such as poor health, housing, and employment opportunities as well as emotional constraints associated with past dispossession and past trauma. First Nations family therapists are especially sensitive to these issues. They also become skilled at dealing with the shame such constraints frequently bring. We believe there is much that non-First Nations therapists can learn with respect to both recognising and managing issues such as these which inevitably limit prospects for growth and change.

Concluding thoughts

First Nations families remain greatly overrepresented in Australia's health, welfare, and justice systems. Although family therapy has an important contribution to make when acute and urgent support for struggling families is needed, good quality culturally accessible services are generally not readily available to First Nations families and individuals.

Since 2010, the Bouverie Centre, La Trobe University has graduated approximately 180 First Nations family therapists capable of providing such services. The aim has been to train First Nations therapists who can assist families in need through a respectful and sensitive marrying of First Nations wisdoms with Systemic family therapy practices.

Initially taught by non-First Nations family therapists in close collaboration with a First Nations consultant, this Course has paid close attention to the special skills that First Nations students bring to Systemic ways of thinking. Its success can be seen through its very high retention rates as well as highly positive feedback from the graduates themselves. The hope is that the Course will continue into the coming years and that an increasing number of graduates will be in a position to facilitate both short-term positive change in First Nations families and make long-term contributions to the healing of future generations.

In the meantime, much has been learned from First Nations families presenting for family therapy at the Bouverie Centre and from the students themselves about what 'works' when engaging with these families. This means that ways of engaging with First Nations families using Systemic principles can also be learned by those non-First Nations therapists who are willing to approach First Nations ways of knowing with respectful and courageous curiosity.

While the numbers of First Nations family therapists continue to build, mainstream therapists have an opportunity to expand their knowledge base and make an important contribution to First Nations families' short-term and long-term healing. As First Nations people continue to recover and regain a rightful place in Australian society, it is our hope that more family therapists are willing to answer Pearson's (2009) call for bi-cultural fluency. Pearson's call was primarily to his own First Nations people, but achieving such fluency should be a two-way process. A commitment to bi-cultural fluency means that in their work with all families, there is much that mainstream therapists can learn from First Nations relational approaches and First Nations wisdom.

Acknowledgements

The authors wish to acknowledge Alison Elliott, a Wiradjuri woman and family therapist, for her generous permission to use an edited transcript of the therapy session cited in this chapter.

The authors wish to acknowledge the genogram artwork of Tagaluka Gurrang Gurrang Artist and Family therapist Karen Doolan.

The authors also acknowledge Bouverie Family Centre for permission to make use of this session, which forms part of Bouverie's online training for family therapists.

Notes

1 This session has been recorded in full and forms part of the online teaching programme at Bouverie Centre. Therapist's comments have been selected to illustrate key systemic family therapy concepts and to comment on their particular relevance in working with First Nations people. Although the family described in this chapter is based on a known situation, names and certain details have been changed to preserve anonymity. The full dialogue, which forms part of the Bouverie Centre's current online training course, emerged from a role-play in which the grandfather (who is in fact a non-First Nations grandfather) and the 'married up' mother (who is in fact a First Nations 'married up' mother) were asked to relate spontaneously to each other around the dynamics described in the summary.
2 See Bowden's (2020) description of his own role as a grandparent in a mixed-race *Arrernte* family.
3 A large majority of the graduates were mature age First Nations students already working in the field. Some non-First Nations students working in First Nations settings and endorsed by their organisations were also accepted onto the course.

References

ABS (2023) Prisoners in Australia, 2022, ABS, Australian Government, accessed 13 March 2024.

American Psychological Association Presidential Task Force on Evidence-Based Practice (2006). Evidence-based practice in psychology. *American Psychologist, 61*, 271–285.

Australian and New Zealand College of Psychiatrists (1999). *Apology for the role played by psychiatrists in the Stolen Generations.* www.ranzcp.org/clinical-guidelines-publications/clinical-guidelines-publications-library/apology-for-the-role-played-by-psychiatrists-in-the-stolen-generations#:~:text=The%20Royal%20Australian%20%26%20New%20Zealand,practices%20of%20the%20Stolen%20Generations

Australian Association of Social Workers (2004). *Statement of apology.* http://www.aasw.asn.au/document/item/618

Australian Bureau of Statistics (2023). *Census of population and housing – Counts of Aboriginal and Torres Strait Islander Australians.* https://www.abs.gov.au/statistics/people/aboriginal-and-torres-strait-islander-peoples/census-population-and-housing-counts-aboriginal-and-torres-strait-islander-australians/latest-release#cite-window1

Australian Human Rights Commission. (2010). *Bringing them home: The "Stolen children" report (1997).* Sydney: Australian Human Rights Commission.

Australian Institute of Health and Welfare. (2022). Child protection Australia 2020–21. Retrieved from https://www.aihw.gov.au/reports/child-protection/child-protection-australia-2020-21

Australian Psychological Society (2017). *Apology to Aboriginal and Torres Strait Islander People from the Australian Psychological Society.* psychology.org.au/community/reconciliation-and-the-aps/aps-apology.

Boszormenyi-Nagy, I. (1984). *Invisible loyalties: Reciprocity in intergenerational family therapy.* Abingdon: Taylor & Francis.

Bowden, M. (2020). *Unbreakable rock. Exploring the mystery of Altyerre.* Churchill, VIC, Australia: Alella Books.

Carlson, D. (2020). *The art of not knowing: Uncertainty as possibility.* www.Xlibris.com.

Centre for Twenty First Century Humanities (n.d.). *Colonial frontier massacres in Australia 1788-1930.* University of Newcastle. https://c21ch.newcastle.edu.au/colonialmassacres

Commonwealth Closing the Gap Annual Report (2022). https://www.niaa.gov.au/news-centre/indigenous-affairs/commonwealth-closing-gap-annual-report-2022

Duncan, B., Miller, S., Wampold, B., & Hubble, M. (Eds.) (2016). *The heart and soul of change: Delivering what works in therapy* (2nd ed.). Washington, DC: American Psychological Association.

Goldner, V. (1992). Making room for Both/And. *The Family Therapy Networker, 16,* 55–61.

Madanes, C. (1981). *Strategic family therapy.* San Francisco, CA: Jossey Bass.

Marmot, M. (2009). Closing the health gap in a generation: The work of the commission on the social determinates of health and its recommendations. *Global Health Promotion,* Supp ((1), 23–27. https://doi.org/10.1177/1757975909103742

Mays, E. (2020) Re-examining Australia's hidden genocide: The removal of aboriginal children in Australia as an act of cultural genocide. *Australian Indigenous Studies, 5.* https://epress.lib.uts.edu.au/student-journals/index.php/NESAIS

McCulloch, S., & McCulloch Childs, E. (2017). *McCullochs' contemporary aboriginal art the complete guide.* Richmond, VA: Australian Art Books.

McLeod, J. (2013). *An introduction to counselling.* Maidenhead, Berkshire: Open University Press.

Moloney, B. (2014). A black and white model for teaching family therapy: Empowerment by degree. *Australian and New Zealand Journal of Family Therapy 35,* 261–276 doi: 10.1002/anzf.1066

Moloney, L. (2016). *Defining and delivering effective counselling and psychotherapy.* Melbourne: Australian Institute of Family Studies.

National Indigenous Australians Agency. (2018). *Closing the gap: Retrospective review/National Indigenous Australians Agency.* Barton, ACT: Commonwealth of Australia, Department of the Prime Minister and Cabinet.

National Indigenous Australians Agency. (2022). *Closing the gap: retrospective review/National Indigenous Australians Agency.* Barton, ACT: Commonwealth of Australia, Department of the Prime Minister and Cabinet.

Pearson, N. (2009). Radical Hope: Education and equality in Australia. *Quarterly Essay 35,* 1–106.

Rosenzweig, S. (1936). Some implicit common factors in diverse methods of psychotherapy. *American Journal of Orthopsychiatry, 6,* 412–415.

Ungunmerr, M. (1993). *Dadirri.* Miriam Rose Foundation www.miriamrosefoundation.org.au

Wampold, B., & Imel, Z. (2015). *The great psychotherapy debate: The evidence for what makes psychotherapy work.* New York, NY: Routledge.

Chapter 13

Dialogical Reflecting Processes and Practices in Family Therapy

Judith M. Brown and Lisa Dawson

Introduction

Reflecting processes and practices have been an integral part of the development of differing approaches to family therapy since the early reflecting teams were introduced in the 1980s by Norwegian psychiatrist Tom Andersen. Although they grew from a rich systemic tradition of therapists working together, Andersen's ideas were a pivotal shift, away from the Milan model of family therapy, with its observing and hypothesising team behind the one-way screen. Harry Goolishan, who developed 'collaborative language systems' therapy (Anderson & Goolishian, 1988), was a great influence on Tom Andersen and was the first to refer to Andersen's work as a 'reflective process', recognising it as a way of being beyond technique for therapists (Weingarten, 2016). Over time, reflecting processes informed family therapy worldwide as they were folded into various collaborative approaches by means of reflective practices.

This chapter will focus on one such approach, that of the *Open Dialogue* model of mental health care and its *dialogical practice*, which comprise ways of being, knowing, doing, and experiencing in meetings with individuals, couples, family, or the wider system. Dialogical practice aims to provide the conditions for a *therapeutic process* that best supports dialogue in the meeting. *Reflecting processes* play an integral part, and they are operationalised in *dialogical reflecting practices*. These include *reflections* and *reflecting conversations* that occur between two or more co-therapists throughout the meeting.

The chapter comprises six parts. Firstly, we will offer a brief description of Open Dialogue and dialogical practice in Part One. Part Two gives a summary of the history and development of reflecting processes and practices, before shifting our gaze to the dialogical approach. Part Three will consider *dialogical ways of being*, the philosophical underpinnings that inform dialogical ideas and concepts relevant to the dialogical reflecting process. Part Four will consider *dialogical ways of knowing*, the theoretical constructs through which to understand dialogical reflecting processes and practices. Our gaze then again shifts in Part Five, to focus specifically on *dialogical ways of doing* reflecting, including the context, set-up, and particular details and nuances. Finally, Part Six will consider the *dialogical ways of experiencing*, the therapist's cognitive, emotional, and somatic experiencing which are pivotal to reflecting processes and practices. We have included some clinical vignettes to illustrate and integrate these aspects of dialogical practice.

For those whose work is informed by a dialogical approach, differing ways of engaging with reflecting practices bring richness to the therapeutic process and this chapter does not purport to be prescriptive. However, we will include points of precision

DOI: 10.4324/9781003490104-14

about dialogical reflecting that are crucial to creating and maintaining a safe dialogical therapeutic process for dialogue. They are grounded in the dialogical ways of being, knowing, doing, and experiencing, from which we all continue to develop in this way of working.

So, to begin, we will share a bit about our memories of how we began learning about the dialogical approach to family therapy.

Judith: Casting my mind back. I am in Finland in 2011, sitting in meeting after meeting, observing the Finnish therapists. Co-therapists reflect between each other during every initial open network meeting and every subsequent family therapy meeting. It seems a natural flow on from the dialogue that is taking place. The reflecting doesn't seem a big deal, nor prepared for, nor strategic. When it happens, the therapists simply turn their heads to gaze only at each other, to share their human response to what the family is talking about in the meeting. The family, on the periphery, seem to be used to this way of working. Over time, the Finnish therapists include me in reflecting. Since most of the meetings are in Finnish, I offer tentative words about the wonderings, emotions, and bodily feelings that have come up for me within the flow of the Finnish conversation. I later recognise that having no understanding of language and meaning increases my curiosity and hones my other senses, allowing feelings, bodily sensations, images to arise within me.

Lisa: I came to Open Dialogue through a research opportunity. As a family therapist, I was familiar with traditional reflecting teams and had heard of Open Dialogue but was unfamiliar with the approach itself. Once I started to gain some experience in dialogical work, I was struck by the simplicity and yet complexity in working in this way, as well as the potential for the holding of human experience in a respectful and authentic way. It felt clear to me early on that when using a reflective dialogical process, another layer of richness and meaning was added to the therapy. There was a felt sense that was shared in the room that 'something more' was happening in the conversation, as compared to a usual therapy meeting. Like ink spilled in water, now that I've started working and thinking in this way, it's been hard to go back. I now notice moments where I can be more dialogical or less dialogical. In the moments where I am less dialogical, there is a tension there now. I find myself in an ongoing and continual process of what it means to be dialogical.

Part one: What is open dialogue and dialogical practice?

Open Dialogue is both an approach to organising mental health care and a therapeutic approach, which gradually developed in Western Lapland, Finland in the 1980s. The Open Dialogue approach initially emerged as a model for crisis care with people experiencing psychosis. It grew out of the Finnish optimistic, resource-oriented 'needs-adapted' approach to the treatment of schizophrenia (Alanen, Lehtinen, Räkköläinen, & Aaltonen, 1991), which recognised the importance of including the family in treatment (Räkköläinen, Lehtinen, & Alanen, 1991). Open Dialogue can be considered as a shift in therapeutic approach and is distinct from traditional biomedical approaches to mental health care. Thus, mental health crises are understood as inherently systemic and relational (existing between people) rather than individualistic (located solely within an individual). Accordingly, the goal of dialogical approaches is not to treat disease but to promote the conditions for dialogue between people in which shifts can occur.

Dialogical practice is a psychotherapeutic way of being, knowing, doing, and experiencing, which developed over time from the Open Dialogue approach. Its aim is to create safe conditions for engendering and staying with dialogue, often around difficult or not-yet-said conversations. In dialogical practice, therapists use nuanced and sophisticated psychotherapeutic skills to create and maintain an unfolding dialogue, in which everyone can hear each other and be heard. Dialogical reflecting practices play a crucial part in this endeavour and are characterised by therapists being attuned and responsive to the family and to themselves, being sensitive to content and process throughout the meeting, and staying with difficult conversation or high emotion.

Open Dialogue is based on seven principles (Seikkula & Olson, 2003), which are concerned with two overall issues: firstly, how care is organised and delivered and, secondly, the ways of dialogical practice. Although they are separated for clarity, they are part of a recursive process. The principles primarily concerned with Open Dialogue as a model of care (Principles 1–5) focus on organisational aspects, with the aim of developing a responsive, open, and seamless integrated care model. The principles primarily concerned with ways of dialogical practice (Principles 6 and 7) support and emphasise the psychotherapeutic process.

1 *Immediate help*: Services respond to immediate needs. In the Finnish context, the first network meeting[1] takes place within 24 hours of first contact with mental health services.
2 *A social network perspective*: The person's social network is invited to participate in family therapy meetings from the first contact with mental health services.
3 *Flexibility and mobility*: Treatment and psychotherapy are adapted to the specific needs of each individual and may take place in the clinic or at the person's home.
4 *Responsibility*: When health care services are contacted, the professional who takes the call has responsibility for the first family therapy meeting, which is joined by the team.
5 *Psychological continuity*: If possible, at least one person from the initial team continues to be involved throughout the family's engagement with the service.
6 *Tolerance of uncertainty*: A cautious approach to treatment and psychotherapy is taken, where options are discussed tentatively and at length before making decisions. Meetings are planned from meeting to meeting, and ways of progressing are unfixed and open-ended to be needs-adapted.
7 *Dialogism*: During the family therapy meeting, the open-ended focus is on listening to all the voices present, to build new understandings between the different participants.

To achieve these Open Dialogue principles, care is organised around a series of therapeutic meetings. Informed by a systemic conceptualisation of a 'problem', members of the person's network are necessarily invited to participate and may include family, friends, or other professionals. In this way, the meetings can involve the personal and professional network, thereby including a relational and social context.

While there are potentially many ways of having a dialogical family therapy meeting, it usually involves a person and their family network, with two therapists who facilitate the meeting. What is essential is to create conditions that support dialogue, in the understanding that change in a participant's behaviour emerges from the dialogue (Seikkula & Arnkil, 2006). In this way, the dialogical approach might be considered less strategic than other forms of family therapy. Listening and responding to all the voices in the meeting is emphasised, without privileging any one voice. The therapist is but one voice in the room. Sometimes the term polyphony is used to describe the goal of eliciting multiple voices and perspectives, whereby responsibility is shared, and decisions are made collaboratively (Seikkula, 2011). Meetings are characterised by dialogical reflecting processes and practices. At certain times during the meeting, co-therapists reflect with each other as the family listens, before asking for the family's response. This multiple reflecting process often contributes to the emergence of new understanding and new ideas for everyone.

Part two: The development of dialogical reflecting processes and practices

> Reflect is a Latin word, re-flectere, that means to bend back. I think of bending back 'something' to what this 'something' was connected to and make the 'bending back' reconnect and impact upon 'what' was originally expressed.
>
> (Andersen, 2008)

Reflecting processes and practices were central to the Milan model of family therapy, in which therapy teams observed the sessions from behind a one-way screen, separate and hidden from the family. At the end of the session, the primary therapist would leave the room to gather the reflections of the team, before returning to relay these thoughts to the family. Over time, this reflecting process took on several forms: the therapy team giving their reflections as the family observed the team through the one-way screen; the therapy team coming into the room with the family at the end of the session to share their reflections; the therapy team being in the room with the family throughout and sharing at the end of the session. In all cases, therapists offered their often-lengthy reflections, as based on hypotheses, positively connoted, to input information into the family system, with the aim of promoting change.

Tom Andersen's reflecting team and reflecting talks

The *reflecting team* of Tom Andersen emerged from his growing urge for greater transparency and thoughtfulness in how therapists spoke about and worked with families. Sensing himself at a crossroads, which manifested in bodily discomfort and doubt, Andersen understood that 'a way to go on' would naturally emerge in time (Andersen & Jensen, 2007; Andersen, 2008, p. 159). The reflecting team was initiated in Tromso Norway in 1987 when the team began to observe the family through the one-way screen, followed by the family observing the teams' *reflecting talks* at the end of the family therapy meeting. Later developments saw therapists and families sitting together in the same room. Most frequently, the therapists shared their conversation together at the end of the meeting, in the presence of the family who listened (Andersen, 1987). Less often, reflections were shared during the meeting. Andersen encouraged therapists to reflect on 'what they heard and NOT about what they thought about what they heard' (Roberts, 2009, p. 63). Following each therapist's reflecting, the family were given an opportunity to respond to the therapists' words. These reflections upon reflections changed the way that therapists and families worked with and experienced each other.

Much has been written about Andersen's reflecting teams, including their conceptualisation, explanation of their structure, and what they seek to offer therapists and families. Three groups of papers are evident: firstly, those published in the 1990s when reflecting teams were being introduced to family therapy; secondly, those published at the time of Andersen's death in 2007, when attention to the practice of reflecting teams was encouraged (Brownlee, Vis, & McKenna, 2009). A summary of these is beyond the scope of this chapter.

The third group of most recent papers are limited in number and explore the experiences, strengths, and challenges of reflecting teams to families and therapists. It is to note that these research papers are based on the traditional reflecting team with the one-way screen. Reflecting teams are found to be useful in increasing family connectedness (Browne et al., 2021), at times of impasse (Hicks, Kustner, & Constable, 2021), and to engender multiple perspectives (Harris & Crossley, 2021). Challenges include the family's discomfort at being observed (Harris & Crossley, 2021) and their uneasiness with the unfamiliarity of the process (Tseliou et al., 2021). Hicks, Kustner, and Constable (2021) find families' responses to reflections differ according to their fit with individual family members. Families report that the most helpful reflections share expert knowledge, repeat what the family has said, or highlight positives; less helpful reflections contain too much information, offer new ideas, use metaphors, or share the therapist's emotion or experience.

Given that reflecting teams with the one-way screen have been commonly used in family therapy for decades, there is a surprising lack of qualitative or quantitative research on their usefulness in clinical practice. Therapist development in the practice of systemic reflecting teams has often been in the context of live supervision during systemic family therapy training. For therapists who seek to learn more about, Tom Andersen's paper on reflecting teams, *Reflecting Processes: Acts of Forming and Informing* (1995), is recommended.

Open dialogue and dialogical practices of reflections and reflecting conversations

In the early stages of the Open Dialogue approach, reflecting processes and practices continued to develop, influenced by Tom Andersen who was external supervisor to the Finnish team. Therapists always reflected during *and* at the end of the family therapy meetings. These extended opportunities helped to create, continue to build, and maintain the dialogue throughout the meeting. This dialogical therapeutic process has a *relational* focus on process and use of self, while also including an *interactional* focus on content and use of skill. Reflecting processes and reflecting practices are operationalised in the form of dialogical *reflections* and *reflecting conversations*. They vary slightly, but both involve therapists turning towards one another and reflecting on their response to the conversation in the family meeting. In this chapter, both forms are referred to, most often under the term 'reflecting'.

Reflections refer to two or more co-therapists openly reflecting with each other at discrete points throughout the family therapy meeting, as initiated by therapists. Reflections are often based on each individual therapist's human response to listening to the family, perhaps something that resonates with them or moves them. In an alternating process, each therapist shares their own reflection in turn while the other listens. For example, Therapist 1 may say, 'When Father said he is feeling depressed, I noticed a heaviness in my chest', followed by Therapist 2 who may say, 'I don't know why, but I have an image of a boat in stormy seas'. In this form of reflecting, each brief reflection stands alone, and therapists do not comment on their co-therapist's reflections. However, reflections may lead the way to *reflecting conversations.*

Reflecting conversations, also termed reflective dialogue (Seikkula, 2002, p. 269) or re-flective talk (Seikkula & Arnkil, 2006) also occur at any time throughout the meeting. They have a conversational quality, as therapists briefly think together about what the family has shared or perhaps how to go on in the therapeutic process. In a sequential process, therapists' wonderings, feelings, and curiosities are layered upon each other. For example, Therapist 1 may say, 'I am wondering whether father wants us to provide a solution to daughter's mental health difficulties', followed by Therapist 2, 'Perhaps it is not feeling safe enough at the moment to keep talking about daughter', and followed by Therapist 1, 'I wonder how we can talk with the family about how to make it feel safe enough for us all to talk some more'. In reflecting conversations, therapists are responsive to the talk between them; however, they are not an opportunity for therapists to talk 'about' the family.

Literature on dialogical reflecting practices is limited. However, one explanatory docu-ment and two recent studies are of note. Olson, Seikkula, and Ziedonis (2014) give a clear overview of dialogical practice, including description and direction on reflections. Florence et al. (2020) find families initially perceive dialogical reflecting as 'weird' (p. 1777) but subsequently recognise their role in slowing the meeting and making it easier to hear and be heard in difficult conversations. Sidis, Moore, Pickard, and Deane's (2022) exploration of therapist's experiences of reflecting points to increases in curiosity, not-knowing, tenta-tive wondering together, respectful collaboration, physiological attunement to self and other, staying present.

As with systemic reflecting teams, therapist development in dialogical reflecting pro-cesses and practices has primarily occurred within worldwide training events, which are congruent with philosophical and theoretical underpinnings (Parts Three and Four) and clinical foundations (Parts Five and Six). Much of the content of this chapter has been in-troduced to us whilst being trainees in such trainings. However, we also include ongoing learnings from subsequent clinical experience, facilitation of training, self-reflection, and ongoing collegial discussions.

The aim of reflecting in dialogical practice is always the same: to manage the therapeutic process with the aim of shifting from monologue towards a *genuine dialogue* in the family therapy meeting. It is possible for genuine dialogue to exist as persons meet with ease to speak and hear all the voices or with everyone struggling to speak and listen to each other in difficult conversations. In genuine dialogue, each person is wholly present to themselves while staying connected to the other.

> The essential element of genuine dialogue, therefore, is the 'seeing the other' or 'expe-riencing the other side'.
>
> (Friedman, 1976, citing Buber, 1957)

Part three: Ways of being based on philosophical underpinnings

Dialogical practice is *a qualitative way of being with people*, which emerges from a way of being with ourselves. We bring ourselves to the family therapy meeting as both a profes-sional and a human being, acknowledging and utilising our professional knowledge and experience, while also acknowledging and utilising ourselves as a human being. We can be moved and impacted by others' words and experiences, we have our own lives and lived experiences, and can access and share our emotional responses to what we are hearing from the family in the meeting. We do not try to mask our humanity, but rather will share it, as appropriate. It is a signal that 'I am human too. Let's figure this out together'. There is a 'withness thinking' rather than an 'aboutness thinking' (Shotter, 2005, p. 585), which informs the ways of *being with* people as opposed to *doing to* people.

This dialogical way of being seeks to *create the safe and respectful conditions to move towards dialogue*. The centrality of dialogue in all human relationships, from the very first beginning of life through to its end, is the essence of Bakhtin's (1984) dialogism and Buber's (1937) I-Thou relationship. Dialogue forms the foundation for 'how to go on together' (Wittgenstein, 1953), moment by moment, meeting to meeting. Dialogue is more than conversation. It feels qualitatively different. Dialogue is safe, connected, potentially meaningful, and presently attuned, in words or silence. To best provide the conditions for dialogue requires us to manage the dialogical therapeutic process. At the same time as being with others moving towards or within the dialogue, we remain deeply aware of our facilitator role and position as the professional in the room. At all times we are attending to the processes in the room and managing safety to keep the dialogical space open. While there is a prioritising of listening to all voices, we necessarily manage this process if one voice creates unsafety for others. Listening to all voices does not mean tolerating unsafety.

A dialogical way of being provides *a space that allows for multiple voices to be heard*, to find words to be spoken often for the first time (Seikkula, Laitila, & Rober, 2012). Creating therapeutic safety is crucial to this process so that people can allow themselves to be vulnerable and brave in the dialogue. The process aims to avoid objectifying those experiencing mental health crises or other difficulties, to reduce the distance between the 'client' and the 'professional'. It hopes to flatten hierarchies that have existed in traditional ways of working with people who are seeking mental health care or other forms of psychotherapy. In mental health care, the inclusion of those with lived experience as peer workers is common in the dialogical approach. A 'not-knowing' stance (Anderson & Goolishan, 1992) also helps us to bridge the gap between 'client' and 'professional'. It asks for humility and tolerating uncertainty in considering that, while there are many benefits to professional wisdom, we do not have all the solutions for all the complexities of human experience that we encounter in practice. We are invited to consider the unique perspective of every member of the family and wider network and to attune to the words and the stories of all the voices more closely and curiously.

The dialogical way of being *seeks response rather than solutions*, allowing us to facilitate and experience a certain way of listening and responding. It asks us for self-awareness and the capacity to deeply listen – to others and oneself – since we are always open to learning about both. This 'generous listening' enables us to speak as a listener (Hoffman, 2002, p. 245, citing Lyotard, 1996). We recognise that we all have outer voices that we share with others, and inner voices[2] that are not expressed in words, although they may emerge in embodied responses (Seikkula, 2008). As outer voices may be in dialogue, inner voices may also be in dialogue. In being dialogical we hope to engender a process that is differentiated from usual communication, where we begin to attune to the outer voices as well as the inner voices of ourselves and the family.

A dialogical way of being *opens a space for reflection*. The therapeutic process tends to be slow, allowing participants time to feel and to reflect on what others are speaking, and to listen to their own inner dialogue. For us as therapists too, it gives space to reflect on what we are hearing and to attune to our own inner dialogue throughout the family therapy meeting. It gives a space too for everyone to reflect on what is between their own outer and inner dialogues (Vytogsky, 1988). The slow pace enables a focus on present moments, a welcoming of pause and silence. In the moments between the spoken words, cognitions, emotions, or embodied responses may arise, to be experienced, noticed, leant into, and given a response. There may be a sense of being in the flow, intersubjective moments of 'mutual tuning-in in relationship, the experience of the "We"' (Zaner, 1961, p. 81), and a shift or new knowing may emerge (Brown, 2015, 2017).

In these ways, we may say that we are *'being'* dialogical, rather than 'doing' Open Dialogue. This way of working often appeals to people's values, offering deep stability and security in integrating the professional and the personal in the work. Yet, there is a continual process, a never-endingness in being dialogical, akin to the unfinaliseability of dialogue (Bakhtin, 1984). We are never 'done' becoming dialogical. We might find ourselves being more and less dialogical but there is no final destination. When people have worked this way for a while, they may have the experience of becoming more dialogical in their life generally. That is, it is not necessarily something that is 'turned on' for the therapy meeting, but a way of being in their life and their relationships.

Summary: Dialogical reflecting processes and practice are informed by a *dialogical way of being*, through which we more consciously tune into this way of working. It includes bringing ourselves as persons and professionals, seeking to keep the dialogue open, making space for all voices, tolerating the uncertainty of not knowing, generous listening to our own and others' outer and inner dialogues, slowing down, being with, and sensitivity to moments of mutuality. These inform what we offer when we respond with dialogical reflecting, which is always at the service of engendering dialogue.

Precision point

- The premise of dialogical practice is sharing human experiences (Seikkula & Arnkil, 2006, p. 105) within a dialogue in the meeting, as supported by dialogical reflecting processes and practices.

Dialogical practice

- How is it for me to share a part of my real human response to what I am hearing from the family?

Reflecting on the therapeutic process

- What would it be like to slow my process down and allow for moments of pause or silence? What would emerge?

Reflecting on reflecting

- An image of an opening and closing camera aperture: Will my reflecting, and how I speak it, tend towards opening or closing the dialogue at this moment?

Part four: Ways of knowing as theoretical understandings

Dialogical practice is *a way of knowing*, which informs how we safely manage the therapeutic process to best provide the conditions for dialogue. Dialogical reflecting processes and practices are part of that process. Their evolution reveals the influence of family therapy theory in the shift from the therapist as an observer of the family in seeking to implement first-order behavioural change to the therapist and family co-constructed system of language and meaning seeking second-order change. Dialogical reflecting processes and practices extend these theoretical understandings to the understanding of co-therapists as 'being with' the family and each other. Throughout the family therapy meeting, there may be monologue or dialogue at differing times. The dialogical space for sharing understandings may be more or less on the way to being open or closed. This moment-to-moment 'being with' best provides the conditions to move from monologue to dialogue in the family therapy meeting, from which change or a shift may emerge. Theories, constructs, and concepts that underpin the practice of 'being with' come from rich and varied research and clinical scholarship on psychotherapy, neuroscience, developmental psychology, and intersubjectivity and centre on how human beings meet and respond to each other. It is never only one person's activity, but always influenced by that which came before:

> This is where the dialogical begins ... the fact that such actions are neither yours nor mine, but truly 'ours', but also the fact that something unique with its own qualitative character is created amongst all involved in the interaction.
>
> (Shotter, 2010, pp. 24–25)

Providing the conditions for dialogue involves *providing safety*. The way we manage the therapeutic process impacts how safe the family network feels in the meeting. When we as therapists are fully engaged, with therapeutic presence, the physiological safety of those in the meeting is activated (Geller & Porges, 2014; Porges, 2022). It can 'make the unpredictable feel safe enough' (Trimble, 2002, p. 276), allowing persons to down-regulate their evaluation of risk and initiate the social engagement system (Porges, 2022). Our dialogical co-therapy reflecting recognises this bidirectional communication of nervous systems between all in the room (Geller & Porges, 2014). Seeking the family's response to the therapists' reflecting within the session supports research findings that the family's experience of the therapeutic presence is pivotal for change, rather than that of the therapist (Geller, Greenberg, & Watson, 2010).

Providing the conditions for a shift or change as a result of dialogue involves *listening*. The concept of listening as a vital relational act has been well conceptualised in the family therapy clinical literature. We are encouraged to listen deeply to families' stories and respond in ways that show that we have heard 'and been moved by them' (Crago, 2006, p. 168). This type of listening involves hearing, noticing, attending to, being curious, and processing the client's story, while also focusing on and being curious about our own responses (Burnham, 2005; Rober, 2011). A dialogical approach calls for 'listening with integrity' throughout the therapeutic process, to respond to those who have spoken (Trimble, 2002). This quality of listening is present before we reflect, it informs the content and process of our reflecting, as well as our return to listen again to the family's response.

Providing the conditions for dialogue involves *the intersubjective process* as the core of being human. It is this quality of meeting that is sought, to best support dialogue wherein change or transformation may occur at levels beneath awareness. Interdisciplinary literature describes such meeting as a 'mutual self-other-consciousness' (Trevarthen & Aitken, 2001), implicit relational knowing (Lyons-Ruth, 1998), a meeting of subjectivities (Muth, 2009; Stern, 2007), and communication between consciousnesses (Seikkula & Arnkil, 2006). Schore's extensive scholarship on the key role of intersubjectivity in the therapist-client relationship is now evidence-based (2021). Moment-to-moment emotional and embodied responses are now recognised as emerging from the psychobiological attunement of therapists with the family, and with each other (Schore, 2010; Stern, 2007). Dialogical reflecting processes and practices are congruent with this scholarship and evidenced in our responding to moments that move us, offering mental imagery, sensory, or cognitive content as 'an internal representation of an interpersonal experience' (McGown, 2015, p. 131).

Providing the conditions for dialogue involves *co-regulation of each individual and the group* to maximise the capacity for all in the meeting to listen and be heard. Mutual or co-regulation between the psychological and physiological states of two persons enables arousal levels to remain comfortable (Butler & Randall, 2013). In dialogical practice, it is the co-regulation in co-therapy that allows us to stay attuned and open while containing the intensity of emotion that may arise (Seikkula & Trimble, 2005). Reflecting as an overt process of co-therapy co-regulation is repeated throughout the meeting and plays a crucial role. Our individual reflecting on self not only serves to coregulate therapists but also serves to increase the family's capacity to self-regulate (Quillman, 2012).

Providing the conditions for dialogue recognises the unfolding of *embodied present moments*, a form of human experience that is increasingly a focus of scholarship. It considers the moment-to-moment quality, form, and experiencing of embodied communication and response (Stern, 1985), embodied synchronicity and intersubjective rhythms of movement (Trevarthen, 1980; Trevarthen & Aitken, 2001), somatic phenomena (Shaw, 2004), and the role of mirror neurons (Rizzolatti & Craighero, 2004). In the therapeutic process, the inclusion of the implicit (not in awareness) and the explicit (often verbal) is seen as unpredictable (Stern, 2004). In dialogical practice, this lack of predictability is welcome, but not always comfortable. We manage such a therapeutic process by our awareness of both process and content, to engender the embodied intersubjective process between all in the meeting that is increasingly found to be essential to effective therapy (Quillman, 2012).

Providing the conditions for dialogue involves *moments of meeting*, in which each person is mutually drawn into a meeting with another, without a specific purpose or sense of control. It is described as a key 'moment of meeting' within a series of present moments from which implicit change emerges (Stern, 2004), the 'I know (feel) that you know (feel) that I know (feel)' (Stern, 2007, p. 42). Such an implicit experience where persons are 'wholly subject and object' (Skærbæk, 2004, p. 93) often has a special quality, openness, and spaciousness where people can be alone and together, often in silence without speaking, questioning, or interpreting (Stern, 1998, 2004). In dialogical practice, the emergence of moments of meeting is influenced by the interplay between inner dialogue within persons and outer dialogues between persons (Lidbom, Boe, Kristoffersen, Ulland, & Seikkula, 2014). Emotions, feelings of belonging, trust, physical relaxation, relief, and love may arise (Seikkula & Trimble, 2005), perhaps experienced differently by those in the meeting

(DeTurk & Foster, 2008). Tom Andersen (2008) describes moments of one person being moved by the other being moved. A dialogical understanding is that moments of meeting involve the mutual creation of ideas and understandings (DeTurk & Foster, 2008), a 'shift in implicit knowing' (Stern, 2004, p. 145), 'an entirely other way of knowing' (Friedman, 1976, p. 163), a knowing of the third kind (Shotter, 1993), and a dialogical knowing (Brown, 2017). A change, shift, or new way to go on together may open.

Summary: Dialogical reflecting processes and practice are informed by a *dialogical way of knowing*, which forms the basis of this way of working. It includes providing safety, listening deeply, the intersubjective process, co-regulation, embodied present moments, and moments of meeting. These inform what we offer when we respond with dialogical reflecting, which is always at the service of engendering dialogue.

Precision point

- The premise of dialogical practice is that therapeutic change involves a shift from mono-logue to dialogue (Trimble, 2002, p. 275).

Dialogical practice

- A remembering of the words of John Shotter: 'Don't ask what is contained in the words, ask what the words are contained in' (personal correspondence, 2014).

Reflecting on the therapeutic process

- Providing the conditions for dialogue involves us balancing process and content within the meeting. We privilege the process between people, particularly when the content threatens to override or overwhelm the therapeutic process.

Reflecting on reflecting

- How regulated am I before speaking my reflection to the co-therapist? Can I pause before speaking, to discern if it will increase the family's sense of safety?

Part five: Ways of doing in the family therapy meeting

Dialogical practice is *a way of doing* in the family therapy meeting, which is at one with its philosophical and theoretical foundations. At the core of dialogical practice is the therapist's facilitation of reflecting processes and practices, by means of reflections and reflecting conversations. The following section will detail the context of co-therapy, setting up, the leading into, the during, and what follows reflections and reflecting conversations.

Context of co-therapy

The use of dialogical reflecting most often occurs within the context of co-therapy. Co-therapy has been evident since the inception of family therapy and there has been ongoing debate about its challenges and advantages. Recent research into co-therapy in the dialogical approach has found that dialogical co-therapy goes beyond multiple perspectives or binocular vision (Bateson, 1979), growth and well-being of therapists (Palazzoli, Boscolo, Cecchin, & Prata, 1990), and simple technique (Gehart, 2018, referring to Andersen). Rather, it is primarily about 'how they [therapists] are together, that is, the quality of their communication' (Hornova, 2020 p. 338).

Co-therapy is the most common context for dialogical reflecting during family therapy meetings. The dialogical co-therapy relationship involves two or three therapists working together with respect, trust, honesty, and openness, offering a model of relationship that enables and models dialogue with each other and with those in the meeting (Brown, Kurtti, Haaraniemi, Lohonen, & Vahtola, 2015). We respect each other's multidisciplinary perspectives as equal and differing expertise; trust in the attunement and 'being with' each other as much as possible; and have honesty in knowing ourselves and our ways of working together; the openness of our reflecting responses is safe and judicious. The co-therapy relationship engenders a process of co-regulation between co-therapists, as we encounter families' (and our own) thoughts and feelings. This is crucial when we may become stuck, anxious, or lose curiosity for a variety of reasons, often in relation to the families' (and our own) feelings of uncertainty, powerlessness, complexity, and tragedy of the work. Any difficulty within the co-therapy relationship is discussed immediately after the meeting.

Setting up

There are important considerations in the set-up of a dialogical family therapy meeting. Before the meeting, we identify who in the room will be participating in the reflecting and who will be in a listening position. If there are more than two professionals, for example, three, we may determine that two will reflect and one will be in a listening position, or all three may reflect. To have at least one person in the listening position is encouraged (Seikkula, 2002). Before the meeting, we also identify if one therapist will primarily facilitate the therapeutic process in the meeting or if this will be shared with a co-therapist. This therapist will usually take the lead in welcoming the family, introducing the participants, deciding when to reflect, and taking responsibility for attending to the processes in the room. Facilitating requires the appropriate therapeutic training and skills to manage the therapeutic process. The professional background (i.e., psychologist, social worker, nurse, doctor, etc.) does not necessarily determine who is best placed for reflecting in any given meeting. Often professionals who might not take on a facilitating role may have much to offer in a reflecting position. Deciding who will reflect provides opportunities to hear from multiple voices from different professional backgrounds, utilising the strengths of a multidisciplinary approach.

Before the meeting, we prepare the meeting room. Having the chairs in a circle with nothing in the centre (i.e., not sitting around a large table) can create optimal conditions for entering into dialogue (see Figure 13.1). Extra chairs should be removed for the correct number of participants, with therapists who will reflect together sitting next to each other. Ensuring there is enough time and space to enter into a dialogical family therapy meeting will depend on the family and team; however, an hour and a half is usually needed for the first meeting and an hour for subsequent meetings. Since the practice of reflecting is not familiar to most families, we introduce the idea at the beginning of the first meeting,

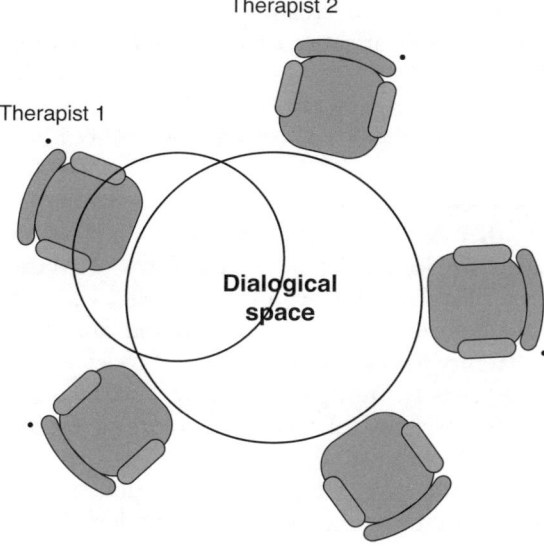

Figure 13.1 Therapist 1 is managing the therapeutic process in the meeting. Therapist 2 is in the observer/listener role.

settling any unease to increase the family's capacity to listen (Harris & Crossley, 2021). We might say:

> *During the meeting it's often helpful for me and for you too, to hear some of my colleague's thoughts, and for me to share some of my thoughts with her. Things that might have come up for us, as we have been listening to your family. It's a chance for you to sit back as we reflect together, to have some space and listen quietly. Just for a while. We will always ask if that is OK with you. As you listen to us sharing, you might notice things coming up for you. It's OK to sit with them quietly. When we've reflected, we'll come back to you and ask what you've noticed in yourself as we were reflecting.*

1.   Leading into therapist reflections

The practice of dialogical reflecting is interspersed throughout the family therapy meeting, often in the early stages, mid-meeting, and towards the end so that the family does not need to take in lengthy information at the end of the meeting. Reflections and reflecting conversations are an opportunity for the family to hear from multiple voices, and for therapists to attend to and manage the therapeutic process. They are not used to strategically drive change but are part of an iterative process where therapist reflections on family conversation, leads to family reflections on therapist reflections, with the hope of creating the conditions for dialogue. We use judgement in reflecting, with the view that it is always offered in service of the dialogue between all in the meeting, from which change can occur.

Reflecting creates *opportunities to manage the therapeutic process*. As therapists, we gradually learn to sense when to initiate the pause for reflecting. Generally, reflections or reflecting conversations are useful for creating openings to dialogue, or when dialogue is shutting down. We may reflect at times such as: after gathering everyone's individual worries about what brings the family to the meeting, when anxiety or emotions in the meeting need to be expressed both/and contained, when voices are negated or silenced by dominant voices, when we need time to pause and reflect about how to go on, just before the meeting comes to a close.

Reflecting can *create a shift in the room*, where the felt experience between people is qualitatively different, either during or after a reflection. This is often a result of slowing down the pace, which we may initiate in order to shift the conversation from monologue, allow co-therapists to regulate themselves, or co-regulate each other and the family. A slowed down pace, both before and after reflections and during the meeting in general, allows for greater opportunity for everyone to feel and to let affect be present. Reflecting also has a role in lowering anxiety during the meeting, and in containing intense emotion. In this way, there is less opportunity for thoughts, emotions, or bodily responses to compromise our thinking or that of the family.

Reflecting *enables pauses and silence* throughout the meeting. Dialogue is a differentiated process from usual communication. We want it to feel different. We want to allow pauses and silences and for the process to feel unrushed. Leaving space and not filling the gaps between words with words creates space for the unknown and for something different to rise to the surface. We are often trying to support people to find the words for something they have never said before. Our role is purposeful, in managing the dialogical therapeutic process to engender the time and space needed to find such words. Reflections and reflecting conversations are integral to this process.

Vignette 13.1:   Reflections and reflecting conversations can create a shift in the process.

Lisa:

Ruth and Isaac were parents of a 15-year-old who was struggling with her mental health. They were attending parent-only meetings to help support their daughter's recovery. Both parents had experienced trauma in their past and seemed to struggle in processing the information they were receiving from the therapy team about what was needed and how to attune to their child. Therapy meetings tended to be very chaotic, and Ruth and Isaac also seemed to spend a lot of time diverging from the topic of conversation at hand. The pace of the conversation was fast and pressured. The therapists noticed that they themselves internally felt anxious sensations when in the room. The therapists decided to use reflections to disrupt the chaotic pace and slow things down.

When there was a pause in the dialogue, one of the therapists jumped in, 'It's been really helpful to hear about how the weekend's gone and hear where you're up to. I wonder if it would be ok for us to reflect on what we've heard you say so far?'

One of the therapists said slowly and calmly. 'You can then have a break from the talking and just listen to us or listen to your own thoughts'. The therapists then turned to each other.

One took a deep breath and sighed, 'There's so much going on for Ruth and Isaac at this moment. I just need to catch my breath and gather my thoughts'*, before proceeding to reflect on some core ideas the parents had spoken about. She also reflected on the process in the room, 'I'm noticing that my heart is racing as I've been listening today. I'm feeling a quickness with my breath. Everything feels very busy. I wonder if others in the room are feeling the same?'

The co-therapist responded, 'I wonder if Ruth and Isaac have felt like this while talking to us today? And if this is a familiar or unfamiliar feeling?'**

Ruth and Isaac sat still and appeared to be listening closely. After the reflecting and the family's response, the affect in the room significantly shifted. There was more stillness, more gentleness, and more deliberateness with how people were speaking to each other. Everything was slower. The reflecting appeared to assist the therapists in regulating themselves and, in turn, in co-regulating the parents and enhancing their self-reflective capacities.

* Reflection; **Reflecting conversation

Precision points

- The premise of the family therapy meeting is to provide the conditions for safety so that the not-yet-said may be possible in time.

Dialogical practice

- Change or shift emerges, not from outside people, but from the dialogue between people.

Reflecting on the therapeutic process

- What would it be like to sit with uncertainty without an outcome, but trusting in the unfolding dialogical process?

Reflecting on reflecting

- Is my reflecting too usual, too unusual, or appropriately unusual for the family? (Shotter, 2007, citing Andersen).

2. During therapist reflections

The content of reflections and reflecting conversations are always chosen from many possibilities, since it is neither possible nor helpful to reflect on all that has been said. We must make choices about what (and how) we reflect. A guiding principle is that reflecting is offered to the family, as a pause for them to reflect on the outer group conversation as well as their own inner conversation. We can ask ourselves – what might be helpful now, what might further open up the dialogue? This means sometimes managing our own urges to reflect on ideas that seem important or interesting to us but perhaps offer little to the family. Reflecting is not a space for talking about the family or what the family do not want to talk about. Nor is it a criticism, a definitive statement or opinion, a summary, or a re-phrasing of what others have said. Reflecting is always offered with a spirit of generosity and with respect and kindness. Theoretical knowledge and clinical opinion are rarely included, since they tend towards talking objectively 'about' the family, rather than sharing our human response 'with' them. If we have been thinking of such things, we ask the family whether they would like to hear this thinking. Often, clinical opinions about the next steps will be shared in the last 10 minutes of the meeting.

Therapists *initiate reflecting at differing points* during the family therapy meeting and always ask the family for permission to reflect. In their current form in dialogical practice, reflecting usually involves two or perhaps three therapists openly reflecting with each other in the presence of the family. During the reflecting process, we turn to each other and take turns to speak about our responses to the outer dialogue and/or our own inner dialogue that may have arisen while listening to the family (see Figure 13.2). If a family member(s) speaks to the therapist(s) or another family member during the time of reflecting, they are gently reminded of the explanation that was given before the meeting started. With families that are overwhelmed or in crisis, this may need to happen more than once. The therapist's reflecting offers the family a pause from the intensity of a conversation and supports down-regulation, the openness of the therapists increases engagement with the family, and the co-regulation between co-therapists can help co-regulate the family. These aspects encourage more dialogue and more reflection.

Reflections and reflecting conversations are *most useful to the family when brief*. We are speaking with a view of helping people to listen and the family will tune out if reflecting

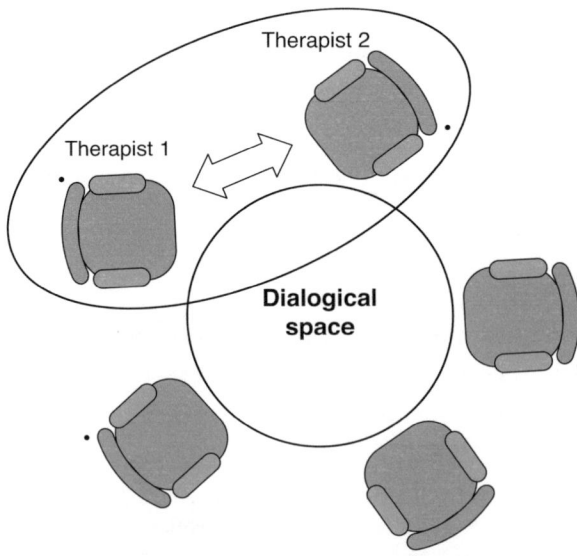

Figure 13.2 If the family agrees, therapists turn their gaze, body, or chair towards each other. Reflections between Therapists 1 and 2. Therapists look only at each other while the family listens.

is lengthy or overly full. The therapist who initiates the reflecting often waits for the co-therapist(s) to reflect before reflecting, to enable them to shift from the facilitator to the reflecting role. There is never a rush to reflect and a pause before anyone speaks is recommended. Reflecting is most often one to three sentences from each therapist and, in total, rarely takes longer than three minutes. As noted previously, reflections and reflecting conversations look slightly different. During reflections, our words stand alone as our individual response to our own process of listening to the family. We may alternate between reflections two or three times before turning back to the family. Reflecting conversation is more like a shared pondering, a leapfrog of responding to each other's thoughts, a layering, for example, on the therapeutic process, a theme from the family conversation, or in relation to how to next go on in the meeting. Sometimes both forms of reflecting ebb and flow into each other, but brevity is important.

Either form of reflecting *invites the family into a different quality of listening*, since there is no need for their immediate response. The family and other members of the network are physically present while listening 'from the outside' to our reflecting. We use family members' names when reflecting, instead of turning and speaking directly to them. The family are freed from the usual social demands of being in a (sometimes difficult) conversation, such as being compelled to respond to the speaker with eye contact, or other verbal or non-verbal actions. Such self-managing takes cognitive effort, which detracts from deeper listening. Listening from the outside gives distance, enhancing everyone's capacity to listen to their own inner dialogue, perhaps to hear their own words said back to them, to sense their experience in a way that is more difficult to attune to when speaking.

In dialogical reflecting we take the time and space to *listen to our own inner dialogue* before speaking. Often much is said, felt, and experienced by therapists in a dialogical family therapy meeting. Our responses to the family may be embodied (sensory), affective (feeling), cognitive (wondering, thinking, 'voices' of self or others), or intuitive (e.g., metaphor, image). Not everything that is spoken or felt needs to be reflected on. Nor should it be. Rather, we are encouraged to listen deeply to our own inner dialogue, as well as to the outer conversation of the family. 'What is coming up for me?' can be a helpful question to silently ask oneself. Tuning in to our own inner dialogue and bringing this judiciously into the open (part of the 'Open' in Open Dialogue) provides another layer of reflecting. We decrease the distance between ourselves and the family and provide a template to others in the meeting by also 'doing the work' of reflecting on our inner response, as we are asking them to do.

Vignette 13.2:   Reflections give space for the not-yet-said.

Judith:

Jamie is seven. His foster carers present to mental health services with an interpretation of events.

Mother: He is disruptive, just wants his own way. He is bullying me. The other kids are scared of him. He thumps the wall, wants his own way.

Therapist 1: What would Jamie's worry be? A worry that perhaps is causing big feelings for him?

Father: (*angrily*) No idea. I was worrying when she (wife) was crying.

Jamie: (*with increasing intensity*). Can I have my drink please? Can I have my book please? Can I have my lunch please?

Mother: I want help with him. I want help with him. I want help to stop him hitting the walls. I need something more for him. We don't know how long we can keep doing this. We tell him that if he doesn't behave that we will get the police to keep him safe.

Jamie, perched alone on the chair opposite, has become quiet. He folds himself into his body and dissolves into tears. The confusion and the emotion of the unsaid have been expressed. The foster care placement is at risk of breaking down. The carers are considering it. Jamie knows it. He has experienced it.

The co-therapists look at each other. They engage in the shortest reflection.

Therapist 2: I am tearing up.
Therapist 1: Me too.

Silence. No one moves. They turn back to the family to seek their response.

Therapist 1 (to Mother): What are you noticing right now?

Silence again.

But there is a slight shift in Mother's affect. She recounts a memory of her biological son with depression at a similar age, speaking of her struggle to get help for him.

Mother: He was diagnosed with depression. Has Jamie got depression?

She begins to cry. She reaches out to Jamie, and he moves to her, climbing up on her lap. He sits being comforted. Or perhaps he is doing the comforting. Finally, we can start to talk about what has been Jamie's big worry and also that of his carers.

Reflecting *emphasises being in the present moment*, which entails staying with the words and message of those in the family therapy meeting moment-to-moment. Instead of having a pre-considered statement, we try to have an authentic conversation in the here and now. We avoid statements that are leading, interpreting, explaining, or telling, or diagnostic statements. There is a goal of allowing emotions to rise to the surface, to respond to bodily responses, and to listen to one's own inner thoughts. Slowing down the pace of the therapeutic process is usually necessary to achieve such aims. We use pauses and moments of silence during the outer conversation to help everyone in the room (including us) to attune to their (and our) inner dialogue. During the meeting, we do not try to hold rigidly onto responses that arise, since this will impact our listening. Rather, we just let them come and go until the time comes for reflecting. We trust in the process that when we reflect, it will be what is uppermost in that moment. It is helpful to speak the reflection or reflecting conversation in the present tense, in accord with staying in each moment. For example, 'this seems important' (present tense and tentative), rather than 'that was important' (past tense and definite).

Reflecting is always *offered in a tentative, wondering, curious way*, from a 'not-knowing' position. Not knowing refers to the attitude and belief that we do not have access to privileged information and can never fully understand another person. We always need to learn more about what has been said or not said, 'the therapist is humble about what she or he knows' (Anderson, 2005, p. 502). Reflections and reflecting conversations are offered cautiously and not presented as firm truths. They are not about giving advice, solving or interpreting people's lives and problems. We are not declaring a single truth but making room for other truths. The use of language is highly considered, and the choice of words emphasises the language of wondering and curiosity. This stance can invite more responses from a family. 'Owning' our reflections in the I-voice is one way of adopting a not-knowing stance, where the tentative reflection is clearly acknowledged as belonging to each therapist and open for discussion. We might say:

> *I'm not sure if this is right or if I have understood Alex in the way she meant, but when she was speaking it brought to my mind an image of a river and of Alex being thrown into it and trying to keep her head above the water.*

Precision points

- Reflections allow the family to listen to the outer reflections of the therapists, while also having the opportunity to listen to their own inner conversation.

Dialogical practice

- Reflecting is not about interpreting someone's experience, nor a space for 'talking about' the family, nor for talking about what the family do not want to talk about.

Reflecting on the therapeutic process

- Does my reflecting speak to the content (what is happening) or the process (how it is happening) of the current family concerns or the family therapy meeting itself?

Reflecting on reflecting

- An image of sitting in a single chair, on the edge of the space between myself and the family: Does my reflection come from objective knowledge, my subjective self, or perhaps it has emerged from the intersubjective space between myself and the family?

3.   After therapist reflecting

After reflecting, it is important to hear from every person in the family therapy meeting by inviting them to briefly respond to the therapists' reflections or reflecting conversation (see Figure 13.3). We do not reflect on our listening to the family without providing

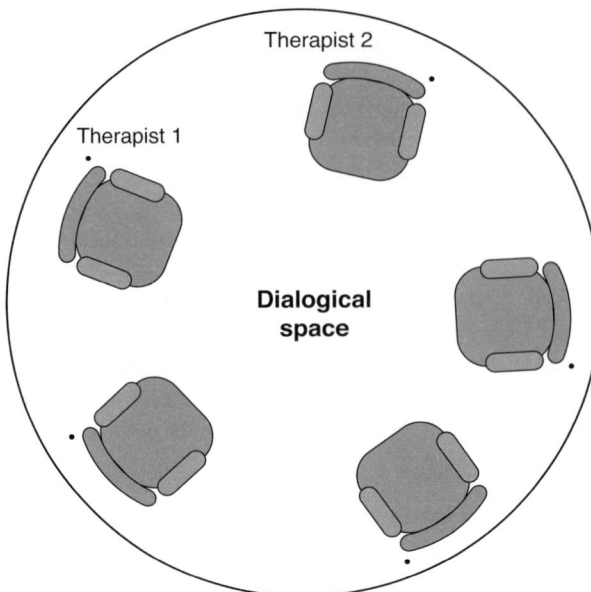

Figure 13.3 Therapist 1 asks the family for their response to what they have just heard. The family responds while therapists listen.

them a space for a response. This process invites self-reflection and reflections on reflections, creating an iterative approach to further deepen dialogue. We might ask family members '*As my colleague(s) and I talked together just now, where did your thoughts take you?*' or '*What struck you about our words? What did you notice?*' Family members are given an opportunity to speak to parts of the reflection that did or did not resonate for them. If a family member moves to repeating or introducing other content, we signify we have heard them, while also redirecting them back to the process, 'Is there anything more that came up for you when listening to our talk?' The family responses to our reflecting offer ongoing feedback throughout the family therapy meeting. Just as each co-therapist welcomes the differing focus of their colleague's reflections and reflecting conversations, so too we welcome the differing responses of the family. The goal in dialogical practice is to allow for a space that includes different voices and differing responses, not to achieve agreement.

The *differing family responses to therapists' reflecting are welcomed* and we briefly gather responses from every family member before continuing the meeting. Sometimes a part of our reflecting resonates with the family, who may say, 'You've got it right, that's exactly how I feel'. At other times a family member may not understand a part of our reflecting and may say 'I didn't get that image'. Some reflections may not land with the family, and this is part of tolerating uncertainty while trusting in the therapeutic process. We are not wedded to any part of our reflecting. Sometimes, despite our best intentions, parts of our reflecting might miss the mark, perhaps inadvertently minimising, polarising, simplifying, or misunderstanding something. If a reflection does not resonate or is challenging for the family to hear, it becomes another opportunity for curiosity, for acceptance of differing views, and an opportunity for richer dialogue. We may ask, '*What do we need to better understand? What words are better to use here?*' Sometimes it is these reflections that progress us further, allow us to model curiosity, and perhaps open again to a joint dialogue. It is crucial to gather responses from all family members before moving on together in the meeting.

Summary of dialogical reflecting process

1 Prepare family that reflections may happen in the meeting, 'We may share some thoughts together as we go along. All you have to do is just listen and then we will check in with you'.
2 Before reflecting, therapists ask permission of the family to reflect. 'Would it be ok if we reflected on what we have heard you all say so far?' Therapists turn their chairs, or their bodies, or their gaze towards each other to reflect with each other.
3 Those who are reflecting look at each other only, not at the family, and use the names of family members instead of turning and speaking to them.
4 Therapists reflect on their individual responses to what they have heard the family speak about in the meeting so far.
5 Therapists might reflect on their inner dialogues, their thoughts, feelings, or bodily responses that have come up for them.
6 Reflections and reflecting conversations are slow and tentative, and as much as possible, spoken in the present tense from the I-position.
7 After the reflecting, the therapists turn back to the family and invite them to each briefly reflect on the reflections.
8 The process of reflecting might repeat one, two, or three times throughout the meeting.

Precision point

- All family members are always given the opportunity to respond to the therapists' reflection and reflecting conversation.

Dialogical practice

- If a family member begins to talk of something other than their response to the therapist's reflecting, we gently remind them that we need to hear from everyone before we move on.

Reflecting on the therapeutic process

- How do I stay with the process of gathering and just listening to everyone's responses, without asking questions until all voices have spoken?

Reflecting on reflecting

- An image of weaving several threads to each person: Often it is necessary to ask each person more than once about their response to therapists' reflecting, 'Is there anything else that you noticed as we were reflecting'.

Part six: Ways of experiencing to inform reflecting

Dialogical practice is *a way of experiencing* in the family therapy meeting, most particularly relating to the therapist's experiencing. It has an important role in dialogical practice. As with the doing of practice, a congruence with dialogical ways of knowing and ways of being is necessary to understand and operationalise dialogical reflecting processes and practices. Therapist experiencing and the use of self in family therapy has been long accepted (Rober, 2005; 2011). In dialogical practice, reflections and reflecting conversations are based on our listening to the family and may be related to cognitive, affective, or embodied experiencing of this listening (Rober, 2011; Rober, Elliott, Buysse, Loots, & De Cort, 2008). In reflecting, we may consider emotions, words, images, or metaphors that arise for us and may link them to a specific point in the conversation, such as, 'When Mother said she is frustrated, I felt a heaviness in my chest and wondered about that'. Although we offer a characteristic dialogical format in this chapter, there is no 'one way' to reflect. The content and words used in reflecting are unique to each therapist. Thus, their possibilities in day-to-day clinical practice are unlimited, due to the myriad of interactions that emerge moment-by-moment between the therapists and family as the work unfolds.

Therapists use *professional wisdom and discretion about what is shared* in dialogical reflecting, with the emphasis always on only sharing safely what is at the service of the dialogue. We do not share every thought or feeling we have and do not share thoughts and feelings that are unboundaried, inappropriate, unprofessional, or solely about ourselves. What we do share is our simple human response to our experience of listening to the family. When such experiences are shared, they are often small but meaningful. Less is more. If we are moved to share from our own personal experience, we do so carefully by keeping the focus on the family, after discerning the benefit for the dialogue. For example, a reflection might be as simple as sharing, 'As a mother, I was moved just now'. Or we may have a reflecting conversation about a shared process (without content). For example, Therapist 1 may say, 'As a mother myself, I can understand the worry that these parents have. It makes me think about my own children and what I would put on the line to help them', with Therapist 2 responding, 'Your words make me think about the ever-changing relationship between parents and children over time'. We share our response to being with people in a way where humanity is shared. Accessing and sitting with our own emotional response models emotional responsiveness and containment to the family. This can create emotional safety for everyone in the room and create opportunities for others to bravely access their own emotions, either quietly or sharing them with others.

Reflecting appears to be sourced in the therapist's *experiencing at subjective or intersubjective levels*. Our subjective experiencing is often more cognitive. Reflecting that may emerge often wonders or notices or tentatively understands something in response to the words of the speaker, akin to a left-brain process. We could call them subjective reflections. Our intersubjective experiencing is often more affective or embodied and seems to emerge when the therapist's humanity somehow joins with and has been touched in some way by that of the family, in the space between them. Reflecting that may emerge at such times is often in the form of metaphor, image, or song, akin to a right-brain process. We could call them intersubjective reflections. Both are equally dialogical. Trying to reflect in a certain form is counterproductive to the dialogical process. We cannot construct them, but awareness and waiting for their emergence are useful to the therapeutic process.

Sensitivity to therapist experiencing may be increased by *attending to the family's own stories and language*. Tom Andersen used the metaphor of listening to client's words and collecting them into a basket. He encouraged therapists to reflect only on what is heard, not what is seen, in the understanding that emotions and gestures are part of a person's inner dialogue, which perhaps has not yet been given words (Andersen & Shotter, 2003). Given enough safety and time, emotions of gestures may emerge in the dialogue as words. In the interim, specific words from the family may be used in our reflecting, as opposed to layering with our own language and interpretations. Words that seem to be meaningful can be repeated as well as words that seem to arouse bodily responses, emotions, or affect in the therapist or family members. While seemingly simple, repeating of a single word either in reflections, reflecting conversation, or dialogue can extend the dialogue further.

Attunement to the therapist's experiencing is increased by *a focus on embodied and intuitive responses* to the family. We are aiming to attend to all aspects of ourselves, including the emotive, affective, creative, imaginative, and intuitive parts of us that cognitive processes alone can struggle to access. Reflecting in an embodied way situates our responses in our body. We may speak about where something is felt and what happens in our own body when listening to the dialogue. Noticing what happens in one's own body increases the therapist's use of self in the room. In this way, reflecting can be an opportunity for family members to themselves wonder about their own embodied experiences. We may also reflect on images, songs, words, metaphors, or other right brain content that may arise when listening to the family. We describe our responses in ways that create more openings for others to respond. For example, images may be easier for some family members to respond to, since not everyone listens or thinks in verbal or linguistic ways. For others, embodied and intuitive responses can create richness or nuance that is not available using words alone.

Ways of reflecting summary

1   Using client words

- Repeating words used by the family that resonate or move.
- 'I heard [these words] being spoken'.
- 'A word that stood out to me was…'
- 'I noticed that this word […] was used many times…'

2   Therapist inner dialogue

- 'I felt…'
- 'I wondered…'
- 'This resonated with me because … [or] I'm not sure why…'

3   An embodied response

- 'I noticed [this sensation]…'
- 'I felt … in my body when…'

4   Using images
- 'It brought this image to my mind…'

Precision point

- Therapists are always judicious with what they share in reflecting. They reflect from *within* their own inner dialogue, not *about* an interpretation of another's outer or inner dialogue.

Dialogical practice

- A remembering of Tom Andersen (Andersen & Shotter, 2003) speaking about body language, 'If I see something [an angry fist] that is not followed by a word, I do not mention it ... the word is belonging to the outer talk and his hand to the inner talk. He doesn't want to tell me ... maybe this is not the moment yet'.

Reflecting on the therapeutic process

- Trying to hold onto what we may think of as a 'perfect' or 'good' reflection until the time comes for reflecting is counterproductive to listening and staying with the dialogue.

Reflecting on reflecting

- Trust in the process and movement of the inner dialogue. There will be something to share when the time comes to reflect.

A pause or maybe a shift when we reflect

At the beginning of this chapter, we wrote that the ideas contained herein are not prescriptive, nor finalisable – in keeping with the dialogical approach. In coming to a pause, we have offered some of our ideas about dialogical reflecting processes and practices, specifically related to reflections and reflecting conversations. The fourfold foundation of dialogical being, knowing, doing, and experiencing offers an opportunity for therapists to begin to engage with, and perhaps include reflecting or reflecting conversations in their own clinical practice.

Specifically, reflections and reflecting conversations are one dialogical practice that can powerfully shift the way that we and families experience the work together. Importantly, they offer a space in the family therapy meeting that can be generative of dialogue. Dialogue can lead to moments where change, shift, or new knowing may emerge through human meetings. Such moments are often characterised by a sense of everyone being most within themselves, yet most with each other. They often point to a way to go on, not only within the meeting itself but also perhaps beyond the meeting. Opening to possibilities.

> Maybe ... the time has come to let what we have to say take its shape more from what comes from ourselves and feels natural, rather just from what the theories and techniques tell us?
>
> (Tom Andersen, 1992, p. 91)

We cast our mind back to the beginning of writing this chapter together. As we began by sharing our reflections, so too we will pause by again reflecting on our experience of the dialogical process of writing together.

Lisa: We have tried to write this chapter as an iterative, dialogical process between us with phone calls and ideas shared as the text developed and changed. Through the process, I have been reminded yet again of how complex the 'simple' idea of reflecting can be and yet how it can also remain simple. I have also been reminded that the journey of becoming dialogical is never-ending and how much I have learnt through this process of writing together. And of how much I still have to learn. The writing has also reconnected me with my goal of continuing to try and create dialogical spaces for the families I am working alongside.

Judith: I remember a moment. Sitting at my desk, I am vaguely aware of the outer world to my right through the window, yet my gaze is fixed ahead upon the intensity of my computer screen. We are on the phone. As writers together, we and the chapter too, are still in the forming stage. As we talk, we enter naturally into a reflecting conversation. It feels like a familiar dialogical process, comfortable, and I trust in the ebb and flow of ideas. Neither of us attaches to any one idea as the solution. Rather, the ideas emerge from the listening space between us. Yet, the process is slowly generative, and we find the next way to go on with the writing. For now, I am reminded that it is not what we do, but how we are with each other in the dialogue that is important. Yet again. On hanging up the phone, my gaze shifts and comes to rest on the sunlit greenery and pink camellias just outside my window. Before returning to the writing … the same, but different.

Notes

1   *Network meeting* is the term that was originally used in the Finnish context and is widely used when referring to Open Dialogue in mental health settings. In keeping with the family therapy context of this chapter however, the term *family therapy meeting* is used to refer to all meetings in all contexts where dialogical practice is used. It refers to the initial meeting or subsequent meetings in all contexts with individuals, couples, families, and the wider systems.
2   Often referred to as the inner conversation (Rober, 2005)

References

Alanen, Y. O., Lehtinen, K., Räkköläinen, V., & Aaltonen, J. (1991). Need-adapted treatment of new schizophrenic patients: Experiences and results of the Turku project. *Acta Psychiatrica Scandinavica, 83*, 363–372.

Anderson, H. (2005). Myths about "not-knowing". *Family Process, 44*(4), 497–504.

Anderson, H., & Goolishan, H. (1992). The client is the expert: A not-knowing approach to therapy. In S. McNamee & K. J. Gergen (Eds.), *Therapy as social construction.* London, England: Sage.

Anderson, H., & Goolishian, H. A. (1988). Human systems as linguistic systems: Preliminary and evolving ideas about the implications for clinical theory. *Family Process, 27*, 371–393.

Andersen, T. (1987). The reflecting team: Dialogue and meta-dialogue in clinical work. *Family Process, 26*, 415–428.

Andersen, T. (1992). Relationship, language and pre-understanding in the reflecting processes. *Australian and New Zealand Journal of Family Therapy, 13*(2), 87–91.

Andersen, T. (1995). Reflecting processes; Acts of informing and forming. In S. Friedman (Ed.) *The reflecting team in action* (pp. 11–37). New York, NY: The Guilford Press.

Andersen, T. (2008). Reflecting talks: My version. In K. Jordan (Ed.), *The quick theory reference guide: A resource for expert and novice mental health professionals* (pp. 427–444). New York, NY: Nova Science Publishers.

Andersen, T. & Jensen, P. (2007). Crossroads: Tom Andersen in conversation with Per Jensen. In H. Anderson & P. Jensen (Eds.), *Innovations in the reflecting process*. London, England: Karnac Books.

Andersen, T., & Shotter, J. (2003). Tom Andersen and John Shotter in Joint Action. London UK Conference 2003. KCC Foundation, UK.

Bakhtin, M. (1984). Problems of Dostojevskij's poetics. In C. Emerson (Ed. & Trans.), *Theory and history of literature*. (Vol. 8). Minneapolis, MN: University of Minnesota Press.

Bateson, G. (1979). *Steps to an ecology of mind*. San Francisco, CA: Chandler.

Brown, J. M. (2015). Wherefore art 'Thou' in the dialogical approach: The relevance of Buber's ideas to family therapy and research. *Australian and New Zealand Journal of Family Therapy*, *36*, 188–203.

Brown, J. M. (2017). A dialogical research methodology based on Buber: Intersubjectivity in the research interview. *Journal of Family Therapy*, *39*, 415–436.

Brown, J. M., Kurtti, M., Haaraniemi, T., Lohonen, E., & Vahtola, P. (2015). A North-South dialogue in open dialogues in Finland: The challenges and resonances of clinical practice. *Australian and New Zealand Journal of Family Therapy*, *36*, 51–68.

Browne, D. T., Norona, J., Busch, A., Armstrong, K., Crouch, S., Ernst, T., Darrow, S., Smith, J. A., & Ihle, E. C. (2021). "Is it us or is it me?": Family experiences of connectedness following a reflecting team intervention. *Journal of Marital and Family Therapy*, *47*(3), 727–748.

Brownlee, K., Vis, J., & McKenna, A. (2009). Review of the reflecting team process: Strengths, challenges, and clinical implications. *The Family Journal: Counselling and Therapy for Couples and Families*, *17*(2), 139–145.

Burnham, J. (2005). Relational reflexivity: A tool for socially constructing therapeutic relationships. In C. Flaskas, B. Mason, & A. Perlesz (Eds.), *The space between: Experience, context and process in the therapeutic relationship* (pp. 1–17). London: Karnac Books.

Butler, E. A., & Randall, A. K. (2013). Emotional coregulation in close relationships. *Emotion Review*, *5*(2), 202–210.

Crago, H. (2006). Beyond blame and shame: Three levels of family work. In H. Crago, *Couple, family and groupwork* (pp. 151–171). Maidenhead: Open University Press.

DeTurk, S., & Foster, E. (2008). Dialogue about dialogue: Investigating intersubjectivity in interview research. *Qualitative Research Journal*, *8*(2), 14–27.

Florence, A. C., Jordan, G., Yasui, S., & Davidson, L. (2020). Implanting rhizomes in vermont: A qualitative study of how the open dialogue approach was adapted and implemented. *The Psychiatric Quarterly*, *91*(3), 681–693. https://doi.org/10.1007/s11126-020-09732-7

Friedman, M. (1976). *Martin Buber: The life of dialogue* (3rd ed). London, England: The University of Chicago Press.

Geller, S. M., Greenberg, L. S., & Watson, J. C. (2010). Therapist and client perceptions of therapeutic presence: The development of a measure. *Psychotherapy Research*, *20*, 599–610.

Geller, S. M., & Porges, S. W. (2014). Therapeutic presence: Neurophysiological mechanisms mediating feeling safe in therapeutic relationships. *Journal of Psychotherapy Integration*, *24*(3), 178–192.

Gehart, D. R. (2018). The legacy of Tom Andersen: The ethics of reflecting processes. *Journal of Marital and Family Therapy*, *44*, 386–392. https://doi.org/10.1111/jmft.12289

Harris, R., & Crossley, J. (2021). A systematic review and meta-synthesis exploring client experience of reflecting teams in clinical practice. *Journal of Family Therapy*, *43*, 687–710.

Hicks, S., Kustner, C., & Constable, C. (2021). The helpfulness of reflecting teams in family therapy. *Journal of Family Therapy*, *43*(4), 711–727.

Hoffman, L. (2002). *Family therapy: An intimate history*. New York, NY: W.W. Norton.

Hornova, L. (2020). Dialogical co-therapy. *Australian and New Zealand Journal of Family Therapy*, *41*, 341.

Lidbom, P. A., Boe, T. D., Kristoffersen, K., Ulland, D., & Seikkula, J. (2014). A study of a network meeting: Exploring the interplay between inner and outer dialogues in significant and meaningful moments. *Australian and New Zealand Journal of Family Therapy*, *35*, 136–149.

Lyons-Ruth, K. (1998). Implicit relational knowing: Its role in development and psychoanalytic treatment. *Infant Mental Health Journal, 19*(3), 282–289.

McGown, L. (2015). A qualitative study of the therapist's spontaneous mental imagery and its impact on therapeutic process. *Counselling and Psychotherapy Research, 15*(2), 128–136.

Muth, C. (2009). How to teach intersubjectivity. *Journal of Social Work Practice: Psychotherapeutic Approaches in Health, Welfare and the Community, 23*(2), 201–213.

Olson, M., Seikkula, J., & Ziedonis, D. (2014). *The key elements of dialogic practice in open dialogue.* Worcester, MA: The University of Massachusetts Medical School.

Palazzoli, M. S., Boscolo, L., Cecchin, G., & Prata, G. (1990). *Paradox and counterparadox: A new model in the therapy of the family in schizophrenic transaction.* Northvale, NJ: Jason Aronson.

Porges, S. W. (2022). Polyvagal theory: A science of safety. *Frontiers in Integrative Neuroscience, 16,* 871227.

Quillman, T. (2012). Neuroscience and therapist self-disclosure: Deepening right brain to right brain communication between therapist and patient. *Clinical Social Work, 40,* 1–9.

Räkköläinen, V., Lehtinen, K., & Alanen, Y. O. (1991). Need-adapted treatment of schizophrenic psychoses: The essential role of family centered therapy meetings. *Contemporary Family Therapy, 13,* 573–582.

Rizzolatti, G., & Craighero, L. (2004). The mirror-neuron system. *Annual Review of Neuroscience, 27,* 169–192.

Rober, P. (2005). The therapist's self in dialogical family therapy: Some ideas about not-knowing and the therapist's inner conversation. *Family Process, 44*(4), 477–495.

Rober, P. (2011). The therapist's experiencing in family therapy practice. *Journal of Family Therapy, 33,* 233–255.

Rober, P., Elliott, R., Buysse, A., Loots, G., & De Cort, K. (2008). What's on the therapist's mind? A grounded theory analysis of family therapist reflections during individual therapy sessions. *Psychotherapy Research, 18*(1), 48–57.

Roberts, M. (2009). Writing and the reflecting processes: A dialogue with Tom Andersen and Peggy Penn. *Journal of Systemic Therapies, 28*(4), 61–71.

Schore, A. N. (2010). The right brain implicit self: A central mechanism of the psychotherapy change process. In J. Petrucelli (Ed.), *Knowing, not knowing, and sort-of-knowing: Psychoanalysis and the experience of uncertainty* (pp. 177–202). London, England: Karnac Books.

Schore, A. N. (2021). The interpersonal neurobiology of intersubjectivity. *Frontiers in Psychology, 12,* 648616. doi: 10.3389/fpsyg.2021.648616

Seikkula, J. (2002). Open dialogues with good and poor outcomes for psychotic crises: Examples from families with violence. *Journal of Marital and Family Therapy, 28* (3), 263–274.

Seikkula, J. (2008). Inner and outer voices in the present moment of family and network therapy. *Journal of Family Therapy, 30,* 478–491.

Seikkula, J. (2011), Becoming dialogical: Psychotherapy or a way of life?.*Australian and New Zealand Journal of Family Therapy, 32,* 179–193. https://doi.org/10.1375/anft.32.3.179

Seikkula, J., & Arnkil, T. E. (2006). *Dialogical meetings in social networks.* London, England: Karnac Books.

Seikkula, J., Laitila, A., & Rober, P. (2012). Making sense of multi-actor dialogues in family therapy and network meeting. *Journal of Marital and Family Therapy, 38*(4), 667–687.

Seikkula, J., & Olson, M. E. (2003). The open dialogue approach to acute psychosis: Its poetics and micropolitics. *Family Process, 42*(3), 403–418.

Seikkula, J., & Trimble, D. (2005). Healing elements of therapeutic conversation: Dialogue as an embodiment of love. *Family Process, 44*(4), 463–475.

Shaw, R. (2004). The embodied psychotherapist: An exploration of the therapist's somatic phenomena within the therapeutic encounter. *Psychotherapy Research, 14*(3), 271–288.

Shotter, J. (1993). *Cultural politics of everyday life.* Milton Keynes, England: Open University Press.

Shotter, J. (2014). Personal correspondence.

Shotter, J. (2005). Understanding process from within: An argument for 'withness'-thinking. *Organisation Studies*, *27*(4), 585–604.

Shotter, J. (2007). Not to forget Tom Andersen's way of being Tom Andersen: The importance of what 'just happens to us'. *Human Systems: The Journal of Systemic Consultation and Management*, 18, 15–28.

Shotter, J. (2010). Movements of feeling and moments of judgement: Towards an ontological social constructionism. *International Journal of Action Research*, *6*(1), 16–42.

Sidis, A., Moore, A., Pickard, J., & Deane, F. P. (2022). "Always opening and never closing": How dialogical therapists understand and create reflective conversations in network meetings. *Frontiers in Psychology*, *13*, 992785.

Skærbæk, E. (2004). It takes two to tango – One knowledge production and intersubjectivity. *Nordic Journal of Feminist and Gender Research*, *12*(2), 993–101.

Stern, D. (1998). The process of therapeutic change involving implicit knowledge: Some implications of developmental observations for adult psychotherapy. *Infant Mental Health Journal*, *19*(3), 300–308.

Stern, D. N. (1985). *The interpersonal world of the infant: A view from psychoanalysis and developmental psychology*. London, England: Routledge.

Stern, D. N. (2004). *The present moment: In psychotherapy and everyday life*. New York, NY: W.W. Norton & Co.

Stern, D. N. (2007). Applying developmental and neuroscience findings on other-centres participation to the process of change in psychotherapy. In S. Braten (Ed.), *On being moved* (pp. 35–47). Philadelphia, PA: John Benjamin Publishing Company.

Trevarthen, C. (1980). The foundations of intersubjectivity: Development of interpersonal and co-operative understanding of infants. In D. Olson (Ed.), *The social foundations of language and thought: Essays in honor of J.S. Bruner* (pp. 316–342). New York, NY: W.W. Norton & Co..

Trevarthen, C., & Aitken, K. J. (2001). Infant intersubjectivity: Research, theory and clinical applications. *Journal of Child Psychology and Psychiatry*, *42*(1), 3–48.

Trimble (2002). Listening with integrity: The dialogical stance of Jaakko Seikkula. *Journal of Marital and Family Therapy*, *28*(3), 275–277.

Tseliou, E., Burck, C., Forbat, L., Strong, T. and O'Reilly, M. (2021), How is systemic and constructionist therapy change process narrated in retrospective accounts of therapy? A systematic meta-synthesis review. *Fam. Proc.*, *60*, 64–83. https://doi.org/10.1111/famp.12562

Vytogsky, L. (1988). *Thought and language*. Cambridge, MA: MIT Press.

Weingarten, K. (2016). The art of reflection: Turning the strange into the familiar. *Family Process*, *55*(2), 195–210.

Wittgenstein, L. (1953). *Philosophical Investigations Trans. G.E.M. Anscombe*. Oxford: Blackwell.

Zaner, R. M. (1961). Theory of intersubjectivity: Alfred Schutz. *Social Research*, *28*(1), 71–93.

Chapter 14

The Final Session

Roxanne Garven and Paul Rhodes

Introduction

"If therapy is to end properly, it must begin properly…".

(Haley, 1976)

This quote, from Jay Haley (1976), encapsulates the preparatory work that contributes to good endings with families. Good endings are continually supported when family therapists, for example, elicit the family's hopes for the work, reframe problems relationally, find the family's preferred ways of being with the problem, and listen for and amplify unnoticed behaviours and perspectives that reflect signs of change.

Once arrived at, final sessions in family therapy provide unique opportunities. A good ending can offer long-lasting therapeutic effects, helping families to consolidate and perpetuate changes made in behaviours, belief systems, and relationships. When families take full credit for their own successes, they can plan and prepare for future challenges, celebrate with meaningful rituals, and may choose to share their expertise with future clients. The purpose of this chapter is to present some specific guidelines for conducting the last session and to provide a detailed transcript to demonstrate their use.

How do you know when it's time to finish?

The first and most obvious reason for initiating a last session is that the presenting problem, and the distress it has brought, is no longer present or has decreased in intensity. At times, however, the completion of therapy might also be indicated by a change in the way the problem is viewed, rather than simply by its amelioration. This can be unique to family therapy, given that the focus of therapy is much wider than the presenting problem. Therapy does not just aim for behaviour modification, but for a more significant and potentially sustainable shift in the rules and relationships that govern behaviour. Systemic family therapists differentiate between first- and second-order change (Watzlawick, Weakland, & Fisch, 1974). In first-order change, the therapist and family focus exclusively on responses to the presenting problem. In second-order change, attention is directed to the family's attempted solutions, rather than simply to the problem itself. Focussing on the full gamut of family interactions supports the long-term sustainability of change.

Imagine a family, for example, struggling with the disrespectful and oppositional behaviour of a teenage son. The father may attempt to resolve the problem by becoming angry

DOI: 10.4324/9781003490104-15

and setting very severe consequences, leading to constant conflict and distress. The son may regularly turn to his mother for support, who pleads successfully with her husband to be conciliatory in his behaviour. This is a regular pattern. The father's attempt to deal with the son is seen as first-order, being linear and directed at the son's behaviour in isolation. A second-order solution would aim to disrupt and change the triangulation between family members, supporting a strong marital relationship, one that could provide effective boundaries for the son. In this example, the focus of therapy must be temporarily shifted from the presenting problem to attempted solutions. Family members must be supported to question long-standing patterns of interaction before the initial problem can be dealt with. The end of therapy is best initiated only when a degree of second-order change has been achieved.

How to conduct the last session

Six specific tasks to support the therapist conducting the last session are given in Table 14.1. These tasks are not necessarily intended to be employed rigidly or in this order. Some are appropriate for most last sessions, and others, such as the use of rituals or asking families to consult with others, may be used less frequently. It is also important to note that it can be useful to gradually fade the frequency of sessions prior to the last. Weekly sessions might be moved fortnightly, monthly, or even quarterly to foster the families' self-reliance prior to the last session.

1.   Plot progress to date and emphasise the agency of the family

The most important principle when reviewing progress is to explore how family members have contributed to change. Without this, families may view progress as fragile, inexplicable, and disconnected from their own motivations and efforts or place undue credit on the efforts of the therapist.

It should be noted that the questions below are derived from solution-focussed therapy (De Shazer, 1991; De Shazer & Berg, 1992), given its emphasis on reinforcing the efficacy and strength of the family. There is also a degree of overlap between the questions below and those employed in Chapter 3 on deviation amplifying for the second session of therapy. In the session two, these questions are employed to amplify small gains to create momentum for change. In the last session, they are employed to consolidate more significant changes and support their sustainability into the future.

Table 14.1 Six potential tasks for the final session

1 Plot progress to date and emphasise the agency of the family
2 Predict and plan for future "hiccups"
3 Prepare for the wider systems response to progress
4 Design a ritual to mark transitions
5 Circulate the expertise of the family
6 Discuss and dissolve the therapeutic relationship

Ask each family member to describe the changes they have seen over the course of therapy:

On a scale of 1 to 10, with 10 representing the problem having its strongest hold over all of you, and 1, representing no hold at all, where do you think you were when we first met? And today?

This scaling exercise leads to other areas of enquiry, such as:

"How did each of you do this?", "What intentions and hopes underpinned these decisions?", "How did you push through challenges that came your way"?

What do you think have been your most important achievements over the past x months?

What achievements are you most proud of seeing in others?

Which do you think have been the most significant or hard-won achievements?

Develop the connection between these changes and the direct intentions and efforts of the family:

What did you do to contribute towards these changes?

How did you decide to do that?

What advice were you giving yourself at the time?

What were your intentions behind these efforts?

Identify the individual and family resources responsible:

How did you/other/the family manage to achieve this given all the challenges and stresses involved?

What skills and knowledge did you/others/the family rely on?

What does it say about your/others/the family's strengths?

What does it say about your/others/the family's values/priorities?

Ask family members to advise their old selves:

If your old selves were in the waiting room and I asked them to come in, what advice would you give them about how to get to your current position?

What would you have to say to them to give them the confidence that they have what it takes to make this change?

Use the two-video camera questions; "If I was watching an old recording of the time when the problem was in your lives, what I see? What would I see with today's recording of your family's life?"

2.   Predict and plan for future "Hiccups"

The aim of this step is to sensitise family members to the possibility of a relapse in the presenting problem, or the interactions that maintained it. The term "hiccup" is used to reinforce the stability of their achievements, whilst normalising future incidents.

> *What would be the earliest signs that might alert you to the possibility of a hiccup in the future?*
>
> *What are some of the ways of making sense of this behaviour that might best equip you to respond to it effectively?*
>
> *What have you learned during the past x months that you would employ to manage future hiccups?*
>
> *If I offered you a million dollars to ensure that the problem returned over the next month, what exactly would each of you have to do?*

3.   Preparing for the wider systems response to progress

In a final session, it can be helpful to ask families how progress will affect their interactions and relationships with members of the wider system, including relatives, friends, and other professionals. These conversations can mediate against any pressure from others to return to prior behaviours or provide families with access to future support and affirmation. Family members can be asked to decide whether it would be helpful to inform others of these changes, to predict how others might respond if they notice the change and to plan interactions if needed. The therapist can also discuss the nature and purpose of their formal correspondence with other professionals, including the referring agent.

4.   Design a ritual to mark transitions

Family rituals can be employed to mark the family's transition, serving as a powerful symbol of change and of the persistence required to overcome problems (Imber-Black, Roberts, & Whiting, 2003). On some occasions, rituals will not simply correspond with the amelioration of problems but also with developmental transitions in the family, including the onset of adolescence, the constitution of a blended family, or the empty nest. Rituals can also serve as emotional rites of passage, including overcoming the legacy of trauma, coming to terms with an illness, or learning to live with a disability. On most occasions, the family serves as the best resource in the development of rituals, ensuring that they are most meaningful, culturally relevant, and representative of the transformation in the life of the family.

Examples from our own clinical practice include a children's party held to celebrate a young boy who had suffered from social anxiety, a meal shared by family and professionals for an adolescent recovered from anorexia nervosa, a mother taking her daughter for a piercing on her transition into becoming a young woman, and a school speech about Autism, written by a father for a son dealing with a history of bullying and depression.

5. Circulate the expertise of the family

Another powerful way to mark the completion of therapy is to ask the family if they would like to act as consultants for families facing similar challenges. This practice, derived from narrative therapy (Sparks, 1997), involves asking the family to return for one session in the future, to tell their story to a new family and then be interviewed by them further about their experience. This method serves to support their transition from clients to experts and provides an avenue for them to give back, consolidating their knowledge and providing hope to new families. Lobovits, Maisel, and Freeman (1995) also describe a host of other means to recognise the expertise of families at the end of therapy. Families can be asked to contribute to handbooks designed for particular problems (e.g., The Temper Tamer's Handbook, The Fear Facer's Handbook, and How to Cool Off and Be Cool). Epston (2001) has also published interviews, artworks, and poems of clients on the internet, serving to recognise their "insider knowledge" and provide solidarity to others.

6. Discuss and dissolve the therapeutic relationship

The focus of the five steps so far has been on the consolidation of the efficacy of the family through their recognition of their own achievements and expertise. It is also important, however, to provide the family with an opportunity to reflect on their relationship with the therapist and to facilitate the dissolution of this bond. One method for achieving this is to turn the tables and allow the family to interview you and your experience supporting them (White & Epston, 1990). Some questions in our own practice have included.

What was the most challenging thing you found in helping us?

Do you ever get upset when you hear about people's problems?

Why do you like doing this job?

Where do you get your ideas from?

Did you think we could do it?

It is important for the therapist to respond candidly, discussing their role honestly, including any doubts, confusion, or distress they might have experienced. This serves to further flatten the hierarchy between the family and the therapist and prepares them for a final farewell. An alternative approach is simply to ask the family for feedback on their experience of therapy, including the therapeutic relationship. Like any relationship, this may have gone through its stresses and misunderstandings, each of which can be discussed briefly to allow some resolution. The family may also choose to discuss the significance of this relationship and to express their gratitude and any feelings of loss they may be experiencing as therapy comes to an end.

Case study

Sally is the mother of two children, referred by her General Practitioner because of distressed relationships with her two children, Amy, 14 years, and Luke, 12 years. The children had been disrespectful towards Sally, failing to do their homework or chores. Sally responded angrily on many occasions, with interactions deteriorating to mutual verbal abuse and tears. Sally is a single parent who has been diagnosed with depression. She has been separated from Adam for four years and the children see their father regularly. The therapist has conducted six sessions and Sally and the therapist have agreed to finish therapy after session seven. Sally, Luke, and Amy attend the last session.

1.   Plot progress to date and emphasise the agency of the family

Ask each family member to describe the changes they have seen over the course of therapy.

Therapist:	What do you think have been the most important things you have achieved together in the past four months?
Sally:	Me learning not to yell, I've just come to the realisation that it doesn't help, that I'm teaching them to be like me and we all end up so upset. I feel like I've got a bit of control back, not just of themselves but that I'm not flying off the handle all the time.
Therapist:	Amy? Luke? What about you? What do you think has been achieved?
Amy:	I agree with mum, we're all a lot calmer. I can talk to mum about school and stuff and I'm not yelling back and things are better.
Luke:	Yeah, but we have to do more now, like jobs and stuff.
Therapist:	What about the depression Sally? What effect have these changes had on how down you were feeling?
Sally:	I just used to think nothing would ever change, that since the divorce it all went wrong, that it was my fault. Now I'm getting on top of it. I can see what to do and I do feel depressed sometimes but it's not as bad. I'm just glad I still have my kids and that we are getting on and they are still seeing their father.

2.   Develop the connection between these changes and the direct intentions and efforts of the family

Therapist:	Looking back, can you recall a time, Sally, where it maybe was touch and go, you could have given up on the changes, but you didn't, and took a stand to change things?
Sally:	Yes, for me, it was around the time when Amy's teacher rang to tell me she was behind on her work. I was so angry. I wanted to really yell at her, ground her, stop the internet access. I felt like giving up on this, that it was going to be too hard.
Therapist:	And what was it about that call, do you think? Looking back on it, what was the worst thing?
Sally:	I felt ashamed; I felt the teacher was judging me, that I was a bad parent.
Therapist:	So, how did you decide to push through and not give in to those feelings?
Sally:	I think I knew that if I yelled at Amy, it would all go back. I didn't want to yell at her anymore. I have realised it makes things worse.
Therapist:	So, what did you do? What happened to the sense of being judged and the shame? What sort of influence did they have on you?
Sally:	I went for a walk, and I thought about it, that I am not a bad parent, that Amy is responsible for her work. So, I came home and spoke with Amy about it.

Therapist:	Amy, did you know about this, about your Mum nearly giving in but deciding not to?
Amy:	No. Just heard this now.
Therapist:	And, what difference does it make to you, Amy, your Mum not giving in to the yelling and talking to you instead?
Amy:	Lots! I don't feel so defensive, angry with her, and I don't try to avoid her.
Therapist:	Do you think your Mum has noticed that, Amy, you avoiding her less? I am curious how she'd respond to you if she had noticed?
Amy:	I think she has. I think she's less angry with me, when I do something, she doesn't like … Beforehand, she would have got really angry.
Therapist:	Amy, what's your guess about what your mother was hoping to achieve by not yelling and thinking about the call from the school, before she spoke to you?
Amy:	I guess she was trying to make sure we don't go back to how it used to be, to keep the fighting from happening.
Therapist:	Sally, what are your thoughts about what Amy has just been saying?
Sally:	Yes, I am trying to get less angry and she's right. I am doing it because the old ways didn't work. If I yelled, she'd yell back. I want us to have a good relationship and I want her to learn to sort problems out without yelling and abuse.
Therapist:	Luke, and for you, what's that been like?
Luke:	It's great coming home from school and there's no tension in the air. Amy's not trying to avoid Mum. I feel more relaxed. I don't worry about Mum so much now. I used to really worry that their fights would push Mum into her bedroom again like it used to.

3.   Identify the individual and family resources responsible

Therapist:	What do you think it says about your family, Sally, that together you were able to get through this, to find another way of relating to each other?
Sally:	Well, I wasn't brought up like this; there was lots of yelling and certainly lots when Adam was around. I guess we are trying to do something new, to make our own little unit, start from scratch.
Therapist:	What are the values you want this unit to be defined by?
Sally:	Just respect, not losing it, staying calm, we need to learn how to get on and be more mature about it.

4.   Predict and plan for future "Hiccups"

Therapist:	Just to be a devil's advocate, let's say that bits of the old problem come back, what do you think would be the first sign of this happening?
Amy:	The yelling, Mum feeling bad about everything, little things blowing up.
Sally:	Yes, I'd say it would have to be the yelling, Amy and Luke getting out of hand.
Therapist:	Luke? What do you reckon?
Luke:	I'd know – Mum spending more time in her room.
Therapist:	Ok, let's say some of those begin to happen, how would you like to see yourselves respond to them so that they didn't get the upper hand?

Sally: I think it would be good if we could all pull each other back, help each other out. I'd like to see myself encouraging everyone to talk first, to start being open about what they are feeling and asking them what they want.

Therapist: Amy? Luke? So, if your Mum encouraged you to talk and as well asked you questions about what you were feeling, would that be a good thing or not?

Amy: Yes, as long as she didn't go on about it and force me to talk. I might not want to talk then or want to tell her.

Therapist: Oh, so then, what would be more useful for you, and how would you let her know?

Amy: Well, I'd want to tell her, without shouting, that maybe I wanted to talk later, and for her to be happy with the amount I've told her, to not grill me.

Therapist: Why would that be important for you, Amy?

Amy: I would feel she trusted me and that she was more relaxed, not so anxious.

Therapist: And, Amy, you also said, "without shouting", why would you want to do it that way?

Amy: Because shouting does not work, and I want Mum and I to get on.

Therapist: OK, Sally, let's say, you do this. How do you think Amy will respond to you?

Sally: Well, firstly, I think it's lovely hearing Amy say she wants us to continue getting along. But I think she'd respond to me in a calmer way, if I don't pressure her. She has a point. I can see that.

Therapist: And in the past, Sally, your view of Amy wanting to be left alone, during or after a fight, how did you use to feel about that?

Sally: I used to think she was wanting to control me, by leaving me out in the cold. Now, I understand that she doesn't want to control me; she wants space to cool off and to be on her own for a while.

Therapist: It's quite a different way of looking at it. What did it take to see it like this?

Sally: I had to think that it was possible that she wasn't doing it deliberately to hurt me, that also, I had to take it less personally.

5.   Preparing for the wider systems response to progress

Therapist: Amy, how have these changes affected your Mum's interactions with her Mum, if at all?

Amy: They have. Mum used to phone Nan a lot, especially after a fight and she'd be crying, and sometimes Nan would come over and Luke and I would feel nervous, thinking Nan would start to blame us and tell us off. So this doesn't happen anymore. I mean she phones her, but they are normal calls now.

Therapist: I guess this is a good thing, but I wonder, in what way do you think it is good, Amy?

Amy: Well, it's good because Nan doesn't have to worry so much now, and Mum can be more independent, and we don't have to have all this fuss around us.

Therapist: Is there anyone else who you think has noticed these changes or who should know about them?

Sally: My doctor, but he already knows, because you have contacted him, haven't you?

Therapist: Yes. Anything different between the two of you now, because of these changes?

Sally: I ring him less! But also, we're talking about coming off the antidepressants and he's telling me how well I'm doing, which is always nice to hear.

6.   Designing rituals or a ceremony

Therapist: If you were to think of something that was a special way of remembering what you have all done to move away from these problems, what would it be?

Luke: Let's go somewhere and just have fun, not worry about everything, just have a good time, remember you always promised us to go to Jambaroo (Theme Park) mum? We've never gone; you always said we would. Why don't we go there and say we're not going to yell anymore?

Therapist: Sally? Amy?

Sally: Sure, I know I haven't been much fun and the kids have been through a lot, that's a good idea, Luke.

Amy: We'll send you photos.

7.   Circulate the expertise of the family

Therapist: I wonder if you would be interested in doing one other thing as well, please feel free to say no if you want, but how willing would you be to come back in the future if I see a family in a similar situation, to tell them your story and what you've achieved; it would be a one hour meeting and I'd just interview you with them listening and they could ask you a few questions?

Sally: Really, we'd love to do that, wouldn't we, kids?

Amy: Maybe just mum. I'd be a bit shy. I'm busy at school too. I'll let you know when it comes up, but mum could do it.

Therapist: Ok, I'll let you know when it comes up.

8.   Discuss and dissolve the therapeutic relationship

Therapist: Before we close this final meeting, I wonder if you have any questions you'd like to ask me, we could turn the tables and you can ask me questions? Like what it was like for me? How I work?

Luke: Why do you always ask questions? You have lots of questions and always come up with different ones.

Therapist: Well, we are taught to do it this way, so we try and help a family to figure things out for themselves. If we just gave advice all the time, it might not fit; each family is different and it's better when they make their own minds up.

Sally: What about yourself, have you got your own family? Does it mean you always sort things out?

Therapist: Yeah, I have two kids of my own, aged 6 and 8; sometimes it helps but generally I have all the same things go wrong as everyone else, same arguments, same behaviour, and stuff and I have to learn to work through it too.

Sometimes when you've been talking, I've thought of my own family, what it was like a couple of years ago when we had our own tough times, but we seem to get through things too and keep coming out the other end.

Amy: Really? Ha, I always thought you had like the perfect family and perfect kids and stuff.

Therapist: No. Well, it looks like our final hour has come to a close; it's always a bit sad when this happens, how are you all feeling about it?

Sally: I just want to thank you for everything you've done; you have helped me so much, to get on my feet, thanks for everything you've done.

Amy: We'll send you photos from Jambaroo.

Conclusion

The final session of family therapy can provide a specific and unique opportunity for extending the gains made in therapy and support the families' final graduation from clients to experts. In this chapter, six possible tasks have been presented for this session, tasks which aim to leave the family with a sense of pride in their achievements, plans for future challenges, and lasting memory of their transition. These tasks consolidate the central role the family has made in driving change, whilst providing an opportunity for reflection on the therapy itself and their relationship with the therapist.

References

De Shazer, S. (1991). *Putting difference to work.* New York: W.W. Norton & Co.

De Shazer, S., & Berg, I. (1992). Doing therapy: A post-structural revision. *Journal of Marital and Family Therapy, 18,* 71–81.

Epston, D. (2001). Archive of resistance: Anti-anorexia/anti-bulimia. Retrieved June 3, 2009, from https://narrativeapproaches.com/resources/anorexia-bulimia-archives-of-resistance/

Haley, J. (1976). *Problem solving therapy. New strategies for effective family therapy.* San Francisco, CA: Jossey-Bass.

Imber-Black, E., Roberts, J., & Whiting, R. (2003). *Rituals in families and family therapy.* New York, NY: W.W. Norton & Co.

Lobovits, D., Maisel, R., & Freeman, J. (1995). Public practices: An ethic of circulation. In S. Friedman (Ed.), *The reflecting team in action: Collaborative practices in family therapy.* New York: Guilford Press.

Sparks, J. (1997). Voices of experience: Inviting former clients to rejoin the therapy process as consultants. *Journal of Systemic Therapies, 16,* 367–375.

Watzlawick, P., Weakland, J., & Fisch, R. (1974). *Change: Principles of problem formation and problem resolution.* New York, NY: W.W. Norton and Co.

White, M., & Epston, D. (1990). *Narrative means to therapeutic ends.* New York, NY: W. W. Norton & Co.

Index

Note: Page references in **bold** denotes tables and with "n" endnotes.